SHOCK TRAUMA

PAT JENSEN

Willow River Books
Calgary

This novel is set in southern Alberta and many of the scenes and places described will be familiar to both residents and visitors. The events described, the LIFE-STAR helicopter program, and all characters exist only as fiction in the imagination of the author. Any resemblance or similarity to real events, real helicopter programs and real people is purely coincidental.

SHOCK TRAUMA
A Willow River Book

Cover Design by Carolyn Filter, Toronto, ON
Cover Graphics by Karol Fodor of Digital Art Inc., Calgary, AB
Photography by Rob Bryden, Airdrie, AB
Desktop Publishing by Kathleen Ennis, Calgary, AB

First printing:	June 1997
Second printing:	October 1997
Third printing:	February 1998
Fourth Printing	January 2002
Fifth Printing	January 2003
Sixth Printing	May 2004

Canadian Cataloguing in Publication Data
Jensen, Pat, 1957 –
Shock Trauma

ISBN: 0-9681956-0-1

I. Title.
PS8569.E59S56 1997 C813'.54 C97-900606-6
PR9199.3.J42S56 1997

For information:
Willow River Books, 131 Sunmeadows Cres SE, Calgary, Alberta, Canada.

Printed in Canada

"A fast-moving, energetic page-turner filled with cutting-edge insider's information, SHOCK TRAUMA takes you behind the scenes of contemporary lifesaving heroics. A highly fascinating life-and-death atmosphere tempered with humor and scintillating romance. Evocative of E.R."

Rick Mofina, Calgary Herald.

"Pat Jensen knows out-of-hospital rescue medicine. She's been there and done it. She's also a superb story-teller, and she creates word pictures that you can almost hear and smell. I really enjoyed this book."

James O. Page, Publisher
JEMS magazine
(Journal of Emergency Medical Services)
Carlsbad, California

"Just the right amount of gore, humor and action… a great read!"

Kathleen Ennis
Independent Businesswoman

"A testament to one woman's achievements against horrendous odds. Fast-paced and highly readable, SHOCK TRAUMA soars from start to finish with an intricate blend of drama, romance and humor to keep it airborne."

Mary M. Cutbill
Freelance Editor

"An exciting story that absorbs the reader into the real-life drama, passion and romance of air medicine rescue work."

Lane Casement
Chief Operating Officer
STARS

"Air rescue tale's a fascinating read… riveting."

Canmore Leader

"Novel captures drama of air-rescue work."

Calgary Herald

This book is dedicated to the men and women of EMS...

on behalf of the countless patients who have felt the magical touch of a firefighter's caring hands...

had their fears calmed by a police officer's comforting words...

their pain eased by a paramedic's expert medical skills...

their tears acknowledged with compassion and reassurance by a flight nurse's confident smile.

And to my husband Gordon,
whose love and understanding kept me sane
and helped me stay focused on the big picture.

CONTENTS

1
A RUSTLING OF ANGEL WINGS

Given its speed, momentum and the almost frictionless rain slicked rails, the fully loaded freight train was going to need at least a mile of track in order to come to a complete stop... a distance that unfortunately would place its lead locomotive 2000 feet beyond the overturned cattle truck, the crushed car, and the twenty or so cows and six people still hopelessly trapped inside the crumpled wreckage.

A guttural wail curdled the crisp night air. With the train bearing down on them and the rusted blood soaked section of angle iron still protruding grotesquely from the man's back, Dave and Kyle abandoned EMS protocol as they forcibly dragged the injured man from the twisted pile of metal that had once been the truck's cab.

Silently watching as the medics hurriedly carted their still screaming patient toward the waiting helicopter, Angie had never been more frightened in her entire life. Only a mere fifty yards away now, the freight's skidding, shrieking steel wheels spit an angry cloud of sparks and fire into the surrounding darkness. She could almost feel the heat from the engine's four blazing headlights as they bore down upon the teetering cattleliner and the car wedged tightly beneath.

All of a sudden, as if some powerful unseen force was at work, the massive trailer magically began to right itself. With twenty-seven heifers still trapped inside, a sickened Angie could hear the terrified animals frantically scrambling to keep their footing as the manure splattered floor tilted beneath them.

Momentarily pausing at a heart stopping 45 degree angle, the bottom heavy trailer abruptly over-balanced, sending its steel-belted tires crashing back to earth with a ground shuddering bounce. Finally free, the two-door Cutlass and its four entombed occupants lurched with a jolt backwards up the highway.

Hidden in the murky darkness, the oil rig workers were putting their very lives on the line in a final courageous attempt to drag the car clear of the tracks using their pickup truck's front mounted winch. It was going to be close.

Feeling her rib cage throb as if her pounding heart was about to explode, Angie found herself staring numbly at the empty Morphine syringe in her hand... and as the brilliant lights of the oncoming train reached out to seemingly swallow her alive, the terrified look in the rookie flight nurse's unblinking eyes was that of a deer caught in headlights.

Dear God... why hadn't she listened to her mother and become a dental hygienist instead?

Mere months earlier, Angie Y. Jackson's mundane existence had started off just like any other workday with an ear shattering blast of country-rock music from her clock radio.

Fumbling for the snooze button, the blurry eyed nurse's first impulse was to book off sick. Blinking cobwebs from her still half asleep brain as she mulled the idea over, she instead wearily crawled out from under the warm covers and headed for the bathroom. As the morning sun poked its sleepy head over a cloudless eastern horizon, its warm June rays found Angie gnawing on a half-frozen poptart as she frantically searched her cramped apartment for her hospital parking pass.

Knowing in her heart that nine other women were no doubt doing more or less the same thing, the nurse stumbled out the door and headed for her car. On the tail-end of a God-awful four day stretch, she and her co-workers had only to make it through one more 12 hour shift before being rewarded with an entire glorious weekend off.

As a Calgary based critical care nurse, the Intensive Care/Coronary Unit at Mountainview Hospital was the facility in which Angie had chosen to ply her high-stress trade. Affectionately known as the Rockpile, its newly renovated ICU/CCU was state-of-the-art. Spread out in a large semi-circle with a nursing station at either end, fourteen of the twenty rooms were privates with sound-proof sliding glass doors. In addition, ceiling-to-floor curtains afforded some degree of privacy for the unit's frequently stripped-naked, wired for arrhythmia, intubated, ventilated and occasionally conscious clientele.

By 7:10 a.m., nine of the ten nurses had arrived for work. After lining up for a steaming cup from the Mr. Coffee machine, they flopped down around the table in the report room. Sipping on their brew, the bright eyed nurses idly chatted among themselves as they studied the large wall-mounted patient report board.

"Mrs. Gried is still alive? And they've put her on dialysis?" one of the older nurses exclaimed. "We had to defib her five times yesterday. It was so awful. You could smell her skin burning. That poor sweet soul is ninety-one years old. Her lungs are gone. Her heart's gone. Her kidneys are gone. Her mind is gone. When are the intensivists ever going to accept the fact that death is a natural part of life? Why can't patients die in their sleep anymore?"

At precisely 7:15 a.m., the Assistant Nursing Unit Supervisor marched in to take her seat at the head of the table. Following a curt hello, Connie Harrington, noticing an empty chair at the far end of the table, did a quick head count of the nurses present. Coming up one short, she scowled at a note taped to her clipboard.

Connie's opinion of herself matched her appearance. Tall and slender with dark auburn hair pulled back in a perfect French roll, even her spotless lab coat reflected the fact that she was a professional career woman on the way up. Her goal was not simply to attain Unit Supervisor status. Heavens no. Rumour had it she was after a much loftier calling, the soon-to-be vacated "Assistant Director of Nursing" post.

Listening as the charge nurse gave account of the unit's nocturnal activities, Connie frequently glanced up from her clipboard to glare at the large round clock on the wall. Not a happy camper this morning, she was letting everyone know it. The slow, steady cadence of the taped report was in harsh contrast to Connie's frenzied scratching of numerous notes to herself. Keeping their thoughts to themselves, the day shift nurses could not help but swallow hard as they watched their exalted leader grind her ball-point pen into the acrylic table top.

Ten minutes into report, the room's far door eased noiselessly open. Clad in baby blue scrubs and white running shoes, a nurse tiptoed around the crowded table to the empty seat on the corner. No one took any notice. No one that is, but Connie.

Nervously twisting the gold nursing school ring on her little finger, late comer Angie Jackson instantly felt Connie's frosty gaze upon her. With nearly twelve years of critical care experience, there was no denying that the fair-haired Ms. Jackson was a fine nurse. She had the talent. She had the experience. At age 35, however, she had something else... a terminal case of ICU burn-out.

Twelve years of keeping people alive had left their toll. The never-ending pressure of caring for critically ill patients. The stress of knowing a simple medication error could cost a life. Where a good day was when nobody was carted out of the unit feet first. More than anything, however, it was the ethics of it all. Rather than saving people's lives, Angie often felt she was merely prolonging their dying. Although she had tried to chalk it up to nothing more than an overactive imagination, she was positive she had once heard the rustling of angel wings as she cared for a patient being kept alive by artificial means. God did not like to be kept waiting.

Today, Angie's muddled thoughts were elsewhere as night report dragged on. After kicking the tires of her lifeless Chevette, she had been forced, yet again, to awaken her neighbour so he could jump-start it for her. Lately, it seemed, that damned vehicle had been jumped more often than she had!

Yes, the day had started on a less than auspicious note and with Connie in charge and every bed in the unit filled with a patient pounding on the gates of heaven, the shift was headed straight for the bedpan hopper... and it wasn't even 7:30 a.m.!

Struggling to pull herself together, Angie listened as report continued. Bed eight was a new admission during the night. A Mr. Roger Alcott. Age 69. Diagnosis: right upper lobe pneumonia. A long-time smoker and poorly controlled diabetic, he was also suffering from the ravages of chronic kidney failure and anaemia.

The charge nurse's report included a short blurb regarding Mr. Alcott's wretched blood gases and the personal opinion that she did not think he would last until noon without having to be intubated.

"He's confused, combative, has an oxygen saturation of eighty-six percent, won't keep his mask on and is starting to pick at the air. He pulled his foley catheter out, balloon inflated and has since been incontinent four times of a large amount of blood-tinged urine. Security had to sit with him most of the night or he would've pulled all his lines out!"

A distorted smile creased Connie's face as she scratched another little note on her clipboard.

As the charge nurse's taped report mercifully came to an end, Angie glanced up at the patient wall board. The remaining 19 patients residing in the ICU/CCU were in no better shape than Mr. Alcott. An acetaminophen ingestion, four chronically vented respiratory failures, a GI bleed, a stroke, two throat cancer surgeries, a post-partum haemorrhage and three motor vehicle accidents. Five acute MIs and a dying cardiogenic shock rounded out the unit's depressingly diverse patient load.

With report over, it was Connie's job to assign patients, coffee breaks and Code beeper duty. An icy smile curling back her painted lips, she saved Angie's assignment for last.

"Since you missed report and the patient you had yesterday was transferred out, I'll bring you up to speed on the situation. ICU is jammed wall to wall. As such, CCU was forced to accept two vented patients during the night. I've asked Janey to start phoning for extra staff, but so far it's not looking very promising. Until she finds someone, we're just going to have to hump it. Bed seven is a vented acetaminophen ingestion... a Mr. Shaw. He's comatose and on a mycomyst infusion. He shouldn't be a lot of work. Just your basic Q two hour turn and suction. As well, I'm giving you Mr. Alcott in bed eight. From the sounds of it, he could be a handful. As you'll be way too busy to get your initial assessments done in time for first break, and with you having been on second yesterday, I've put you on third coffee. Any questions?"

Having heard enough, Angie's clenched teeth were half way through her tongue when Connie handed her the Code beeper as well. Sweet Jesus! Carrying the beeper meant that Angie would have to respond to all Code 99's called in the hospital during her shift. A Code 99 was paged over the hospital's public address system when a patient was found to be in cardiac or respiratory arrest.

There was also an unwritten rule that went along with the Code beeper: if you save them... you keep them. In other words, if the revived patient survived long enough to be brought back to the unit, the Code nurse would inherit their care. For this reason, the charge nurse usually assigned the Code beeper to the nurse with the lightest patient assignment. That would not be the case today.

Fighting to keep her emotions in check as she stuffed the Code beeper into her scrub's chest pocket, Angie was just about to head off toward the CCU nursing station when Connie's voice forced her to pull up short.

"Angela, I'm not through speaking to you yet. This showing up late for work is becoming habit forming, don't you think? Fourth time this month."

"It's my darn car," Angie struggled to defend herself. "I went out to start it this morning and the battery was dead again. I had to get my neighbour out to bed to jump it for me."

"I'm sure I'm speaking for your poor neighbour when I suggest you stop off at Canadian Tire on the way home tonight and check out their automotive department. Better yet, you might try stopping off at a car dealership. One more thing, Kris Hill finished her orientation last week but knowing how you like to teach, I took the liberty of buddying her with you. She's got the fresh MIs in beds one and two and I've already spoken to her about checking with you if she has any questions. This won't be a problem, will it?"

Mutely shaking her head, Angie watched as Connie turned on her heel to stride briskly down the hall toward her office. Listening to the happy click of her heels on the linoleum, Angie knew that her supervisor was smiling.

Her brown-spotted scrubs a testament to the kind of shift she had put in, the night nurse sitting at the desk expressed disbelief upon hearing Angie state she had both bed 7 and bed 8 as a patient assignment.

"You've got Shaw and Alcott! Man, you really must've peed in Harrington's cornflakes this morning. Sheryl Powers had Mr. Shaw last night, but one of her kids is home sick with the flu so she wrote up report and left early. In a nutshell, Shaw OD'd on acetaminophen three days ago and has basically cooked his liver. He's unconscious, not assisting the ventilator and his skin is turning a lovely shade of yellow. As well, all that charcoal we've been diligently pumping into him has his bowels working overtime. Sheryl and I changed his bed just before she left, but it just keeps oozing. I'll never get this crap off my uniform. Anyway, Shaw will be the least of your problems. Mr. Alcott in bed eight has been trying to crawl out of here all night. Damn near succeeded, too. He's a pneumonia, end-stage cirrhosis and is growing staphylococcus in his blood cultures. Security had to leave at six-thirty. Somebody was down on parking level three, breaking into cars. The guards are still looking for the culprit. If you ask me, they won't be back. Playing cops and robbers is much more fun than trying to hold down a drunk who's soaked to the gills with pee. I'm afraid you're on your own girl. I can't believe Connie gave you both of them."

"I love my job. I love my job," Angie muttered under her breath as she ran off an ECG printout on her two patients. As she was taping them to their respective flowsheets, Becky Dexter, another day shift nurse, reached out to take the tape dispenser from her.

"Ange, if it will make you feel any better, I did a quick poll and the general consensus is that Connie must have the weirdest menstrual cycle of all time. She's got PMS every flipping day and you know the old joke, "What's the difference between a terrorist and...." Becky paused in mid sentence.

Angie heard it too. A deep, throaty, vibrating sound... as if a 747 was about to touch down on the roof of the hospital.

"Oh no!" Angie let out a moan as the pager in her scrub pocket started to beep. "The last time those guys landed here was because their patient was trying to croak on them!"

Like *M.A.S.H.*'s Radar O'Reily, she sensed what would happen next.

"Code 99... Emergency. Code 99... Emergency."

Cutting across a back hallway, Angie charged down the stairs to the emergency department. Huffing and puffing, she headed directly to the trauma room where several ER nurses stood waiting.

Using their stretcher to burst open the trauma room doors, the bigger of the two medics was fighting to hold pressure on the patient's right groin. With the heel of his latex gloved hand buried wrist-deep in jellied blood clots, it still wasn't enough to stem occasional spurts of bright red arterial blood from arcing high into the air.

As the doctor and his team immediately went to work assessing the patient's airway, inserting a central line, drawing gases and trying to figure out why this person was trying to die on them, lab and X-ray personnel hovered quietly in the shadows, awaiting their turn.

Like she had done countless previous times, Angie grabbed the metal clipboard off the top of the crash cart so she could record the events as they unfolded around her. As the ICU nurse involved, it was her job to instantly interpret the type of cardiac rhythm the patient was in, keep accurate account of all the various treatments given by the other members of the Code team and chart all vital signs. For legal purposes, every action had to be recorded and it had to be written down in the correct sequence.

It was only after several minutes of frantic scribbling that Angie was finally able to sneak a peek in the direction of the two male medics. One blood-splattered, mustachioed individual, having given his report to the emerg physician, had since returned to the helicopter to fetch their patient care log. His clean shaven partner, meanwhile, had elected to stay behind to bag the patient while a respiratory tech suctioned out the man's airway. As Angie was giving his finely tuned body the once over, the big strapping paramedic looked up and, lifting his bushy eyebrows in mock surprise, flashed her a mischievous grin.

Angie Jackson's shift had finally taken a turn for the better. The gorgeous male leaning against the other end of the stretcher was none other than that infamous scourge to nurses everywhere... Russell P. Andrews. More importantly, he also happened to be the very best friend Angie had ever had.

"We have a twenty-six year old male for you," Russ began his report. "Was riding his Harley to work when he made a very unwise left turn in front of an oncoming station wagon. Unconscious with probable head, neck and spinal injuries. His upper trachea was crushed so we were forced to perform a cricothyrotomy in order to maintain an airway. Worked real well at first. Had his oxygen sats up to one hundred percent.

About ten minutes out, however, his sats suddenly plummeted into his boots and his heart rate started climbing. Kyle was having a bitch of a time trying to bag him so we elected to divert to the nearest medical facility instead of continuing on to Parkland Memorial."

The Code team crowded around the deathly pale biker. The Harley's clutch lever had ripped open the right groin, severing the femoral artery hidden deep inside. As well, intravenous fluid that the emerg resident had purposefully infused into the man's belly was now draining back a pale pink, indicating there was internal bleeding going on somewhere inside. The only good news came when the attending physician got a few moments to study the man's cervical spine film. While the X-ray showed a compression fracture of C-5, there was no visible displacement of the spinal cord... and hopefully no paralysis.

Strapped to a wooden spine board with a rigid plastic C-collar around his neck, an ugly purple bruise had already discoloured the poor fellow's entire right cheek and temple area. The force of impacting with the roadway had torn the full-face helmet from the man's head and fractured both the nasal and cheek bones. The right eye was completely swollen shut.

"There was so much resistance when Kyle was bagging him, I needled his chest to rule out a tension pneumo. All we got back was some dark blood though. I couldn't listen to his lung sounds in the helicopter, but he was shocky as hell and his neck veins were flat so I'm pretty sure he's bleeding into his chest. I'm willing to bet that's why his oxygenation is so poor."

As Russ gave his report, the doctor was already busy tapping his fingers against the patient's mottled chest. Quickly straightening up, the doc called for a chest tube tray. Slicing open an inch and a half long incision in the man's chest, the doctor jammed his left index finger down into the hole to further widen and deepen it. From a sterile, blue-wrapped bundle spread out on a nearby stand, a nurse handed the resident a long plastic tube shaped like a knitting needle. Using a cork screwing motion, he forcibly shoved the chest tube between the fourth and fifth ribs until he felt a distinct pop.

Copious amounts of dark red blood immediately began to gush from the tube; even before it could be attached to suction. With his right lung now able to re-expand and two units of O negative blood pouring wide-open into the IV lines, the young man's vital signs and oxygen saturation grudgingly began to improve.

Redirecting his attention to the patient's groin, the doctor carefully guided a long metal kelly clamp down into the wound. A single spurt of blood splashed the doctor across the chest as he struggled to clamp off the half-inch diameter artery. Snapping the kelly into place, the physician called out to one of the emerg nurses, "Diane, have the unit clerk phone over to the Grey Nuns and find out who's on call for cardiovascular surgery. Tell her I've got a lacerated femoral artery here and unless we want this guy's leg to eventually turn black and fall off, he'll need prepped for a vascular repair immediately."

As the man's condition had stabilized, Angie stepped out of the way so Russ and his partner, a tall, dark and very married medic by the name of Kyle Stevens could help the respiratory technician and one of the emerg nurses wheel the patient over to CT for a brain scan. With nothing left to do now but finish off her charting and get back to her unit, Angie carried her notes and numerous ECG strips over to the counter so she would have more room to work.

Half way to X-ray, Russ came to the realization that it didn't take four people to push a stretcher. Announcing to Kyle that he would meet him back at the helicopter, Russ hustled his buns back to emergency. Noiselessly tiptoeing through the trauma room doors and seeing Angie's back turned, the purely romance-minded medic couldn't resist the temptation to tenderly plant a kiss on the velvety nape of his girlfriend's neck.

Dracula would have received a warmer reception. Sometime during screaming for help and flailing at her unseen assailant, Angie sent her precious Code sheet flying into a sink used for disinfecting instruments. Frantically fishing her now savlon-soaked paperwork out using a pair of forceps, the emotion-weary ICU nurse appeared ready to burst into tears.

"It's okay!" Russ found himself apologizing as he plucked the dripping document from her grasp. "I've had this happen to me lots of times... we'll just pop this puppy in the microwave and...."

"Andrews... you... you...." Angie found herself struggling for words as she snatched at the soggy unreadable mess, "if you really want to help me... THEN DON'T HELP ME!"

As the handsomest male she had ever hooked up with stared remorsefully at the floor, Angie immediately regretted her words.

"I'm sorry. It's not your fault. It's just I'm having a bad day and I've got a splitting headache and when Parkland finds out you absconded with one of their precious trauma patients, you'll be lucky if they don't come chasing after all of us with a fully charged defibrillator!"

"I hope they do," Russ replied softly as he gazed upon his favourite RN. "Then we'll have an excuse to run away together."

"Run away with you? Mr. Andrews, I'll have you know I still haven't forgiven you for that prize you tormented me with last month... you remember, the patient who chewed his IV line in half and then escaped down the fire exit wearing nothing but a five thousand dollar telemetry unit and his jockey shorts? Know where the cops finally found him? Trying to flag down a ride on fourteenth street that's where. Told them we weren't feeding him enough and that he'd just stepped out to pick up a sub sandwich! Russ, you must remember the guy. He weighed three hundred pounds! And guess whose patient he was? Mine! And the Assistant NUS has been ragging on me ever since. Told me I should've kept a closer eye on him. For crying out loud, I was down at lunch at the time."

"Torment you! What about me?!" Russ fired back. "The other night we were sent to a bar fight downtown. Our patient was spraying blood all over heck and only after he spit at Kyle and tried to bite me on the leg did he bother to mention the fact that he was HIV positive!"

"He tried to bite you? That's nothing! Yesterday I had a patient go berserk on me on the way back from Nuclear Med. He was a Heroin/Cocaine/Librium overdose and to top it all off, he wasn't even my patient. I was just spelling a friend off so she could take a whiz. The attendant and me were bringing this guy through our unit's double doors when all of a sudden he thinks we're the cops hauling him off to jail. He's fighting and kicking and somehow he gets his foot caught in the siderail. Gives a big kick and flings himself halfway off the stretcher. There we were, trying to wrestle this degenerate back onto the stretcher when the automatic doors suddenly started to close. I'm telling you it was just awful! I got squished between the door and the siderail... nearly collapsed a lung and the girls in emerg said they could hear me screaming all the way down there. Oh, and did I forget to mention that while this was all going on, the guy was woofing charcoal from both ends? It was running off the sides of the stretcher. It was all over the floor. The doors got it... the walls got it... I got it! And it was while I was trying to scrape the stuff off my pant leg that I got this funny feeling. Somehow, I just knew which medic had brought him in. I checked the guy's chart. Want to hazard a guess whose name was scrawled on the ambulance sheet? Four major hospitals in this city to chose from and yet you seem obsessed with bringing all the nut cases here. I've had it with you expecting me to look after every 'weed and feed' weirdo that you and your faithful buddy

Tonto scoop out of the ditches at all hours of the day and night. It's got to stop! Do you hear me Rusty? It's got to stop!"

Angie's rendition of a nurse in need of a Valium climaxed as she none-too-playfully grabbed her friend by the collar of his navy blue flight suit.

"For God's sake, woman, that's what I live for!" was his near-asphyxiated response as he struggled to pry her hands from around his throat. "I always try to bring the worst cases here because I know that your gentle hands and soft voice will comfort their hearts and souls and mend their broken bodies!"

Angie had always told Russ that he should have been an actor. As her tired facial features slowly melted into an exasperated smile, she found herself reaching up to fluff some life back into his helmet-flattened curls.

"As you may have detected, I'm having a bad day, but I'm off tomorrow. Would you care to risk getting together later for a pizza or something?"

Russ winced. "I can't. Kyle and I volunteered to cover till eleven tonight so the night crew can go to our station barbecue. Hey! Why don't you come over after your shift and tag along with us for awhile? Maybe then you'll understand what it's like to live on the cutting edge of life!"

For some absurd reason, the idea actually appealed to her, but she still gave Russ a wary eye. "Will I be expected to do anything physical or will I be along strictly for moral support?"

"That depends on your morals. But if you want to get physical with me after the shift's over, that's another story!"

Feigning disgust, Angie pushed Russ' ever-creeping hand away from her rear end. "You guys are all alike. You all have insatiable egos, you're all sexually deprived and you're all on the make."

After sharing a much-needed chuckle, they gave each other a big comforting hug. "So do we have a date for tonight or what?" the medic persisted.

"You know most normal guys would take a girl out for dinner and a movie when they went on a date?"

"Uh, but you know I'm not normal."

"Oh I know that!"

"So... is it a date?"

"What the heck," Angie finally gave in. "I can't think of anything I'd rather do tonight than ride around in the back of a hot, smelly ambulance while you and your testosterone-riddled partner cruise the city streets in search of fresh roadkill!"

2
HIGHWAY TO HEAVEN

Russ and Kyle were busy restocking their ambulance with supplies when Angie finally blessed them with her presence.

"I really didn't think you'd show," Russ smiled.

"Wouldn't have missed it for the world." Angie stifled a yawn as she rested a pale cheek against the freshly-washed ambulance's cool metal exterior. Watching as the medics continued with their restocking, Angie was reminded of something that had been on her mind all afternoon.

"Tell me, if you guys are stationed out of this fire hall, how the heck did you end up with a chopper flight today?"

Russ and Kyle grinned. "It's called being in the right place at the right time," Russ grunted as he stuffed a handful of suction catheters into an overhead compartment. "We'd just dropped a patient off at Parkland and were enjoying a leisurely cup of coffee and a jelly doughnut in the nurse's lounge when we overheard a nurse complain that she and a trauma doc were waiting for the rescue helicopter to pick them up so they could fly out to a scene call near Priddis. Their emerg was just a zoo today and right then, they had patients backed up all the way to admitting. The flight nurse really didn't want to go because she'd been airsick on her last trip and the resident kept grumbling about how EMS choppers tended to crash and burn, so we kindly volunteered to go in their place."

"Coffee, doughnuts, having someone fly you around. Yep, this being a paramedic sounds like a tough way to make a living, alright!" Angie lamented.

"Yeah, it's a dirty job, but somebody's got to play the hero!" Kyle piped up. "By the way, how's that patient we brought in doing?"

"His CT of the head looked okay. The surgeons fixed up his leg; removed his spleen. He's still in a coma, but he withdraws to pain. With any luck, he'll be back riding his 'hog' in a month."

Nodding in agreement at Angie's update, the two medics slowly climbed out of the vehicle to give their cramped muscles a stretch.

"How about a backrub?" Russ asked with a flirtatious wink. Angie was smiling at the thought when a loud series of tones erupted over the PA system. They had a call.

Sliding open the side door of the ambulance, Russ quickly ushered

Angie inside. With Kyle buckling himself in behind the wheel, Russ hopped into the passenger seat and radioed dispatch for further information. "Medic twenty-six, you have a motor vehicle accident with injuries near De Winton. Take Highway two south... further location info will be relayed as it comes in."

While Kyle maneuvered his speeding ambulance through traffic, Russ thumbed through a binder of road maps. In the back, fingernails embedded in the edge of her seat, Angie twisted her head so she could look through the front window, now pock-marked with light rain.

As the city limit sign receded in the side mirror, dispatch came back on the line: "Single vehicle roll over, one mile west of De Winton on secondary road five-five-two. Multiple patients involved. One female in active labor. Okotoks EMS not available. High River ALS ground unit responding. Police and fire department already on-scene."

Angie began to make mental notes about what medical equipment they might need. God knew what they were going to find at the scene, and it was this fear of the unknown that was making her heart thump like a kettle drum. What would they find? Would she know what to do? This was not going to be the nice, controlled environment she was accustomed to... with internists and specialists fighting for a piece of the patient. This time, there would be only three of them out there—two over-sexed paramedics and a burnt-out nurse.

Speeding down the divided expressway as it bisected the lush, green countryside, all Angie could think was, "What the heck have I got myself into?"

As Kyle turned off the highway onto a gravel road, the dispatcher radioed with more information. "Medic twenty-six, we have an update on the MVA location. Take secondary road five-five-two, keep going till you come to a red barn... RCMP say you can't miss it, it's a big red barn... continue on till you cross a set of train tracks. You should be able to see the flashing lights from there."

Five minutes later they were pulling to a stop next to a jumble of fire trucks and RCMP squad cars. Sporting a paramedic jacket she had found under her seat, Angie jumped out and fell in behind Russ and Kyle as they hurriedly side-stepped down into the ditch and over to where the rural firefighters were kneeling beside something.

Lying in the tall grass were two people: a male and a very pregnant female, both in their thirties. They had been catapulted from a pickup truck which was now balancing on its hood in an adjacent hay field.

Incredibly, between the road and the truck—a distance of a good seventy-five feet—the four foot high alfalfa crop was untouched!

As Kyle and Russ began assisting the couple, a constable gave them a brief summary of the accident. "The husband told us his wife had gone into labor and he was driving her to the Grey Nuns Hospital. He admitted he was traveling pretty fast and when they crested this hill, he swerved to miss some deer standing on the road and lost control of the vehicle. Happened about an hour ago."

"What's your name?" Kyle asked the man who was lying on his back with an obviously fractured left femur.

"Colin Roberts," the man moaned, "but don't bother with me, okay? Please look at Donna. I was driving her to the hospital. She's expecting our first kid and... just make sure she and the baby are alright. Please?"

"It's okay, Colin," Kyle murmured, laying his hand on the man's chest. "My buddy's looking after her. She's in good hands."

Russ and Angie were already hard at work assessing the woman's injuries. Russ took over from the firefighter who had been carefully stabilizing the woman's neck. Thrown as far as she had been, a neck injury was a real possibility. Holding her head firmly between his knees so that his hands were free, he began hooking his portable oxygen tank to a non-rebreather mask setup. As a paramedic with 15 years of street experience to guide him, he knew that the best and easiest treatment he could give a pregnant patient and her unborn child was oxygen... lots and lots of oxygen.

Angie knelt beside the poor woman and was immediately struck by how out-of-place the pregnant woman looked, lying crumpled in the weed-choked ditch. Following the standard ABCs of pre-hospital assessment, Angie first checked for level of consciousness and a patent airway. The patient before her was totally unresponsive to any stimuli, verbal, painful or otherwise. Her airway sounded clear and she was breathing on her own, but her respiratory pattern was far from normal. Each breath was very rapid and very deep.

Angie could detect a moderate pulse in the side of the woman's neck, but could not find any pulsations in either of the woman's arms. This usually meant the patient was in profound shock and probably had a blood pressure hovering somewhere down around the 60-70 systolic mark. A pressure this low could not be tolerated for even a short period of time. Without pressure to circulate blood and oxygen, the body's tissues and cells would quickly begin to suffocate and die.

Winding up her initial assessment, Angie did a quick "Look, Listen and Feel" examination of the woman's chest and abdomen while Russ slipped the oxygen mask into place.

"In my opinion, she's a definite load-and-go!" Angie said. "She's unconscious, the most probable cause being a closed head injury. Her respiratory pattern is grossly abnormal with rapid, deep breaths that seem to be of a neurological nature. She's also got to be bleeding inside somewhere because she's in shock, big time. The only pulse I can detect is a carotid, so her pressure can't be much higher than sixty systolic! The chest looks, feels and sounds okay, but it's her belly I'm worried about. I've palpated a lot of pregnant tummies in my time, but hers is rock-hard, so I think we should forget the formalities and get the heck out of here!"

While Angie had been relating her findings to Russ, she had simultaneously been trying to assess whether the woman's pupils reacted to light. The much abused flashlight she had found in her jacket pocket, however, was refusing to cooperate. "Work... damn it!" she cursed, slapping the flashlight against her thigh. With that delicate technical adjustment, the light blazed to life and Angie quickly carried out her pupil check. She was not happy with what she found. The woman's pupils were equal, but very sluggish to react.

Continuing to support the woman's head with his knees, Russ reached down and gently palpated the bulging abdomen. It was hard. Very hard. "I sure hope to God it's all baby in there and not a ruptured spleen or something," he remarked quietly.

Just then, he felt movement under his hands. "Maybe it is all baby in there, Ange. I just felt the little gaffer kick!" It was a hopeful sign, but Angie and Russ both knew it could also mean the fetus was becoming distressed. Which meant that every second now was an extremely precious one!

The ambulance crew cast tall shadows into the growing darkness as they moved about in front of the fire truck's powerful flood lights. The rain had stopped, but in its place a thick blanket of fog was settling over the area. Creating a ghostly dreamscape, the dense haze flowed across the roadway in endless waves which silently swirled around the EMS vehicles.

Once its sparse vegetation had been trampled flat, the ditch had quickly taken on the appearance of a mobile trauma room. Empty gauze envelopes, blankets, spine boards, neck collars and oxygen bottles littered the ground around each patient. Assisted by a volunteer firefighter, Russ and Angie gently transferred the woman onto a metal scoop stretcher. Strapping her in, Russ positioned a horseshoe-shaped blanket roll around her head, securing it to the stretcher with long pieces of adhesive tape.

Suddenly she convulsed. Though deeply unconscious, Donna's tightly clenched teeth chewed viciously on her oral airway as her arms and legs thrashed against the stretcher's nylon restraints. Russ immediately reached to protect the intravenous site in her arm, yelling, "Draw up some Valium, Ange, and be damn quick about it!"

Angie was frantically stomping on a foot pump, struggling to inflate the MAST, or Military Anti-shock Trousers, which Russ had velcroed into place around their patient's legs and abdomen. "How the heck do you expect to inflate them with her doing the funky chicken like this, girl? For God's sake, whack her with the Valium. Once she quits seizing, I'll show you how to inflate those MAST leg compartments by mouth."

Immediately upon "packaging" their patient to Russ' satisfaction and tilting her on her left side so the enormous weight of her uterus would not collapse the large abdominal blood vessels, Russ and three young firefighters heaved the stretcher and its two hundred and fifty pound load up the steep embankment and into the ambulance. The EMS unit from High River had arrived on the scene and after speaking briefly with Russ, its two-member crew immediately went to relieve Kyle who was in the process of applying a traction splint to the man's fractured leg.

Once inside the warm ambulance, Russ contacted Mountainview's emergency department by mobile radio. Under the bright lights in the back of the ambulance, Angie got her first glimpse of the woman's ashen pallor. Her skin was clammy and moist. Her pupils were growing more dilated with each passing minute. "I can't find the carotid anymore!" Angie cried out as she anxiously probed the woman's neck. "She's got no pressure!"

While Russ was calmly relaying details of the patient's deteriorating condition to the ER doc, Kyle's head poked through the ambulance's open door. "The High River crew said they'd transport the husband, so we can roll as soon as you're ready."

"Wait!" Russ barked as he held up his hand. "Just give me a minute, okay?" The telephone pressed tightly against his ear, he listened for several seconds, then repeated the physician's orders aloud as he received them.

"MAST pants? Already on. Inflate legs only. Keep her on her left side. Saline IV wide open and an obstetrician will be on hand when we arrive.

"Okay Kyle, let's get the hell out of here!" Russ commanded as he hung up the phone. "This little momma's circling the drain!" Slamming the heavy rear doors, Kyle leaped into the driver's seat.

The fog hung like heavy white sheets over the roadway. Kyle had not driven far before he was reluctantly forced to turn off the ambulance's flashing overhead lights. Reflecting off the impenetrable haze, their harsh glare was blinding.

Russ and Angie meanwhile, were totally absorbed in keeping their patient alive. Knowing she had to start a second large-bore IV, Angie was methodically palpating the woman's arms for suitable veins. Simultaneously, Russ hooked up the cardiac monitor and after running off a strip, calculated the expectant mother's heart rate at 160 beats a minute, roughly twice what it should have been!

Accustomed to the spacious emergency trauma room, Angie was finding the ambulance very cramped. With the stretcher filling most of the available floor space, there was little room for her feet. After very nearly yanking out her first IV because it had suddenly quit dripping, Angie was frantically checking her line for kinks when she discovered the real cause—one of her size nine sneakers had inadvertently come to rest atop the soft, pliable tubing.

"She's got zilch for veins. I'm going to try for a blind antecubital," Angie called out as she tore the protective cover off another bag of IV fluid. "Wish me luck."

Russ was pulling a curved blade out of his airway pack. His mind deep in thought, he snapped it into the handle of the laryngoscope.

"Luck? You're the best, Ange. You'll get it. You always do. The extra fluid will hopefully give us a blood pressure. Just be quick about it, okay. I'd like to get her tubed as soon as possible. I'm scared she's going to woof her cookies and choke. I've got the tape all ready, but with the C-collar on, I'll need you to apply some throat pressure so I can visualize her cords." He knelt on the floor and positioned himself directly behind Donna's immobile head.

Barrelling down the road as fast as he dared, Kyle was only half-listening to the commotion going on behind him. Catching a glimpse of several deer standing off to the shoulder, the frightened medic muttered under his breath, "Holy geez, if those deer had been in the middle of the road, there's no way I could've... HOLY SHIT!"

Hunched over the steering wheel, peering into the gloom, Kyle could hear Angie telling Russ to pull the endotrachial tube back just a tad, as she couldn't hear any air entry to the woman's left lung. "Must have it down the right main stem," the medic mused. Just then, something on the road directly ahead captured his undivided attention. The fog did not seem quite right. Instead of a solid white wall, the damp, swirling mist was now drifting in short, regular bursts to the right... to the right... always to the right.

For a split second, Kyle did not have the slightest idea what it might be. Then, all of a sudden, he did.

With no time to shout a warning, he wrenched the ambulance into a savage sideways skid. The terrified medic could only listen as a startled cry from one of his passengers was abruptly cut short by a bone-jarring thud... followed by a chilling silence.

The tires shrieked like an animal being butchered as they ground to a gravel-spewing halt. The unearthly stillness was broken only by a strange, naggingly familiar sound: chunka... chunka... chunka....

It was as if time itself had come to a stop. Finally, Russ thrust his bleeding head between the ambulance's bucket seats. "Christ, man!" he cussed. "What the hell are you trying to do? Kill us all?" All the while struggling to stem the flow of blood pouring down his face from a large cut above his eye, Russ got absolute silence from his usually yap-happy partner.

His large meaty fists welded to the steering wheel, Kyle continued to stare through the bug-splattered windshield at the fog bank before him.

After threatening to check his good buddy for a pulse to see if he was worth killing or not, Russ was just about to give his stunned partner a smack when something floated past the windshield.

"Oh my God?"

Not five feet from the ambulance, monstrous things were emerging from the mist. Ghosts! The huge objects glided past at a dizzying speed, only to vanish again into the dense fog. But they were not monsters, they were not ghosts. They were white anhydrous ammonia railway tanker cars.

3
YOU CAN'T KEEP A GOOD WOMAN DOWN

The phone rang three times before an unsteady hand snaked out from beneath the blankets and fumbled for the receiver. "Hey Angie, it's Russ! I've been trying to get hold of you all day. There must be something wrong with your phone or something. Anyway, I've got some really great...."

Dropping the receiver into its cradle, the hand limply retreated back under the covers. The phone was quiet for a moment before ringing again. After a bit, the answering machine kicked in and Clint Eastwood's virile drawl prompted, "It would really MAKE MY DAY if you would leave your name and number after the beep. If, however, you decide to just hang up and not leave a message, I think you should stop and ask yourself one simple little question: DO YAH FEEL LUCKY TODAY? WELL, DO YAH?"

After the beep, Russ' harried voice came back on the line. "Look Angie, I know you're home. I called the unit and they said you'd booked off sick for a week! Don't you think that's a bit much? I mean all you busted was your nose and you always told me you didn't like the way it looked anyway. Heck, here's your big chance to have that nose you always...."

Angie snatched for the phone. But with neck muscles so stiff and sore she could barely turn her head, her sudden change of position sent the ice bag saddling her swollen nose tumbling into the bed, spilling water and crushed ice everywhere. "Look you... you rodend!" she shrieked into the receiver. "I'll have you know I can'd breed, I've losd my sedse of tasde and every tibe I sneeze id feels like my endire face is going to blow off!"

Angie slowly collapsed back onto the bed. Her head felt like it was splitting apart.

"Hey Ange, I'm sorry," Russ said softly. "I just wanted you to pick up the phone, that's all. I didn't mean it. What I really meant to say was that I'd like you even if you ended up with a nose like Karl Malden's."

"Karl Malden's? Dear God!" Angie groaned as she gingerly repositioned the ice pack atop her bloated features.

"I've got some great news for you, girl! I phoned the Mountainview this morning and that patient we brought in was 'all baby' after all. The docs did an emergency section on her and delivered a healthy nine pound six ounce boy. The CT scan of the mom's head showed only minimal swelling so they're just treating her with steroids and lots of TLC. She's still on a vent, but she's got some purposeful movement in her arms and legs and actually tried to pull out her ET tube last night, so that's a good sign. Hopefully she won't have any permanent deficits. Isn't that great? Hello... Ange? You still there?"

A moan oozed from beneath the melting ice. "Whew! For a second I thought you'd quit breathing or something. Thought I might have to dial nine-one-one."

"You still mighd have to call nine-one-one when I ged through wid you, Mr. Andrews."

"Now, now Ange... steady girl. Remember your Grey Nuns motto-'Semper fidelis... Always Faithful.' Cure the sick. Heal the injured. Be true to your school and all that nurse stuff."

"Russ, if you want sobthing thad's always faidful, buy a dog, 'cause as soon as I have my docdor's permission, I'm coming over to your place to give you a back massage wid my Garden Weasel!"

"My kind of girl... and I always thought you were into leather whips and stuff. I'm getting excited. By all means, please let me know when your doctor says it's okay. But I'm getting off topic here. The reason I'm calling is to see if you'd like to go to a movie with me Friday night?"

Angie was about to utter something derogatory when a trickle of ice water escaped from the nasal pack and dribbled into her ear. The accompanying vocals were not unlike those of an alley cat caught in a fan belt.

"I take it... that's a yes?" came the medic's halting reply. Hustling to change the subject before she changed her mind, Russ quickly added, "Oh, and by the way, my station captain wants you and me and Kyle to meet with him at ten a.m. tomorrow."

"Whad aboud?"

"I suppose he wants to discuss our latest escapade, and he also mentioned wanting to ask us about a new helicopter rescue program starting up this summer." Russ paused for a second. "You know, Ange, Kyle and I really appreciated your help last night. You'd make a damn fine paramedic if you'd just quit bleeding all over the patient."

Sinking into her pillow, Angie closed her puffy eyes as she remembered back. How could she ever forget? Kyle's rapid braking action had hurled her, face first, into the fiberglass partition separating the back of the ambulance from the driver. Stunned, Angie very nearly collapsed on top of the poor patient. Stumbling backward with blood spewing from her nose and mouth, Angie's eyes began to water so badly she could barely see. Cradling her shattered snout with one hand, she blindly groped in one of the sidewall compartments for a gauze dressing.

The sudden stop had slammed Russ' face against the edge of the same divider, splitting his left eyebrow wide open. The medic had actually been very lucky. He had just missed being thrown through the open space between the front seats, and into the windshield.

Kyle quickly came to the aid of his injured passengers. He first did a quick reassessment of the patient... checking for further injury. Fortunately, Angie and Russ had finished intubating her before the accident, and, because she was strapped down, Donna had come through the ordeal basically unscathed.

Kyle then turned his attention to Russ and Angie. By the time the train had rumbled past, he had worked his medical magic and was seated behind the steering wheel again, anxious to get the show back on the road.

Because she could not see what she was doing, Angie was forced to take over Russ' job—helping the patient breathe by forcing 100% oxygen into her lungs with a collapsible Bag Valve Mask or BVM. As she sat slumped in the jump seat, madly bagging life back into her patient, she unknowingly continued to drizzle blood all over the top of the patient's head, all over herself, and all over the once-gleaming floor of the ambulance.

It was left to Russ to check the IV lines, monitor the woman's vital signs and phone the hospital with a patient update. As soon as he had things under control again, he glanced over to see how Angie was holding up. As things turned out, however, it was Angie, not Russ, who was presented with a truly unbelievable sight.

Skipping the usual gauze bandage wrap, Kyle had decided to save precious time by using a maternity pad to bind his best friend's wound. Stuffed under the brim of Russ' baseball cap, the innovative idea had worked surprisingly well. The hat kept pressure on the absorbent pad, which in turn, controlled the bleeding quite nicely. Unfortunately, one of the pad's gauze ties had since pulled free and was now flapping about like a blood-soaked bandanna.

Despite her best efforts to remain calm, Angie was forced to turn away in hysterics. Russ thought she was crying and leaned closer, trying to comfort her. That caring gesture made the gauze tie flap around even more. After awhile, Angie did end up crying. But only because it truly did hurt too much to laugh!

4

ALL THEY REALLY WANTED WERE A FEW GOOD MEN

Brilliant sunlight streamed through the cramped office's lone window and Angie found herself squinting painfully as she, Russ and Kyle waited patiently in front of the fire captain's desk. When the husky firefighter strolled into his office, Russ and Kyle automatically started to rise, but were quickly motioned to remain seated.

William Scott, a 26-year veteran of the Calgary Fire Department, stood behind his desk, quietly surveying the three of them. Russ wore wrap-around sunglasses to hide his blackened left eye, but they failed to conceal the enormous swelling of his cheek and the nylon stitches poking up through his bushy eyebrow. Kyle also wore dark shades and a baseball cap pulled low over his eyes but, rather than a cool dude, he resembled someone about to knock off the corner "7-11" store.

As bad as the two medics looked, Angie stole the show. With eyes puffed and bruised, the sides of her nose were so swollen that they blended directly into her chubby cheeks. The miniature Plaster-of- Paris cast atop the bridge of her nose did little to enhance her appearance, and because she was now forced to breathe through her mouth, Angie Jackson looked and sounded in immediate need of adenoidal surgery.

As the well-packaged captain was introduced to Angie, he deftly skirted the corner of his desk to give her hand a firm shake. "Pleased to finally get to meet you, Miss Jackson. I've heard a lot about you!" He shot a grin in Russ' direction.

Even through blurry eyes, Angie could not help but notice the unspoken exchange. Just what the heck had Russ been saying about her, anyway?

"Okay, let's get down to business, shall we?" Captain Scott began. He looked at the athletic, dark-blond woman. "Angie, I've already been given a pretty good rundown of the accident the other night. That aside, how did you feel about working in the field as a medic?"

Angie glanced at Russ as she cleared her throat. "Uh well, sir, as you know I've done a couple of ride-alongs wid Russ before, bud mostly jusd on routine hospidal to hospidal transfers and to be honesd, I always found them kind of, you know, routine. This last call was the firsd scene call I'd ever gone on. Don't ged me wrong, sir, I don'd mean to say thad I was happy aboud nearly gedding killed and all, bud when we were on-scene, I found I had to think on my feed a lot more, you know, adapt to the siduation. Id was a real learning experience. I guess thad was the pard I liked best."

William, or Big Bill as his crew referred to him behind his back, struggled to conceal a smile as he nodded thoughtfully, watching Angie gently dab with a tissue at her once petite nose.

"That's good to hear, Angie. I'm glad this hasn't affected you in a negative way. It was a situation that isn't likely to be repeated." Bill looked at Kyle as he spoke. The medic nodded tightly, then returned to staring at his boots.

The room was quiet as the veteran firefighter leaned back in his chair, steepling his fingertips together. "I'll tell you the real reason I asked you here today. As you know, the Olympics are less than eight months away and it's a sure bet they're going to put a heck of a strain on the emergency medical services in this city and the surrounding area. With this in mind, Parkland Memorial Hospital and Riverside Medical Center are currently in the process of revamping their air ambulance program.

"Designated with the call sign, LIFE-STAR, the 'Shock Trauma Air Rescue' service will utilize an immediate dispatch system which will allow for a much more rapid transportation of patients than the system currently in use. The way it stands now, when a call is received, the helicopter is first dispatched to either Parkland or Riverside to pick up a trauma doc and an emergency nurse.

"Kyle and Russ here can tell you that some nurses and doctors like to fly in choppers and some don't. Some would like to, but get airsick every time their feet leave the ground. This fact, coupled with the often twenty to thirty minute delay in leaving for a call, has become a real problem which must be corrected if this program is to remain viable.

"What LIFE-STAR program directors would like to do is organize full-time flight teams. Based at the airport, each crew will consist of two pilots, a paramedic, a critical care nurse and an emergency department physician. The program's mandate is to provide the smaller rural hospitals and EMS services with a highly skilled medical team, available to assist in the care and rapid transport of ill or injured patients to Calgary for further treatment.

"Each member of the LIFE-STAR medical crew must be top notch, with ACLS, BTLS and PALS certifications. They will also receive additional training in basic rescue techniques such as sling retrieval, outdoor survival and water rescue.

"This service will cover all of southern Alberta and southeastern B.C. During the actual Games, the unit will also respond to any accidents of a critical nature involving Olympic athletes or visitors at the mountain venues of Nakiska and Canmore.

"Right now, because of a serious lack of government funding, our program's main objective doesn't stretch much beyond the Winter Games, but rumor is that if we can successfully pull this project together, there is every chance that LIFE-STAR will continue to fly long after the Games are history.

"I've been asked to submit a list of possible Air Medical Crew candidates to our recruiting co-ordinator by the end of next week. A training camp will be held later this month to select the five paramedics and five nurses needed to man... uh, operate the program.

"It's going to be tough on your body and your mind!" Big Bill stated emphatically. "No cake walk. You'll often be flying into the mountains and I might as well tell you right up front that the accident rate for EMS med-evacs has been statistically very high in the past. We're going to try to skew the odds in our favor by having two pilots on board for every flight and not over-working them. It'll be risky, dangerous work at times, but for the right kind of person, it could also be extremely rewarding."

Bill turned to face his two medics. "I'd like to submit both of your names. I'll give you a couple of days to think it over. Let me know by Friday." Immediately noting that the best damn nurse in the entire city had somehow been left out of the conversation, Angie gave the captain a questioning, demanding look.

"Don't worry Ms. Jackson, I didn't forget about you. I'd like to submit your name as well. Like I said, I want you three to think it over for a few days and let me know what you decide."

The meeting over, Angie, Kyle and Russ filed out of the office. Tagging along behind like a lost puppy as they headed for the parking lot, Angie bristled as she listened to her paramedic pals babble excitedly about the new program. "Look guys, this Big Bill character forgod I was even alive in there! You could jusd tell he doesn't think I can cud id."

"He's probably right, you know," Russ teased as he stuck his nose in the air. "I mean, what if we had a call and it was your time of the month? I can see it all now... me fighting to keep the patient alive and you unplugging valuable life-saving medical equipment so you could plug in your heating pad!"

Russ barely got the comment out before being forced to run for his life. Struggling to unlock his car door, he tried frantically to ward off Angie who was smacking him mercilessly with her ice pack. "You chauvinistic sleaze bag!" she wailed nasally.

Deciding to make a desperate run for it across the fire hall lawn, Russ could've easily outrun her and made good his escape had he not tripped over a garden hose hidden in the grass. Finding himself suddenly face down, he automatically reached up to protect his neck, but was light years too late as Angie triumphantly straddled his broad back and dumped the entire bag of melting ice cubes down his shirt.

Kyle had made a clean get-away and yelled from his truck window as he sped past the prostrate pair, "Hey Russ, must be a full moon... always drives a woman wild with desire!"

Angie lobbed several ice cubes at Kyle's receding vehicle, then, being careful not to bump her tender, misshapen nose, leaned forward and whispered seductively into Russ' ear, "If only I had my Garden Weasel wid me!"

Without warning, the medic rolled from beneath his attacker and within seconds was on top, pinning Angie helplessly to the ground. With a wolfish leer, he inquired if she would like to see his very own Garden Weasel.

Big Bill, who had been watching the entire proceeding from his office window, wistfully shook his head as the young couple continued laughing and wrestling on the fire station's immaculate front lawn.

If only his wife would jump on him like that.

5

WHERE THERE'S A WILL

Angie did a lot of thinking about the Air Rescue program during the three long weeks prior to the LIFE-STAR selection camp. In total, 34 medics and nurses had been invited to try out for the ten Air Medical

Crew positions. As usual when confronted with a new challenge, one part of her was all confidence, while another part didn't think she had a hope of making the squad. Whatever the outcome, she thought the survival training sounded kind of fun, a refreshing change from the sterile confines of a big city hospital.

Russ and Kyle, on the other hand, couldn't wait for the week-long training camp to start. Having already flown on board the med-evac helicopter, they considered themselves shoe-ins for the job.

The morning of the first day was spent writing four tough exams covering everything imaginable pertaining to the care and air transport of critically ill patients—from knowledge of first line cardiac IV medications like Epinephrine, to rapidly interpreting and correctly treating potentially fatal ECG rhythms.

Angie found that most of the questions dealt with basic textbook scenarios, but rather than being straight-forward in their approach, they tended to make her stop and think a lot. Some scenarios appeared, at first glance, to have only one correct answer, but not when she took a few extra minutes to carefully re-read them.

What the instructors obviously wanted to determine was how the paramedics and nurses approached unusual medical situations. Would their combined knowledge be complimentary, or would they simply end up stepping all over one another's egos?

In-depth studies in Europe and the U.S. had revealed that if a med-evac program had a higher ratio of scene calls vs hospital-to-hospital transfers, a nurse and paramedic made a much better core transport team than, say, a doctor and nurse, or a doctor and paramedic. The research showed that, while physicians were superb at handling a crisis in the ER department where all the medical amenities were close at hand, they were not all that useful when their prospective patient was still embedded in the wreckage of an overturned vehicle. Extrication and packaging were obviously not topics covered in Med school.

A decade in ICU had made Angie an expert in cardiac care, a fact which her glowing test marks would verify. However, to be really successful in this line of work, she was going to need something else—the confidence to act on her own. There would be no doctor on board for routine scene calls, so she would need to believe in her ability to correctly diagnose a problem, and then treat the patient accordingly.

With time of the essence, the Air Medical Crew was expected to do a quick assessment, treat life-threatening conditions, package the patient, and then transport him or her as rapidly as possible to hospital. Often the hospital wouldn't hear from the flight crew until well into the return leg of the mission, and by then it was too late to ask the emerg doc for permission to do some life-saving procedure that should have been carried out thirty minutes earlier. Even though the helicopter was equipped with the most sophisticated mobile radio that money could buy, there would still be times when the paramedic and nurse would be all on their own.

After three numbing hours writing the exams in a muggy, university science theatre, Russ, Angie, and Kyle could not wait to escape into the fresh air. They sat on the lawn of a nearby hamburger joint and, between bites of succulent cheeseburgers and sips of thick, ice cold vanilla shakes, conducted a test post mortem.

"What did you put down for the physiological effects of MAST pants?" Kyle asked Russ. That had been one of the many questions in the baromedical section under the heading: "How does flying at altitude affect a patient and why?"

"It was a simple matter of elimination, Kyle," Russ replied, popping a ketchup-drenched french fry into his mouth. "MAST pants are presumed to supply blood to the vital organs by forcing blood from the legs up into the belly and chest, so the only answer that positively did not belong was the one about them increasing intracranial pressure."

Angie sat back and quietly sipped her shake. The exam results were the furthest thing from her mind. She knew she had done well. With the exception of the baromedical section, they were the same ones she had to write each year in order to stay certified in her unit. No, the exams were not going to be a problem, but something else she had learned this morning would be.

Tomorrow, all the trainees were going to learn water rescue. It was not the fear of failure that had Angie worried; it was the fear of embarrassing herself in front of her peers by drowning.

Angie Jackson could not swim! More succinctly, Angie had trouble facing a shower. As a kid growing up on her parents' farm, she had even hated setting out the lawn sprinkler for fear of getting splashed. As long as she could remember, she had been afraid of water. Since there was no logical reason for it, Angie was adamant that in a previous life, she must have drowned. For all she knew, she could have gone down with the Titanic; there was just no other explanation for her unprovoked hydrophobia.

She had taken beginner swimming classes twice as a child and successfully learned to open her eyes underwater. That was it. As an adult, she had taken a "Terrified of Water" course and, while she did eventually learn to float on her back, if someone splashed so much as a molecule of water on her face, she keeled over and headed straight for the bottom. There was none of this "going down for the third time" stuff—she just sank like a tombstone, and that was the end of it.

While swimming ability was not mandatory, the instructors had made it very clear that in the case of two equally-qualified candidates, the more proficient swimmer would get the nod. After a bit of snooping around, Angie had made the unsettling discovery that part of the water rescue course involved treading water for twenty minutes. Twenty minutes! It might as well be twenty years!

Oblivious to Russ and Kyle's natterings, Angie stretched out on the grass and sleepily pondered her options. Maybe if she sort of floated on her back and pretended she was treading water? No, that wouldn't work. What if someone splashed her or the instructor made her tread water the correct way? Then, another thought came to mind. Should she be trying to cheat at all? After all, this was not a Math 30 quiz. If she could not pass the water course, maybe she didn't deserve to be considered for the team.

On the verge of falling asleep, a positively brilliant idea took shape in her overheated brain. God, it was so simple! Why hadn't she thought of it before?

"What did you put down for your answer, Angie?" Kyle's rough voice roused her back to reality.

"Wha... ?" she asked with a sun-stroked expression.

"You know, the one about MAST pants and how flying in an unpressurized aircraft would affect them. Does it increase or decrease the pressure inside them?"

"I... uh... think I circled both of them," the blurry-eyed blonde babbled as she gathered up her burger wrappings and staggered clumsily to her feet.

"You put what down?" Russ blurted. "Why on earth did you do something dumb like that? There was only room to mark one correct answer!"

When Angie confessed that she had, in fact, answered a number of questions with more than one answer, both paramedics groaned in unison. "You probably flunked out, big time!" Russ announced.

"Well since I've no doubt washed out of the program already, I think I'll just go home, mix myself a Zombie and drink myself into oblivion!"

"You never could lie!" Russ said. "You hate rum! So just where is it you have to go in such an all-fire hurry?"

"I thought I just told you!"

"Hey! How come he gets your leftovers and not me?" the meddlesome paramedic was on his feet now as he watched Angie give Kyle sole custody of her remaining french fries.

"Because his father didn't die of a heart attack at age fifty-eight, that's why! Oh, and by the way, the correct answer was 'BOTH OF THEM! It wasn't mentioned in the question, but since an aircraft has to both take off and land, the pressure inside the pants would correspondingly increase with altitude and decrease upon landing, thus making 'A' and 'B' together the only correct answer.

"And on that thought-provoking... and in you losers' case, probably a somber... note, I'll see you boys bright and early tomorrow morning."

The freshly-slapped expression on both mens' faces left Angie wishing she'd brought along her camera.

6
FIRST IMPRESSIONS

It was after normal operating hours at the university pool, and the hushed sound of water gently lapping concrete softened the silence. Angie noticed none of this as she stuffed her generous curves into a spiffy one-piece aqua blue swim suit, scrounged from her sister. She emerged from the change room like a bird expecting to be eaten, and made for the shallow end of the pool, a zippered bag tucked tightly under one arm.

Staring out over the calm, shimmering waters, she could feel her stomach start to tighten. She knelt down and gingerly stroked the water with her hand. An icy shiver spiraled up her spine.

Remembering a trick from one of her many futile swimming lessons, she headed back to the change room. A brisk shower was supposed to make the frigid waters of the pool seem warmer, but the shock of the freezing shower nearly stopped her heart. As her goose-pimpled extremities imitated rigor mortis, the determined RN stuck it out, coughing and sputtering, for a full minute under the numbing spray.

"Suffocating... gasping for air... what a truly horrible way to die!" her chilled gray matter yammered as she scrambled out of the shower. Reluctantly tossing aside her towel, she hurried back to the pool's edge; it was time for Plan A.

After splashing about in the shallow end for awhile, she picked up the water skiing belt she had brought with her. A gift from an old boyfriend, it released a heartful of memories as she buckled it round her trim, muscular waist.

Countless hours Jeff had spent trying to teach her to swim. Time after time, he would hold her up and time after time, she would start panicking as soon as he let go. Incredibly, in spite of her fear, Angie had looked forward to his lessons. Between near-drownings, Jefferson would hold her close to reassure her. To the love-struck nurse, there was much to be said about cuddling up to a nice warm man who was repeatedly saving her life! In fact, after awhile she couldn't wait to start sinking. The reward for failure just felt too good. Now, all alone in the empty pool, Angie wished she had paid more attention.

What she desperately needed right now was a damn good pep talk. "You can't drown in four feet of water, you idiot!" she scolded. "Settle down. Take some deep breaths." With goggles and ear plugs in place, she clutched the tiled edge and eased onto her back. Suddenly she found herself suspended on the surface of the water. "Piece of cake!" Sucking in a ragged breath, she plowed a clumsy furrow across the shallow end, her painful back stroke resembling a paddle wheeler in reverse.

"Okay, let's try it on the belly, shall we?" she muttered. The ski belt was working miracles. First she tried the simple dog paddle, gradually adding, whenever she remembered, sporadic kicking of the legs. When she found herself, incredibly, on the other side of the pool, she laughed out loud.

On the observation deck high above the pool, a lone figure leaned against the rail. Gazing down, the slim, blond-haired man smiled at the woman jabbering to herself. Finally, he picked up his gym bag and descended the stairs to the men's change room.

Angie was downright giddy. Having ascertained that the ski belt would keep her from drowning, she moved on to phase two of her plan.

Carefully she slit open one of the belt's sealed compartments with a paring knife, then removed some of the Styrofoam hidden inside. Again she practiced her strokes.

Her goal was to determine the minimum amount of foam required to keep her afloat. In the morning she would duct tape the foam blocks to her belly, and cheat her way through the water rescue course. She knew it was wrong, but she had made a solemn promise to herself to take swimming lessons again, just as soon as the training camp was over.

Two foam blocks, she eventually discovered, were enough to keep her head above water. Removing them from the belt, she shoved them down the front of her bathing suit until they were positioned roughly to either side of her navel.

The suntanned stranger, now standing in the doorway of the change room, had been watching with increasing fascination. His first impression was that the poor woman had lost her breast prosthesis. "What a shame," he murmured. "A young female like that, having a double mastectomy. Well, give her credit for getting back into a swim suit. Good for her."

Then he watched her position the foam pads, not on her chest, but around her belly button! "What the hell... " he breathed. As he strained to get a better look, he got another shock. This woman was no former mastectomy patient. She had a damn fine set of all-natural hooters and now, by golly, she seemed to have four of them!

The poor man could only watch, dumbfounded, as Angie pulled her goggles back on, slipped into the water and paddled off. In all his years swimming at some of the finest beaches in the world, he had never seen anyone move through the water quite like that before. With the growing curiosity of an old tom cat, he sauntered over to the pool, took a seat on the edge and dangled his long brown legs in the water.

Angie meanwhile, was attempting the front crawl. Grossly over-confident by now, she brazenly put her face in the water with the intention of coming up for breath every second stroke. She lasted two and one-half strokes.

Having committed the dreadful faux pas of breathing in when she should have been breathing out, the heavily chlorinated water poured into her lungs and Angie's new enthusiasm for swimming transformed instantly to mind-blowing panic. Coughing and gagging, her goggles half-filled with water, she began clawing hysterically for the pool's edge.

The fellow perched at pool-side called out to her, asking if she was alright. Angie never heard a thing. Ripping off her goggles, she squinted painfully, searching frantically for the ladder. She made a final desperate lunge for the middle of the top rung.

Being grabbed by the balls had not even entered 45 year-old Dale Morgan's mind that evening when he decided to go for a swim. Yet, here he was, being molested by a deranged, half-blind, totally deaf female with four breasts. The guys back home were never going to believe this one.

As for Angie, something in the far recesses of her brain was telling her that whatever she had just grabbed hold of in her frenzy... it did not feel like the rung of a ladder. Then her forearm brushed against a warm, muscular thigh. In an instant, it all came together. She was confronted with the awful realization that yes, she definitely had hold of... an adult male.

Not wishing to get up and make a run for it with this mad woman attached, Dale decided to make the best of it. "Find anything you like?" he meekly inquired, his rich Aussie voice elevated a full octave higher than usual.

As if she'd grabbed hold of a high voltage wire, Angie leaped back. Yanking out her ear plugs and rubbing her eyes, she looked up to find herself face-to-groin with a ruggedly handsome man with wavy hair and a large Australian flag on the front of his swim trunks.

"I know it doesn't look like much, "he said, "but back home, we're all rather proud of it."

Her eyes big as ostrich eggs, Angie froze.

"I was talking about the flag... you know, the Australian flag?" He even pointed, but it only made things worse.

Angie heard herself reply: "Uh, you're quite right. It's truly lovely... I would be proud of it, too... uh... oh God!"

Looking down to avoid his gaze, she noticed with horror that her illicit foam blocks had migrated together and now looked like one large breast at the level of her navel. Immediately she sank down and, walking on her knees, crawled to the shallow end. She then made a mad dash for the change room.

She would have stayed in there forever, but it was getting late. Twenty minutes later, praying the poor fellow had departed, she stuck her head out the door. Finding the coast was clear, she scurried for the exit.

Suddenly, a small piece of foam appeared over her shoulder. Letting out a terrified screech, Angie spun around.

"I believe you left this floating in the pool?" Dale said, handing her the foam block.

Wanting for all the world to run back to the change room, Angie instead heard herself mumble a barely audible, "Thank you," as she humbly accepted the man's offering. Hoping that would be the end of it, she turned and walked away, all the while trying to stuff the infernal slab of foam into her equipment bag. Unfortunately, the bag's zipper had hung up on something and she could not get the flipping thing open.

"Here... allow me," the Aussie said as he untangled the zipper and pushed the block inside. "There you go," he added cheerfully as he handed it back to her.

"Look... I'm... uh... so embarrassed. I hope I didn't hurt your... uh... oh my...."

"No harm done," Dale smiled. "You know, I was just thinking... if all the girls in Calgary are as direct in their approach as you are, I just might enjoy living here. Look, I'm new in town. Would you like to go out for a beer or something?"

"You can't be serious! I mean... I don't even know you!"

"Good heavens, woman, after what I've been subjected to tonight, I'm the one who'd be taking a chance! Come on Miss... " Dale paused to glance down at the name tag on her gym bag. "A.Y. Jackson? Wasn't he one of the Group of Seven painters?"

"You've heard about the Group of Seven?"

"Of course. I was an art major in university. But I really think your parents should've named you after the other guy in that group, what was his name... Tom Thomson. Wasn't he the one who drowned? My name's Dale, in case you're interested. Dale Morgan. Happy to make your acquaintance. Now, do I get to find out what the A.Y. stands for, Ms. Jackson?"

"After what's transpired here tonight, sir, that secret is going with me to the grave!"

"Well, from what I've seen of your aquatic ability, that won't be long in coming!" Dale sniggered. "Maybe if you'd let me treat you to a beer, we could discuss your need for such... um... unique floatation devices."

Angie groaned. This guy was just like Russ, he never gave up. In spite of herself, she felt a smile creep across her lips as she headed for the exit with Morgan right in step beside her.

Dale held the door open as they stepped into the brisk night air. His ego bolstered by having talked this spirited young woman into spending the evening with him, he boldly asked his new lady friend a rather delicate question.

"Have you ever thought about maybe using one of those inflatable bras?"

7
LIGHTNING STRIKES TWICE

The next day dawned hot and sunny and the weather office forecast little chance of precipitation. Within the confines of the University of Calgary pool complex, however, it was quite another story. With close to one hundred percent humidity, you could actually taste the moisture in the air. While Angie credited her sweat-soaked appearance to this phenomenon, the real reason was fear. Fear of water... and of being caught cheating.

Clad in her one-piece Speedo, Angie stayed near the back of the group as they waited for the Water Rescue session to begin. Russ spotted her and immediately headed over. "You really seem to fill out that suit today, Ange," he teased. "All those bust improvement exercises must've paid off, eh?" he added, trying to sneak a peak under her firmly-crossed arms. Watching as Angie blushed and squirmed, the nosy medic had another question for his woman. "By the way, I tried to call you around eleven last night, but all I got was your machine."

Never one to be caught off-guard, Angie had a cover-story ready and waiting. "Alright Mr. Andrews! I confess. You caught me red-handed. I was out prowling the town, okay. Instead of sipping cocoa and watching the boob tube like a good girl, I cruised over to the medical book store to check out their selection of stethoscopes. While I was there, I ran into an old girlfriend and we wound up going for a beer. Satisfied?"

As a skeptical Russ was mentally digesting Angie's alibi, the head instructor meanwhile, had emerged from the pool office, followed by a trio of water rescue specialists. One fellow was wearing swim trunks, the other two wet suits with scuba tanks.

Too many heads were getting in their line of vision, so Angie and Russ moved closer to the front. While Rusty hurried ahead, Angie's every step was slow and measured. She was deathly afraid that one of her foam blocks might accidentally detach itself from her belly and decide to migrate.

Suddenly she stopped dead, her jaw nearly dislocating as she stared, transfixed, at one of the men standing at the front of the group.

This could not be happening.

The camp's portly head instructor, Peter Lawson, began the introductions. The first two men were with the special Maritime Rescue unit based at Canadian Forces Base Comox in British Columbia.

"Our third instructor," Peter gestured toward a slim, blond fellow in black trunks with the Australian flag emblazoned across the front, "is joining us from Yellowknife, but he hails from the land down under... Cairns, Australia." Angie shuffled quietly in behind Russ.

"He's an expert in both mountain and water rescue. Served two tours of duty in Vietnam as a chopper pilot and has experience flying in every kind of weather imaginable. I'm particularly proud to say that he'll also be joining our program full-time as our chief helicopter pilot. Please welcome Dale Morgan."

As the color drained from her face, Angie had to remind herself to breathe. This could not be the same guy. Could it? Dale hadn't told her a lot about himself, having only casually mentioned that he was involved with aviation somehow. Angie hadn't bothered to ask much about him, being far too busy trying to protect her own identity. However, having fallen in love with his thick Aussie accent by her third beer, she eventually confessed that she was in dire need of learning to swim. The lifeguard-turned-pilot agreed to help her out... but only if she wagered a dinner date if he succeeded.

The evening had ended on a happy note, Dale seeing her safely to her car and bidding her a gentleman's adieu—saying he was quite looking forward to their next pool encounter. Angie had readily agreed. But that was all ancient history now.

Lawson was droning on. The Air Medical Crew hopefuls had been divided alphabetically into groups which were to rotate through three stations. While one group was being tested for swimming ability, a second would be checked out on various types of underwater gear. The third group's objective was to rescue an instructor who was pretending to drown.

Turning to say something to Angie, Russ was startled to discover her standing directly behind him. "What the heck are you doing back there?"

"Oh... I'm just... you know... admiring the view," Angie lied as she flashed a glance in the direction of Russ' muscular behind.

"Hum," the medic whispered seductively as he attempted to slip an arm around her waist. "Wouldn't you rather see what I stuff the front of my 'Fruit Of The Looms' with?"

"Andrews, you are so crude! Is that all you think about? Sex!" Angie hissed, grabbing a fistful of chest hair.

"Jackson, Andrews... quit molesting each other and get into your groups!" Peter shouted at the flailing pair.

Dale looked over to see what all the commotion was about and, when he saw Angie, burst into a grin.

"Do hurry up, Yvonne. We haven't got all day you know," he called, waving her over to his group.

"Ange? What the hell is going on here?" Russ demanded as his woman started slowly toward Morgan's group. "First, you compliment me, then you attack me, and then some guy you haven't even met yet is calling you by your middle name? What's going on?"

"I'm really sorry, Russ. Must be those darn PMS hormones." Angie mumbled as she continued to back toward Dale's end of the pool.

"PMS... my ass!" the flustered medic bellowed. "Do you know that guy from somewhere?"

Receiving only a feeble shoulder shrug in reply, Russ reluctantly went to join the equipment group.

What the heck was going on? She'd never kept secrets from him before. They were best buddies... weren't they?

Having watched as Angie had endured a multitude of passionate encounters that invariably ended up the same way, on the rocks, Rusty had been her sounding board—her shoulder to cry on.

Not that the studly medic had been a great role model himself. While Russ had always considered himself quite a catch, for some reason, he never seemed to find a girl worthy of taking home to meet his mother.

After each traumatic affair, he and Angie had instinctively run back to one another for moral support... knowing the other would understand. It was that age-old adage: Misery loves company!

Back at the pool, Dale was taking inventory. Out of his motley group of seventeen, ten assured him they were strong swimmers... good enough to swim ten laps with no problem.

"How many of the rest of you think you can swim at least two lengths without drowning?" the pilot curtly inquired. Six more people put up their hands. That left only one. Angie.

Sick at heart, she waited for him to ask, "Is there anyone here who can't swim at all?" Instead, Dale abruptly marched over to where she was standing and squinted dramatically into her right ear. "How long has your ear been like this?" he demanded with an air of great authority.

"All my life, sir?"

The Aussie rolled his eyes. "No, no, how long have you had an ear infection, Miss Jackson?" He said it loudly enough for everyone across the pool to hear.

"Oh! Oh, that? Oh, I've had that about a day or two, sir. I'd really hoped it would've cleared up by now. I do want to pass this course so much and I...."

Dale raised his hand to silence her. "No, I can't possibly allow you to go in the water for at least a week." He glanced around to make sure everyone in his group was listening. "But not to worry. If you're healthy by next Saturday, I will personally retest you on all the areas covered here today."

"Oh gee, sir," Angie sighed. "Thank you so much for giving me another chance."

As Dale stood facing this ditzy babe, his expression betrayed him: "God, she can't swim and she can't act either?"

"So as today won't be a total loss, Ms. Jackson," he said, "I fully expect you to pay close attention while I instruct these so-called swimmers in the fine art of proper stroking."

Ordering everyone into the pool, Dale turned to join them, but not before giving Angie's duct-taped midsection a clandestine flick with his finger. "You can change into your civies if you're quick about it. I wouldn't want you to get tape burns or anything."

At noon there was a short break. Russ found Angie sitting cross-legged on the lawn, in the shade of a big spruce tree. She looked up briefly as he collapsed beside her. Pulling an apple from his lunch bag, he munched loudly as he stared across the vast campus.

It was Angie who finally got up the courage to ask how his day was going; a big mistake. "Oh, my day couldn't be going any better, Ange," he flippantly replied. "Let's see, I was almost asphyxiated when my tank regulator malfunctioned. I nearly drowned twice trying to rescue that damn instructor. But heck, that's enough about me. How's your day been, Ms. Jackson? I've noticed you haven't gotten wet yet. What did you promise Morgan in exchange for letting you skip his class?"

Her cheeks flamed, but Angie refused to take the bait. "For your information, it just so happens that I have an ear infection and Mr. Morgan doesn't want me to get any water in my ear."

"An ear infection? Do you really expect me to believe that crock?"

"Look," Angie spit out her words as quietly as she could, "this is the best thing that could've happened to me. You know I can't swim. I promised Morgan I'd take private swimming lessons every night for the next week. Then, depending on how I do, I'll be retested on Saturday."

The paramedic laughed out loud. "You've always been scared to death of water. You told me you can't even face a shower, for Pete's sake. You've taken lessons before and they didn't help, so just what makes you think you'll do any better this time round?"

Angie chewed on her lower lip a long time. "Because Dale... uh... Mr. Morgan said he'd teach me himself?"

Russ coughed out part of his apple. "What? That guy's been riding my can all bloody day... screaming I can't swim well enough to save myself, never mind someone in trouble... said he just might have to fail me for my own good and now you tell me he's going to give you another week to learn?"

"Look, he knows I can't swim, okay? But I guess he feels sorry for me and he's willing to try and help me pass this stupid course. You should be happy for me!"

Russ' ruddy complexion went violet. "Why should I be happy? He's been threatening to flunk everyone else in the class."

"Andrews, I couldn't care less why he wants to help me. He seems like a decent-enough kind of guy... a heck of a lot nicer than you are right now. If he can't teach me to swim, then nobody can. Did you know he was a member of the Australian Olympic swim team? He was their national breast stroke champion three years running.

"I bet he was!"

Angie got up to leave.

"And another thing... " Russ yelled as he, too, jumped to his feet, "you know this morning, when I said how you really filled out your swim suit? Well, I never could understand why you can't swim. You know how well fat floats!"

That did it. A parting shot about her weight! He knew how sensitive she was about that. Men! When they can't win an argument, they insult you!

For one brief second, she actually felt like coming clean and telling him the whole story, but why did he have to know absolutely everything that went on in her life?

Suddenly, a much better idea took shape in her vindictive little mind. Snatching the partially-eaten apple from Russ' hand, Angie stepped back and with one powerful, overhand throw... fired away.

Her gender-altering assault caught Rusty totally off-guard.

The mouthy paramedic dropped like a sack of rotting cabbage.

8
PRIDE AND PASSION

At six o'clock the instructors brought the Water Rescue class to a gut-wrenching close. Literally. Their nauseated bellies sucked full of pool water, nearly every single trainee had had to rush to the bathroom to throw up... the result of having been ruthlessly dragged underwater by a sadistic Howard Bateman, the so called "drowning victim."

"A drowning victim," he had begun his lecture, "will grab hold of you and in his panic, literally try to climb on top of your head to get out of the water. In the interests of rescuer safety, sometimes it's better to wait until the person loses consciousness before attempting to approach him."

It was a sad fact, but true—more than one would-be hero had gone to the bottom after blindly rushing to the aid of another.

Kyle had been pulled under twice, and tried later to describe the feeling to his wife. "It was like trying to fight off an octopus. Arms everywhere, clutching, grabbing, pushing my head under. For a moment there, I honestly thought that bastard was going to drown me! I really did!"

Even though she had only watched, Angie was also feeling sick to her stomach... with guilt about what she had done to her best friend. It was Russ who had kept her alive after Jefferson Logan departed her world with the tired and untrue line about "wanting to remain friends."

Following her breakup with Jeff, her sole reason for living crumbled to dust. Any further enjoyment of life was over. She had trusted Jeff utterly with all her innermost secrets, her hopes and every one of her dreams for the future. For months following the breakup, Russ watched her knock back many a bottle of cheap wine as they talked long into the night about how rotten Jeff was and what a creep Jeff was and how Mr. Logan was the real loser in the end.

It had been a whole year now, but Angie still caught herself thinking about Jeff every now and then. If nothing else, she had learned something very valuable from the awful experience. Never again would she allow someone to use and abuse her like that. Not ever.

Yes, an entire year had passed. Now here she was, finally beginning to think about the possibility of dating again, when it seemed her nearest and dearest pal was having an emotional crisis of his own. What the heck was eating him? It couldn't be jealousy, could it?

Angie walked out to her Chevette, drove aimlessly around the empty campus, and ended up parking right next to Russ' car again. Resting her head against the steering wheel, she rehearsed what she was going to say. Good God, what else was there to say but... sorry!

Still frantically searching for the right words, she saw the tousle-haired medic emerge from the sportsplex and head for his car. Forced to shift his muscular frame sideways to squeeze between the two vehicles, he purposely turned his head the other way as he unlocked his car and fired his swim bag into the back seat.

Angie stepped out nervously. "Rusty, I don't know what came over me at lunch. I'm really sorry about what happened. It was an idiotic thing to do. I'm so ashamed. Can you uh... can you ever forgive me?"

His reddened eyes glowered down at her from their lofty six foot two inch perch. Voice wavering, Angie tried again. "Come on, we need to sit down and talk about what happened. Everything got way out of hand. How did this whole mess start anyway? I don't understand what's happened to...."

"I may never be able to father kids thanks to you... that's what happened!" his enraged shout interrupted her.

Russ had never yelled at her before. Angie turned away abruptly. She'd be damned if she'd give him the satisfaction of knowing he'd made her cry.

Standing defiantly with arms folded, Rusty stared intently at the pavement. "You want to go for coffee somewhere?" he asked quietly. "There's a little place across the street...."

Angie glanced up just in time to see him brush something from his eyes.

The sombre-faced couple was about to walk across the street when the paramedic reached out and did something he had never done before. He took Angie's hand in his and, carefully interlacing their fingers, gave it a tender squeeze.

9
ROCK-CLIMBING SCHOOL

For the next two days, the training camp moved to the Yamnuska Mountain Centre, a facility renowned for its rock and icefall courses. The staff were all top-notch climbers with major international experience; several, in fact, had been members of the successful Canadian Everest expedition.

Peter Lawson had three main objectives for this segment of the selection camp. "First," he told his instructors, "we'll learn who has the stomach for helicopter work, that is, who tends to get airsick and who doesn't.

"Our second goal is to find qualified people willing to work their butts off to get the job done. Our medical crews have to be very good at what they do, but more importantly, they have to mesh together as a team. There is absolutely no room for a STAR-GOD in this program. The last thing I want are prima donnas who think they're special or somehow above the rules.

"Finally, I want you people to watch for the little things that make a big difference—the ability to absorb new ideas, willingness to share knowledge and, above all, the tenacity to work on weak areas, even if it means spending extra time after class.

"What we're looking for," Lawson concluded. "are the ones who are the very best in their medical field, who work and play well with others while under tremendous pressure, and can do it all in an airborne rollercoaster without tossing their cookies. It's not too much to ask... is it?"

Following the hour-long, crack-of-dawn bus ride from Calgary, the drowsy trainees were shown to their cabins. Hoping to breathe some new life into his sleepy-eyed recruits, masochistic drowning instructor Howard Bateman ordered everyone on a brisk half-mile jog around the lake.

The mountain air, crisp as a bite of green apple, was heavy with the spicy, pungent fragrance of spruce as they sprinted off. Eager to impress, the non-smokers were soon far in the lead, leaving their tobacco-inhaling colleagues huffing and puffing to catch up.

Enveloped in an all-natural "Rocky Mountain High," Angie felt she could run forever. Bounding along, feet barely touching the forest floor cushioned with evergreen needles, Angie was in a world of her own. It had been so very long since she felt this way. Russ was right at her side and every now and then would glance over and flash her a big, cheesy grin.

They had spent the previous evening getting their confused emotions sorted out. First off, misunderstandings were cleared up. Dismissing Dale as nothing more than a friend, Angie confessed to having met him the night before at the pool. Not exactly how she had met him, just that she had.

With that touchy issue finally resolved, their coffee grew cold as they revealed to one another—in fact, to themselves for the first time—how they had both wasted years dating other people. People who could never quite measure up to the feelings they had always had for each another.

While they agreed not to rush things, at least not until this whole training camp thing was over, it was a resourceful Russ who insisted on following Angie back to her apartment. "Just in case you have car trouble or something."

At her apartment door, Angie, her thoughts elsewhere, fumbled through her purse for her key, then dropped it. "Here... let me," Russ said softly. He opened the door and left it slightly ajar. Staring at the floor, Angie had not felt this nervous since seventh grade! Eventually looking up, she found the paramedic holding out his arms.

Standing there in the deserted hallway, Angie's loving arms wrapped tightly around him, the moment of truth had arrived. Russ pulled back slightly to take her trusting face gently in his hands.

While to the casual observer, it may have appeared as if they were attempting to eat one another, Angie and Russ' first official necking session actually started off with a virginal innocence.

Their initial buttery-soft kisses, however, soon led to ear nibbling and breathless, increasingly bold caresses. The couple finally, reluctantly, untangled themselves and, like teenagers on their very first date, couldn't help but grin sheepishly at one another. Russ brushed back the curls from Angie's face and gazed into her blue-green eyes. They had a luster, an inner fire, that he had not seen for a very long time.

Glancing up at her apartment one final time as he drove away, Russ noted the bedroom light was on. He would have given anything to have stayed, to have tenderly held her in his arms as she slept, but he knew it was too soon. For the first time in his lustful life, Russ Andrews was not after a quick roll in the hay. He wasn't after a cheap, one-night stand.

"Oh yes," Angie dreamed lazily as she sprinted along, "a weekend off, a handsome man, falling in love... what more could a working girl want?"

A tremendous roar shattered the idyllic mood; a cherry-red helicopter was passing overhead. On its side, in bold white letters, were the words, "LIFE-STAR 1." Then Angie heard the deep, throaty purr of its engines edge up a notch. Its four mammoth rotors blasted a dark cloud of dust and grit as it set up to land in front of the training center.

"Just being this close to it is exciting. What will it be like to actually go up in the thing?" Angie wondered as she raced Russ back to camp.

Peter Lawson gathered everyone beside the helicopter. "Okay group, this is what it's all about," he said, jabbing a thumb toward the helicopter. "Over the next two days, you will learn how to handle yourselves around a chopper, and how to use all the medical, rescue and communication equipment on board. You'll also learn the basics of rappelling and how to survive in the wild.

"We're going to start off by dividing into groups and then rotating through the different stations. As the temperature is expected to hit twenty-five Celsius today, this morning we'll concentrate mainly on rock-climbing. Once you've got that mastered, we'll teach you how to rappel out of the helicopter without endangering yourselves, your patients or our high-priced pilots. In addition, Canadian Forces Search and Rescue has graciously loaned us one of their FLIRs or Forward Looking Infrared night scopes. This device can quite literally turn night into day and we'll be using it tomorrow during a simulated rescue mission."

Peter then introduced the various climbing, survival, and fire safety instructors. Dale took over after that and introduced the seven other pilots who would fly the helicopter on a rotating basis. Each pilot had more than 3,500 hours of flying experience; several had military training.

Introductions completed, the AMC trainees were divided up and assigned to instructors. Angie headed off to rock climb, while Russ and Kyle followed Dale over to the chopper.

"Okay, first off, this is a BK one-seventeen helicopter," Dale began, his intense stare demanding full attention from his charges.

"The BK's most important feature is its twin engines. Only one is required to maintain the aircraft inflight. It cruises at one hundred and fifty miles per hour and is VFR certified. While it does have some IFR instrumentation which would allow us to fly during reduced visibility, for the time being, we will be operating strictly under Visual Flight Rules.

We use a two-pilot crew at all times. One flies outbound, the other inbound, on each mission. In this way, we keep our flight skills up and fatigue does not become a factor. A few years back, the U.S. had a very high med-evac crash ratio. They found there were three main reasons: having only one pilot on board, fatigue from overwork, and engine failure in single-engine aircraft. Our program is based on theirs, but we have hopefully learned from their mistakes and taken steps to correct them."

Dale opened the clam-shaped rear doors. His students gathered around and peered into the back. The chopper was obviously designed to maximize its limited amount of cargo space. The two main medical crew seats were positioned back-to-back with the pilots' seats. A collapsible, wheeled stretcher took up all the available floor space along the port side, while two more seats directly across from the stretcher could easily be folded up if a second patient needed transport. A bulkhead positioned between the back-to-back seats held the radios and formed a barrier separating the pilots from the medical crew.

"Those heavy black curtains suspended from the ceiling behind the cockpit," Dale explained, "are used at night to prevent light from the rear of the aircraft disrupting the pilots' night vision. On day flights, the curtains keep us from being distracted by the occasional life-and-death drama going on behind us."

Dale and another pilot, Alex Davis, then went through the helicopter, demonstrating how to use the radio and pop out the side doors in case of fire, then discussed general personal conduct while in the vicinity of a helicopter.

A "hot load" meant loading a patient while the engines were running and the rotors turning. The trainees were sternly instructed to always approach the chopper from the front or side so the pilots could see them. They were also warned to stay away from the tail rotor, period.

After making a landing, the pilot would remain in the right hand, "number one" seat, while the co-pilot would quickly hop out of his number two seat and rap his knuckles on the Medical Crew door as he trotted past. After unlocking the rear doors, the co-pilot's sole responsibility was to position himself between the back of the chopper and the dangerous tail rotor.

Upon hearing that "all clear" tap, the medical crew would climb out, remove the stretcher from the rear of the aircraft, pack up any other equipment they might need, and head off in search of the patient.

The Air Medical Crew hopefuls were never to walk behind the co-pilot for any reason whatsoever. A tail rotor in motion was invisible, and with the roar of the engines drowning out someone yelling a last second warning, more than one unfortunate soul had carelessly wandered into the whirling blades. "Tail rotor fatalities have closed-coffin funerals," Dale concluded tersely.

Once everyone had gone over the medical equipment on board, then unloaded and loaded the stretcher a half-dozen times, Dale and Alex demonstrated the FLIR spotting scope. It was a technical byproduct of modern warfare. Used on night maneuvers, it could detect any object that radiated heat... and the more heat emitted, the more clearly it would show up on the viewing screen.

Dale sat down on the landing skid as he demonstrated how to adjust the controls. "I can't really show you how well this thing works in broad daylight, but Alex will be available this evening to let you practice with it.

"Search and Rescue units often use FLIR to help locate missing people. A body, especially a decomposing one, will generally emit more heat than its surrounding area. Pre-dawn or early morning is the best time to use it, as the earth's surface is at its coolest temperature, and any heat-producing object will easily show up."

Dale pointed the scope's sensor at the parking lot to demonstrate how cars sitting in the sun gave off a "hot" whitish glow while vehicles in the shadow of the training center radiated ever deepening shades of "cool" green.

"Remember," Alex added, "this scope can only detect an object giving off heat. A rock outcropping in the sun can get pretty hot, as can an old car fender, so check the situation out very carefully with binoculars before you decide to jump out the door and rappel down. Otherwise, you might find yourselves rescuing a junked Pontiac or a big boulder! Look before you leap!" The boyishly handsome pilot turned things back over to Dale.

"Okay," Dale said, "the next thing we'll cover is how to safely anchor your rappel rope to the floor of the helicopter. The pilots and crew must work very closely together. Having something heavy dangling off the starboard side of the aircraft will throw its delicate center of balance completely off, so, as pilots, we have to compensate in the opposite direction to maintain a level hover.

"Routine slings from the ground will eventually be well within our capabilities. However, for our first year of operation, we'll be happy to leave the difficult patient retrievals to the Mountain Rescue Helicopter

Unit set up by the National Park wardens."

Dale studied the faces around him. "Look people, don't let this whole thing spook you, okay? We haven't even got to the scary stuff yet! Just remember, the wardens are the experts in this field, so our job will just be to stand by and wait for them to deliver the patient to us. We are to assist them in every way possible and act as their backup, but we'll never be asked to do anything that we don't feel completely comfortable with."

Russ and Kyle suddenly turned and looked at each other. A horrible thought had just entered both their minds. "You don't suppose the Yoho wardens have a similar program?" Kyle hissed to his partner. "God wouldn't do something like that to us... would He?"

"Mr. Stevens!" Dale snapped. "Do you have a problem with this?"

"Uh... no, sir! I was just wondering... uh... if you might happen to know any of the wardens involved with this special Mountain Rescue Unit?"

Dale shrugged. "Maybe if you contacted the Parks Service they could..."

Lawson, who was sitting in on the group, interjected, "Captain Morgan, maybe I can help. I'm not sure about all the fellows involved, but I do know that one of the wardens is Jefferson Logan. He used to work as a part-time paramedic in the Calgary area two or three years ago, so some of you might know him.

"For those of you who don't," Peter continued, "Jeff was also a Search and Rescue specialist with the Canadian Armed Forces for a number of years. He left the Force, took his EMT-P training and then joined the National Parks Service as part of their Sling Rescue Unit. He also happens to be one of this country's top mountain climbers and was a member of the Everest expedition. From what I've heard, he's one very talented and unique individual."

Russ screwed up his face as he muttered to Kyle, "He's certainly one unique individual, alright!"

"I need a volunteer to help demonstrate the rappelling harness," Dale announced. Russ jumped to his feet.

"Mr. Andrews! This is truly an unexpected honor."

As Russ pulled on the harness, he positioned himself with his back to the group so he stood face-to-face with Dale. "Morgan, I want you to teach me absolutely everything you know about this rappelling stuff, okay? You'll never find anyone more eager to learn."

Dale stepped up close to loop a climbing rope through the figure-eight rappel buckle on Russ' harness. "Oh, really. And why would that be, I wonder?"

"Because Jefferson Logan is an asshole, that's why," Russ spit back, "and I hope to God that I never have to ask for his help... ever!"

Dale made some minuscule adjustments to the medic's rappel line, stalling to analyze Russ' comments. "This sounds like something best discussed over a couple of cold brews, don't you think?" Dale asked quietly, giving a hard jerk to the rappelling rope secured to the floor of the helicopter. "Maybe then we could also clear the air about a few other little problems you and I seem to be having."

Sizing up his scrawny adversary, Russ replied, "Fine with me. How about tonight... after supper?"

Dale gave a curt nod as he turned his attention back to the group. "Stevens! Get off your duff and get the heck over here. I need someone to play the bloody patient! Let's have a little fun with this scenario, shall we? Kyle, I want you to pretend you're a smart-assed off-duty paramedic. After picking a fight in the bar, you have just had your clock cleaned by a mild-mannered helicopter pilot who, it turns out, happens to be an ex-special forces commando!"

10

ROPE AND OTHER FOUR-LETTER WORDS

After a short mid-morning break, the groups switched stations. Angie's group staggered over to the helicopter and collapsed onto the sun-baked grass. From a distance, they looked like victims of a mass disaster.

Angie had once been thoroughly captivated by the movie, *The Man Who Skied Down Everest*, with all its danger and romance and high adventure. She had even entertained thoughts about taking up mountain climbing—all that good exercise, fresh mountain air, the thrill of the assent, the challenge of athlete against mountain. "What a rush!" she had thought then.

What a bunch of crap!

In spite of her heavy cotton sweats, the rough granite slope had left a bloody, weeping mess of her elbows and knees. On her left hand, a four-inch rope burn snaked angrily from one side of her palm to the other. Worse yet, two hours of frantically clawing for handholds had reduced her guitar-picking fingernails to raw, serrated stumps.

She had learned, however, about harnesses, carabiners, Purssik knots, bolts, and the original four letter word... rope. Mostly about rope. How to tell a safe rope from a damaged one. How far they would stretch. How much they could support. How to tie them. How not to tie them. And how you should always treat them with respect. Never stand on a rope. Never drive over a rope. Never let them get dirty with oil or fuel or anything corrosive. Always check for signs of wear: frayed ends, kinks, depressions, abrasions from rubbing against a rough surface.

And there were sanctions for disrespect! A first offense for simply stepping on a rope was an automatic twenty pushups. A second infraction meant rappelling down the rock face with Howard Bateman right on your tail, broadcasting a blow-by-blow narrative of your progress.

"Look down! What would happen if your rope broke right now? You'd fall, your buddy would probably be pulled down with you, and the climbing victim you'd been working so hard to rescue would be thanking his lucky stars he was still hanging upside down off a ledge somewhere, and not already tied into your line. As your instructor, I would be deeply saddened if I had to watch you fall two thousand feet to the valley floor. Since you'd be dead, I'm the one who'd end up having my ass chewed out by my supervisor. Are you people getting the gist of this conversation?"

If Angie thought her morning had gone poorly, the afternoon schedule of activities proved to be even more physically demanding, and to make matters worse, there had been that little foul-up just as Dale was trying to teach one of the more timid nurses how to rappel off the roof of the cafeteria.

The pilots had painstakingly constructed a replica of the chopper's door and landing skids, then placed it on the roof of the cafeteria. That way, students would actually have to rappel down to the ground once they exited the mock-up. Things went relatively smoothly until June Campbell, a short, cuddly redhead was set to start backing off the roof. After hesitantly stepping through the chopper's doorway, she took one look at the ground thirty feet below and froze.

"No problem, June," Dale called up to her. "You're doing fine, luv. Just back up to the edge, lean out and then let the rope slide slowly through the buckle until it feels like you're almost sitting down. Then just start walking backwards down the wall."

June did exactly what Dale told her to do. She cautiously backed up to the edge of the roof. She let the rope slide slowly through the rappel buckle. She leaned back. She did everything correctly, except for one small detail—she didn't walk down the wall.

One of her looping shoe laces had snagged on a shingle nail and in her struggle to free herself, June forgot all about the rope which continued to slide through her hands. By the time she did notice, she was completely upside down... with her left running shoe still caught on the nail and her right foot now firmly pressed against the underside of the eave.

Peter Lawson picked just that moment to drop by and check on how things were going. Alex was trying to calm the hysterical woman as he desperately hacked at her shoelace with his pocket knife. Peter turned to the stone-faced Australian standing beside him. "Don't tell me, let me guess. This is how you rappel back home in the land down under... right?"

"Uh, no sir," Dale replied. "This is strictly an emergency escape maneuver to be used when... uh... say there was a possibility of the climber being caught in a... uh... rock slide... or something."

It was then that someone yelled, "FIRE!"

Small puffs of dense black smoke could be seen curling up from behind the building. Angie immediately ran to the site of the fire safety lecture, returning with a dry chemical extinguisher. Ignoring their stunned instructors, she and several other nurses dashed off in the direction of the smoke. This was no doubt one of the impromptu drills their instructors had warned them to expect over the remainder of the camp.

They had just spent the better part of the afternoon learning how to properly extinguish cooking woks filled with blazing jet fuel. That was as close to actually fighting a helicopter fire as their instructor wanted any of them to ever get. In fact, his parting words were, "In the event the helicopter does catch fire, you are to forget everything I have just shown you. Believe me, if this chopper crashes and catches fire, you are to abandon ship immediately and run upwind as far and as fast as you possibly can. Do not stay around and attempt to put the fire out... do you understand?"

The nurses sprinted toward the back deck. It was just as they expected—another cooking fire, alright. Someone, most likely an undercover instructor, had been barbecuing some burgers. To make it look really impressive, he had let the fat drip down on to the hot coals... igniting them and engulfing the entire grill with a wall of flame a foot high.

Just as they were taking up their positions, someone wearing a chef's hat came running around the building, shouting and waving them away. "Stand back, we can handle this!" Angie reassured him as she dramatically pulled the pin on her extinguisher and took careful aim. The other two nurses hauled the wildly protesting man out of her line of fire, then, "PSHEEEEW!" A dense yellow powder erupted from the extinguisher as if shot from a cannon. The choking cloud instantly smothered the flames, settling on the grill in a thick, foul-smelling layer. Their instructors would be so proud. What team work.

But with the smoke beginning to clear and the man threatening physical abuse, they made a dreadful discovery. He really was the camp cook and he really had been flame-broiling 47 succulent burgers. That is, until he had gone to see the amazing upside-down rappelling nurse, and Angie and her fire fighting friends showed up.

"Do you know what you've done?" the incensed chef screeched. "I hope you idiots like bloody Kraft Dinner because that's all you're bloody going to get for your bloody supper tonight!"

"Look, guys, this entire weekend has been a complete bust!" Angie lamented to her two buddies as they downed their macaroni later that evening. "I mean, do you know what I learned to do today? Before I learned to put out flaming barbecues, that is?"

Russ and Kyle laughed and shook their heads.

"I learned how to intubate a pig. Can you believe that? Our trauma instructors had a whole bunch of pig tracheas and they made us intubate them and then do tracheostomies on them. Then we all got to learn how to decompress a cow's chest. A skill like that should come in real handy if I'm ever out at my parents' farm and one of Dad's heifers suddenly develops a collapsed lung or something!

"They duct taped some beef ribs onto an inflated inner tube and we had to take turns inserting a needle between the ribs until we heard air escaping. I mean, is all this really necessary? Do you really think that one day, they'll actually let me use some of this knowledge on a real live human patient?"

"Hon," Russ reassured her, "it's the only way the instructors can teach you how to do those procedures. Everyone of us medics had to go through the Basic Trauma Life Support course. Trust me, all these things will come in handy one day."

Angie was not convinced. "After this weekend, if we ever crash into a farmer's barn, and we accidentally land on top of some of his valuable critters, we can all jump out, intubate the pigs, decompress the chests of any cattle who look like they might have developed a tension pneumo from mooing too hard, and then when the farmer ends up chasing us around the yard with a double-barreled shotgun, we'll all scatter like rats, safe in the knowledge that, if his flaming buckshot ignites what's left of our flying gas can, we'll all know exactly what to do. Run like hell... upwind."

"I hate to tell you this," Russ laughed, "but if you thought that was fun, you're going to love the Survival Course. After you learn how to construct a sturdy, all-weather lean-to using nothing but spruce boughs and your shoe laces, you'll be taught how to gut a grouse in one easy motion by standing on its itty-bitty wings, pulling on its feet, and... voila!"

"You will also learn all about grubs," Kyle added, "as in, which ones are safe to eat and which ones will give you raging diarrhea. You'll discover why you shouldn't melt down yellow snow for drinking water and last, but not least, you will be taught how to load and operate a flare gun without blowing away your hand or your foot or your partner in the process."

Angie covered the macaroni remaining on her plate with her napkin.

"Oh, and one more thing," Russ grinned. "In a crash situation, never forget the pilots. Those fearless souls who fly our great red bird and who are probably one hundred percent responsible for the crash in the first place... are, in an emergency, completely edible."

After supper, with day one of the strenuous selection camp winding down, the flight crew hopefuls, depending on which group they had been assigned to, either headed off to their evening classes or back to their rooms to study or in some cases, to collapse into the outdoor hot tub to soak their various aches and pains.

Angie was on her way to the Survival Course when she saw a truly unbelievable sight—Dale and Russ... together... in a camp pickup truck. As they passed, each gave her a big smile and a wave worthy of the Queen, before cruising down the gravel road toward the bustling town of Canmore.

Neither man spoke during the 20 minute trip. When they entered town, Dale pulled up in front of the first lounge he saw.

It had been a long, exhausting day, and with the beer ice cold and their throats parched, they soon had the waitress fetching another round.

"Well, what should we talk about first, Mr. Andrews?" Dale asked.

"You and Jefferson or you and me or you and...."

"It's really quite simple!" Russ interrupted, studying the bubbles clinging to the inside of his beer glass. "Jeff and Angie used to have a thing going. He treated her like crap and dumped her a year ago. It's taken me all this time, but I've finally got her over that loser and willing to take a chance on me and that's how I want it to stay, okay? The last thing I need is for that asshole Logan to mess up her head again."

Dale leaned back in his chair and, after taking a leisurely glance around the smoky, half-filled lounge, added, "Or me?"

"Or you!" Russ confirmed, glaring across the table.

Dale smiled and took a long drink of his beer, draining his glass. "Look Son, I'm still recovering from my own messy little divorce and that's pretty much how I ended up moving to Canada, okay? Because of that, I'm not exactly on the make right now. I didn't know you and Angie had something going. If I had, I'd...." Dale paused.

"I've never been one to steal another man's woman," he started again, "but let me tell you this, Andrews. If by some chance you blow it with her and she comes crying to me, I won't turn her away."

Russ wanted desperately to haul off and pop this egotistical fly-boy a good one when two men in National Park uniforms sauntered past their table.

As Russ turned his scowling attention toward the wardens, and silently watched them order coffee and make small talk with the waitress, the meddlesome Aussie asked, "Is one of those guys Logan?"

"No, but the one on the left looks a hell of a lot like him!" "Look Andrews, if you treat your woman right, I'll never be a threat to you. No man will. But an old flame, now that's something else again. Even when you think the fire's completely out, there could still be a spark under all those ashes. If that's what you fear, then only time will tell and there's not a damn thing you can do about it."

Russ slowly got to his feet. Leaning heavily on the table with both his huge hands, he stared Dale straight in the eye. "You know, Morgan, I really should thump you out right here and now, but since somebody's got to teach Angie how to swim next week, I guess I'm going to have to let you live for awhile. You seem pretty good at shooting your mouth off. Are you any good at shooting pool?"

Dale locked eyes with the man towering over him. "I can hold my own."

Russ gave a short laugh as he walked around the table to rack up the balls. "Oh yeah? Well I'm the reigning EMS city champ so I guess you could say I can hold my own, too."

Snacking on peanuts as he watched the muscular medic flex his shoulders to break, a chilling image suddenly popped into Dale's head. All this talk about pool and holding his own had rekindled vivid memories of his close encounter with Angie at the swimming pool.

If old Rusty ever found out about that....

11
EVEN THE BEST LAID PLANS

The hushed valley slumbered peacefully beneath the ghostly gray monotones of pre-dawn. It would be another two hours before the sun climbed high enough to peer over the ridge of towering mountains bordering the camp to the east. A dense layer of cloud hid the surrounding peaks from view, but every now and then a rain-slicked cornice of cold, gray granite sleepily poked its nose up through the swirling mist.

05:30 found two wide-eyed Flight crew hopefuls nervously huddling to keep warm as they awaited the helicopter's lift-off. An hour before, a pair of instructors had set off from base camp toward a pre-arranged checkpoint a mile to the south. As the "lost hikers" for the morning's Search and Rescue exercise, the instructors' were to sit and wait until the helicopter found them with the help of the FLIR spotting scope.

Angie, as fate would have it, had been assigned to the first team to go up. With Dale and Alex handling the piloting chores, Michael Brown, a paramedic from Airdrie, rounded out the medical crew while Jim Hamilton, a K-Country Provincial Park Ranger would be tagging along to scrutinize their every move.

With each team limited to fifteen short minutes to scan the search area using the FLIR scope, whether they successfully located their targets or not, the neophyte rescuers would then return to base for a performance debriefing with their instructor.

Though it was never openly stated, this first in-flight test was crucial. If a medic or nurse couldn't handle the simple act of riding in a 'copter, they were toast as far as being selected for a helicopter-based rescue program was concerned.

Outfitted in white flight helmets and navy blue flight suits, Angie, Mike and Jim were in the process of buckling in when the BK's port side engine began to whine. Carefully increasing throttle as the four rotor blades slowly began to rotate overhead, Dale continued to feed power to the #1 engine until his triple tach RPM indicator showed 60 percent. With the noise level generated by the screaming turbine making conversation without a headset all but impossible, Captain Morgan added to the thunderous roar by giving his co-pilot the okay to fire up the starboard #2 engine.

Her own heart racing to keep pace, Angie felt the helicopter begin to lift into the air. The eastern sky ablaze with the muted reds and oranges of sunrise, Dale flew due south for about a minute until he was circling over the last known camp site of the missing hikers. "Okay people," Alex's husky voice boomed over the intercom. "Let's see what you've learned."

Upon receiving the go-ahead signal, Michael, a pair of binoculars at the ready, immediately twisted in his seat so he could look out the starboard window. Jim commenced scanning the forest to the other side of the aircraft.

Trying hard to appear ultra-keen as she occupied the sideways facing number three seat, Angie had volunteered to use the FLIR spotting scope first. With a trembling hand on the directional joy stick and the video monitor wedged tightly between her knees, her grid search area consisted of the valley floor passing directly beneath the chopper.

The densely packed spruce and pine trees formed a nearly impenetrable carpet of green, with only a few open areas or chutes where avalanches had swept down from above the tree line.

Angie stared intently at the viewing screen in her lap. As she applied slight pressure to the FLIR's pistol-gripped control stick, the scanning gimbal, mounted to the bottom of the chopper, began to rotate slowly in the same direction.

Nothing. Not a single hot spot anywhere. Where were these guys? Zipping up her flight suit and rubbing her aching eyes, Angie checked her watch and decided to keep it up for another minute before handing off to her fellow trainee. With the examiner watching and analyzing everything she did, she was not about to let eye strain or hypothermia make her come across as a wimp.

As Dale lazily orbited in ever-increasing circles over the target area, it was as they were passing over an old avalanche chute, that Angie finally spotted something... four hot spots... about fifty yards off to the southwest. "I've got something!" she shouted. "Holy cow, I've got hot spots all over the place!"

Dale immediately put the helicopter into a hover above the site. Everyone on board began scouring the forest below for signs of life. "You said we were only looking for two guys, right?" Angie wondered aloud.

"Let me have a look," Jim replied, taking the viewing scope from her. The largest white spot, along with one much smaller a hundred feet away, appeared not to move. The activities of the other two hot spots, however, were bizarre, with the larger of the two objects racing in tight circles around the other.

Dale kept the chopper in a rock-steady hover as Alex keyed the external PA system. "You there on the ground, this is the LIFE-STAR rescue helicopter. Do you require any assistance? Over."

Alex activated the exterior microphone to pick up any responses from the ground. "If it's deer or some other animal, the helicopter should've frightened them away," Dale remarked, shooting a questioning look at his partner. The roar of the rotor blades transmitted over the microphone was deafening, and Dale was reaching to turn the volume down when a blood-curdling sound escaped from the forest below. It was a man, screaming.

Everyone froze as the horrifying sounds carried over their headsets. "HOWARD, IT'S TOO LATE FOR ME... FOR GOD'S SAKE SAVE YOURSELF... MAKE A RUN FOR IT!"

Realizing this was the real thing and not another mindless drill, Michael frantically scrambled into his rappel harness.

Angie, quickly looping a nylon climbing rope through the figure-eight descender clipped to the front of his harness, attached a secondary safety line to his rappel rope. Secured with a Purssik knot, the short piece of cord would immediately jerk Michael to a stop if he accidentally lost his grip on the rope. It was hard to be careful and methodical with the screaming from the ground shrilling relentlessly, jarring every nerve and triggering the strong impulse to just hurry and get someone down there now!

Jim checked Mike's equipment, then anchored the rappel rope to a thick metal ring in the floor. Pulling his helmet visor down to protect his eyes from the harsh rotorwash, the Park Ranger tried to sound reassuring as he cracked open the starboard door. "Mike, don't try anything fancy, okay? Just assess the situation and report back."

Michael bobbed his head. After a quick check that his chest-mounted walkie-talkie worked, the medic stepped out onto the landing skid and started down.

Angie had the distinct impression that the guy was scared spitless. She had seen it in his eyes when she'd helped him on with his gear. To be quite honest, she was scared to death, too. Geez, this wasn't some dumb training scenario. Peoples' lives depended on what they did next... or what they failed to do.

All at once, the screaming stopped. Abruptly silenced in mid scream, the effect was chilling. Sinister. Angie felt her mouth go dry. With parched lips sticking to her teeth, she could only imagine what horror had just occurred in the dense foliage beneath her.

Alex was contacting base camp, telling them to notify Canmore hospital and have a doctor standing by. Staring out his side window, Dale, meanwhile, fought to keep his aircraft from drifting off-line. Knowing that snagging Michael or his rappel rope on a tree could have disastrous consequences for all concerned, the outwardly calm pilot squinted, unblinking, as he watched the young paramedic, spinning slowly, vanish into the tree tops.

"Talk to me, Mike?" Jim called over his radio. "What's happening down there?"

"I'm okay sir... can't see much yet... just going to follow this branch down a little further... OH MY GOD! There's a huge bear down there... maybe twenty, thirty feet directly below me. Looks like a grizzly and it's... HOLY SHIT... IT SEES ME!"

"Mike?" the pilot interrupted. "This is Dale. Settle down. You're doing just fine, son. Have a good look around. Do you see anybody?"

"Easy for you to say, asshole!" The medic's whispered comment was audible over their earphones. Then, "HE'S HUGE... HE'S... Jesus, he's trying to climb the tree... the tree I'm hanging onto. Christ, he's eating the bark... he's tearing it off with his teeth."

"What else do you see?" Dale persisted.

"I DON'T SEE ANYBODY... JUST THE GOD DAMN BEAR!"

Just then, a sudden downdraft grabbed hold of the chopper, sending it plummeting fifteen vertical feet before Dale could react. "WHAT THE HELL ARE YOU DOING?" Mike screamed. "PULL UP... PULL UP... I'M RIGHT ON TOP OF THE... AAAAAAAAAAAAAAH!"

Everyone on board felt it. Felt the abrupt downward tug. Felt the helicopter list slightly to the right. Dale immediately corrected to lift and level the aircraft. No one else moved. The implication was unspeakable. Either Mike had just gained two hundred pounds or something had grabbed hold of his rope.

For many long seconds, the only sounds coming from Mike's radio were incoherent struggling, grunts and curses. Then the strangled cry, "MORGAN... PULL UP AND GET US THE HELL OUT OF HERE!"

With his left hand pulling smoothly on the collective lever, and his feet expertly countering the increasing engine torque with just a touch of pedal pressure, Dale launched his German-engineered aircraft skyward. Once he had Mike clear of the trees, he headed for the nearest avalanche chute. Glancing back at the strung-out medic, the Aussie got the shock of his life. Something was clinging to Mike's back. A big something, clad in the olive green of a Park Ranger.

Slowing to a hover above the wind-swept sixty-degree chute, Alex kept a watchful eye on the whirling overhead rotor blades as Dale gently toed a landing skid up against the steep slope. Instantly engulfed in a billowing rotorwash of choking dirt and grit, Mike and his passenger wasted not one second scrambling on board. Mike collapsed in a breathless heap on the stretcher. From the look of it, he had had more than enough of this rescue shit for one day; maybe forever.

The Park Ranger turned out to be their arrogant swimming/climbing instructor, Howard Bateman. Hurriedly untangling himself from his exhausted savior, the stocky 42 year old EMS supervisor angrily slapped on a headset. "Dale, you turn this God-damned machine of yours around and take us right back to where you picked me up!

"Larry Moyen and I came across a fresh elk kill half an hour ago, and we were trying to clear out of the area when all of a sudden this huge grizzly sow comes ripping out of nowhere. Flattened both of us. I managed to climb a tree to get away from her. Larry wasn't fast enough. Last I saw, he was lying face-down a hundred feet north of my tree. He wasn't moving so I don't know if he's dead or playing dead or what, but that bitch won't leave him alone. Kept trying to flip him over so she could finish him off!

"I tried to divert the attack by yelling at her... got her to come after me instead. She was in the process of eating my tree when 'Hollywood' here showed up."

Even as he talked, Howard was climbing into the spare rappel harness. Yanking the waist straps tight, he ordered Jim to drag the flare kit out from beneath his seat.

Angie suddenly called everyone's attention back to the FLIR monitor screen. As they watched, the big white blotch merged with the smaller of the two immobile heat sources. Both spots then slowly began to move off to the southeast.

"Howard!" Jim shouted. "That second hot spot's too small to be the elk kill. It can mean only one thing... she's dragging Larry down the hill!"

Howard took a long, hard look at the screen. "Howie," Dale said, "if the bear's got him, you can't go down there alone!"

"He's right," Jim said. "You'll need someone to stand guard while you get Larry packaged. How about it, Mike?" He turned to the crumpled form slumped against the wall. "I hate to ask, but I don't have any rappel experience. Do you think you're up for another go?"

"Sure, no problem," Mike muttered, his hands and voice trembling. He started crawling toward the open door.

Angie suddenly reached out and pushed him back. "You've had enough, Mike!" she found herself saying. "It's my turn. I'll go."

A scowl distorted Howard's face. "The hell you say! I'll be damned if I'll let some female be the only thing standing between my ass and a murderous grizzly!"

"I'm going!" Angie repeated as she boldly met Howard's angry glare. To be truthful, she could not believe what she was saying either. Just the thought of backing through that door scared the living crap out of her, never mind what would be waiting for her if she and Bateman did make it safely to the ground. At least part of the reason behind her decision had been Mr. Bateman's condescending, not to mention chauvinist attitude toward her and all the other women attending the camp.

Mike quickly removed his harness and handed it to Angie. Jim helped her on with it and after double checking to make sure she had buckled it correctly, nodded his head.

It was show time. With a flare gun clipped to her harness and a portable radio strapped tightly to her pounding chest, Angie backed out the door. Balancing unsteadily on the narrow landing skid, the nurse glanced between her boots at the blur of forest 80 feet below. None of this was real. Standing out on this skid wasn't real. Preparing to rappel out of a helicopter wasn't real. The enraged grizzly bear hidden beneath those treetops wasn't real.

"Jesus, girl, you and your big mouth have done it again!" Angie whispered to herself as she sucked in a deep breath and stepped into space. Howard, his stubbled face mottled with rage, rappelled out the door right behind her.

Every sense Angie possessed was functioning at 110% capacity. Sight, sound, hearing, touch, smell were all acutely-tuned as her hiking boots broke through that first layer of spruce boughs.

Descending several more feet, she suddenly spotted the bear. It was directly below. The enormous sow was standing over something half-buried in the dirt. Both she and Howard stopped rappelling.

"I see the bear and am preparing to fire a flare at it. Stand by!" Angie radioed as she struggled to steady her aim. She gently squeezed the trigger. As a blinding flash of light exploded three feet to the right of her target, the four hundred pound grizzly bolted into the trees.

"Okay," Howard barked into his radio, "the sow's backed off! We're continuing our descent."

Touching down, Howard ran directly to the dirt-covered mound that was Larry's motionless body. Larry flickered his blood-caked eyelids. "Good Lord, Howie, what took you so long?" he mumbled through what was left of his shattered lower jaw.

Howard carefully began brushing the dirt away. "I'm going to get you out of here right now buddy. Just don't make any noise, okay?"

Starting at the nape of his neck, Larry's balding scalp had been turned completely inside out and was now hanging in a bloody flap down over his forehead. A rucksack stuffed with survival gear had luckily taken the full brunt of the grizzly's fury, shielding the Ranger's back and neck to a large degree. All that remained now of the double-reinforced nylon backpack were the shredded shoulder and waist straps.

By putting his hands behind his neck and laying flat on the ground, Larry had protected his vital areas—face, throat and belly. But as the bear had repeatedly attempted to flip him onto his back, its razor-sharp claws and teeth had inflicted terrible damage. In particular, his buttocks and hamstrings were an oozing mess of torn muscle, multiple puncture wounds and bear-sized mouthfuls of missing flesh.

The bear had simply been protecting her elk kill when the two instructors accidentally intruded into her space. After knocking both men to the ground, the grizzly had chosen Larry to strip-search first. After cuffing him about for a few minutes, the sow grudgingly turned her attention toward Howard. Safely up a tree by then, Howard unfortunately was minus his radio which had fallen from his jacket pocket during the initial attack.

Thinking the bear had gone when it had only been distracted, Larry had made the near-fatal mistake of staggering to his feet and trying to make a run for it. The bear immediately gave chase and with one swipe of a massive paw, sent the Park Ranger flying face-first into the dirt with his scalp dangling over his eyes. The grizzly had been in the process of biting deeply into Larry's unprotected upper back when the helicopter had mercifully returned.

Larry was now struggling to breathe. A multitude of gaping puncture wounds riddled his blood-stained chest. Quickly sealing off the largest hole with the heel of his hand, Howard realized that the lung on that side had already collapsed. Surprisingly little blood soaked the ground beneath the Ranger. That could mean only one thing. Larry's body had been almost completely drained of its nearly six litres of blood.

Angie reloaded her flare gun and stomped out a small grass fire lit by her first flare. While remaining alert for the bear's possible return, she helped Howard carefully log-roll Larry into the Bauman transport bag. By positioning him on his left side, they hoped to keep blood from Larry's badly damaged left lung from spilling over into his already compromised right lung. In addition, the weight of his body would hopefully seal off a number of "sucking" chest wounds—potentially lethal wounds that bubbled air every time Larry drew a breath.

With the Bauman bag now firmly snapped to Howard's harness, Angie radioed Dale to begin his ascent. When their feet left the ground, the frazzled nurse had never felt such relief in her entire, miserable, life. Well, maybe once before, when she had missed a period and thought she was pregnant... but no, this really could not be compared to something like that.

Just as they were entering the thick canopy of foliage overhead, Angie caught a glimpse of the bear lumbering off through the trees. The intruders had been vanquished and now it could take its time burying the elk kill. Bears prefer their meals on the ripe side and Larry no doubt, had he stuck around, would have made a tasty late night snack after a few days tenderizing under a hot June sun.

Howard radioed Dale and ordered him to fly straight back to base camp. Less than a minute later, the Aussie was gently depositing his windblown cargo onto the grass in front of the cafeteria. Anxious camp instructors ran to help out. As if they had practiced the grim scenario a hundred times, they soon had the Ranger loaded for the short flight to Canmore. As the helicopter had room for only three medical personnel, not including the doc, survival instructor Jim Hamilton elected to stay behind.

Flying down the middle of the mountain valley with the Bow River sparkling less than five hundred feet below their skids, the trip took four minutes. An emergency doctor was waiting at the pad with four units of unmatched O negative blood stuffed into a Styrofoam picnic cooler. Once on board, he took one look at Larry and immediately cleared the helicopter for take off.

Dale pushed his aircraft to the max for the harrowing 65 mile journey to Calgary. Traveling at 150 miles per hour, and with the added benefit of a moderate Chinook tail wind pushing from behind, their ground speed was 200 miles per hour. The flight took just over 22 minutes; by ground ambulance, it would have taken an hour.

En route, Angie showed why she was considered one of her unit's best vein sniffers by starting not one, but two large-bore IVs in what remained of Larry's left arm... quite a feat considering he had no visible or palpable vessels due to his severe hypovolemic shock.

Unable to intubate Larry due to the hideous fracture dislocation of his lower jaw, the doc elected to try for a blind nasal intubation. Just as she had learned in her trauma course the day before, Angie watched the physician gently insert the half-inch diameter endotracheal tube into the Ranger's right nostril. Operating strictly by feel, he then quickly advanced it down the back of Larry's throat and into his windpipe. Blood and gore instantly exploded out of the tube, splattering all over the ceiling and flight suits of the once immaculate chopper and its medical crew.

While Howard was helping Mike secure the tube with tape, the doc asked Angie for a chest tube. With no time to inject a local freezing, the physician thrust the foot-long plastic tubing deep into a gaping puncture wound in Larry's ravaged left lower chest. More blood and clots angrily spewed forth as the doctor quickly attached the tubing to a vacuum drainage container. Within seconds, the litre-sized container was half full.

There was no blood pressure to speak of, so a pair of rubberized MAST pants was quickly velcroed in place and inflated. The pressure pants would force whatever blood remained in Larry's legs up into his abdomen and chest cavity. Without blood, the pounding heart had nothing to carry oxygen to the vital organs. Called hypovolemic shock, the condition would rapidly lead to tissue anoxia and death.

Even after 3000 cc's of normal saline and four units of blood had been pumped into him, Larry's pressure stubbornly clung to the 70 systolic mark. A pressure this low made a painkiller like Morphine or Demerol a very risky proposition, but with a brain starving for oxygen, Larry was no longer with the program. Drifting in and out of consciousness, his unseeing eyes had already taken on a lifeless stare.

Alex patched the Canmore doc through to the thoracic surgeon on duty at Parkland Hospital. With an Estimated Time of Arrival of five minutes, the newly revamped LIFE-STAR program was about to bring in its first official patient.

The flight back to camp was a sobering one as Angie mindlessly picked at the blood caked beneath her splintered nails. She had come to the awful realization that this type of call would probably be just another day at the office if she succeeded in being selected for the LIFE-STAR program. She knew she could deal with the physical aspect, but what about the mental? Could anyone be expected to handle this level of stress on a regular basis?

The accident put a real damper on things for the rest of the day, but as soon as the helicopter was hosed out and refueled, flight training resumed. LIFE-STAR was, after all, a rescue program. Their mandate was to pick up patients and transport them to hospital. That was their job. They had performed that job and now it was time to get back to work. There was nothing more they could do for their friend. Larry Moyen was in God's hands now... or more correctly, a trauma surgeon's.

On their return to Calgary that evening, Angie and Russ grabbed something to eat before setting out on a long walk around Glenmore Park. Strolling slowly, hand-in-hand, Angie gave Russ the grisly details of her ordeal.

As her boyfriend responded by sharing some of his innermost feelings about the frightening incident, Angie learned something she had never suspected—he, too, was having second thoughts.

With that less-than-macho confession out in the open, it was just like old times. The two of them comforting each other, giving each other that much-needed pep talk, knowing exactly what it took to bolster the other's tired spirit.

As the harrowing day drew to a close, the young couple snuggled in one other's arms outside Russ' apartment. This time, nature was allowed to take its course.

Midnight found Angie nestled against Russ' muscular chest. Making love with him marked the beginning of a new chapter in her life, a prospect that both excited and frightened her. While she was contemplating what direction their lives might take, the emotionally exhausted nurse was lulled to sleep by the hushed sounds of Rusty's breathing... by the slow steady beat of his heart... and by the gentle patter of rain as it fell softly on the sidewalk beneath the open bedroom window.

12
THE RESCUE RACE

The Rescue Race would be the instructors' last chance to see the crew hopefuls in action before sitting down to make some tough decisions.

The race scenario was as follows: on the way to a call, the helicopter had been forced to make an emergency landing due to engine failure. One of the pilots was killed on impact, the other badly injured. The medical crew's job was to assess his condition, treat and stabilize his injuries as much as possible, then transport him to the nearest medical facility—in this case designated as Parkland Memorial Hospital.

The starting point for the race was ten miles northwest of the city in an area surrounded by gently rolling hills, stately evergreens, and multitudes of high-priced estates. The teams could use any mode of transport to get their patients to hospital. With several nearby roads and plenty of vehicular traffic in the area, the instructors were anticipating no major problems.

To ensure that the patients would not assist the rescuers in any way, the injured pilots would be played by camp instructors. Peter Lawson was giving his henchmen free rein, allowing them to fake as many complications as they deemed necessary during the race... to test their rescuers' medical knowledge and composure under stressful circumstances.

The 3-person team, nurse, medic and patient, had to finish together. Either everybody finished or nobody did. On a final note, having your patient suddenly sit up and announce to the world that he had just croaked was to be considered a very ominous sign, indeed.

Paramedics and nurses had been free to choose their partners, and to no one's great surprise, Angie and Russ had picked one another. After registering their team, the twosome was presented with a paper bag containing the names of pilot-patient combos. Hoping against hope to pull Dale's name, Angie had trouble making her throat work as she read out that Howard Bateman and Alex Davis would be playing their doomed pilot roles. She did not need a crystal ball to deduce which man would be pronounced dead at the scene.

Dale was to play the role of patient with the dynamic duo of Martin Fleming and Brett Harris. Everyone, fellow medics and instructors alike, had already elected them as the team to beat. Martin, a city paramedic, was a provincial-calibre long distance runner, while his emerg nursing pal, Brett, was a body-building fanatic. They were also arrogant and self-centred to the point of being obnoxious.

On the bus ride to the mosquito-infested slough that was the starting point, teams huddled in their seats, striving to concoct a winning strategy. They had each been given a map of the area and were busy making notes as to the direction, type of terrain and distance to the closest road.

Russ knew, as did every other male paramedic who had chosen to pair up with a female, that he was going to have to work extra hard to make up for Angie's lack of upper body strength. He loved her dearly and yet, after carefully studying his map and noting all the hills they would have to navigate, he was starting to have real misgivings. For the first time, he was wondering if maybe his station captain and the chauvinistic Howard Bateman had been right all along... women really did not have a place in Search and Rescue.

While emotionally bolstered by Rusty's pep talk of the night before, Angie was also not totally convinced of her abilities. She was not into all this macho stuff, but she did want to prove that, as a woman, she was tough and could pull her own weight; that she was willing to give it everything she had... and then some.

Her biggest fear, however, was not about her own personal failure, but how it might affect Russ' chances. If she couldn't keep up, it would hold Russ back and possibly even jeopardize his shot at making the squad.

Sitting in the back of that stuffy bus, something weird popped into her head. It had to do with, of all things... *Hockey Night In Canada*. The Edmonton Oilers had been battling their arch rivals, the Calgary Flames, when, between fights, a TV announcer made a comment about Angie's all-time sports hero... the great Wayne Gretzky.

"Gretzky is far from being the biggest player in the NHL and he's certainly not the fastest skater," the commentator had observed. "Even his slap shot is not considered all that hard, and yet, when it comes to being able to think on his skates, 'The Great One' is in a league by himself. He knows how the play will develop before anyone else does. He's always in the right spot at the right time—he never wastes energy chasing a rebound off the boards, he waits and lets the puck come to him. Wayne simply uses the physical tools and intelligence God gave him, and the end result is the finest hockey player this announcer has ever watched play the game."

The more Angie thought about those words, the more it seemed to make sense. Maybe she wasn't the strongest person alive, but she had lots of other things going for her. First, she was smart. That alone should count for something. And second, she had the disposition of a bulldog. As a kid growing up, she had discovered that if she couldn't accomplish her chosen goal, she simply had to come up with a different strategy—Plan B. As her friends could attest, when she set her heart on something, she would never quit thinking, never quit trying, and never quit inventing Plan B's.

The bus pulled over and stopped. After following a pot-holed gravel road for miles as it wound around the base of a thickly-forested hill, a yellow Dead End sign signaled the end of civilization.

It was 7:45 a.m. With the temperature already hovering in the high teens, and without a whiff of cloud marring the sky, it was going to be a scorcher of a day.

The teams drew for start numbers and Team One left at 8 o'clock sharp. Ten minutes later, the blast of an air horn signaled the next twosome to their feet. Like sheep to be shorn... or worse, they obediently fell in line behind their assigned instructors, starting up a narrow cow trail which disappeared into the trees. Martin and Brett, along with pilots Dale Morgan and Jan Elliot, had drawn the number eight starting position. Russ, Angie, Howard and Alex were team number nine.

As they waited, Russ tried to squeeze a little information out of his patient. To his casual inquiry as to whether every patient would have the same type of injuries, Howard's response had been a smirk.

Angie tried a somewhat different approach. With a sugary-sweet smile curling her lips, she eased an arm around Howard's waist and posed a simple question: just how much did he think his miserable life was worth?

"Let's face facts, Howie," she said. "I mean, suppose you're all strapped down on a spine board and we're crossing a raging river or something and maybe one of us slips and you land in the water... face down... and well, Rusty and I were wondering... you know, if we accidentally lost you or something in the water and we couldn't fish you out in time and you eventually resurfaced at, say, the Willowbrook sewage treatment plant... you know... like three days later in one of their huge aeration ponds and... well we were just wondering if we would... you know... get 'A' for effort and pass the course anyway?"

Unfortunately, as Alex would later tell them, Bateman had already decided that because Angie had had the audacity to challenge his authority during Larry Moyen's rescue, he was going to give it to her and her sex-crazed boyfriend with both barrels.

Pausing to give a big overhead stretch, Howie yawned loudly and, after leisurely scratching his hairy belly, announced, "Gee, I think I feel a very unstable C-two fracture coming on."

Watching as the surly instructor sauntered over to where the other patients were lounging in the shade, Angie was not about to be denied the last word. Speaking loudly enough for all the instructors to hear, Angie asked, "Hey Russ, what are your thoughts on euthanasia?"

At 9:30, Air Medical Crew number nine started up the steep cow path. After five minutes of huffing and puffing, Russ and Angie entered a small clearing and were surprised to see a decrepit helicopter lying in the dense undergrowth. Obviously having crashed there a long time ago, stripped of all usable material, the crumpled skeleton was all that remained of the once proud warbird.

Changes had been made to the inside of the wreck so it now had essentially the same seating arrangement as a BK 117. As well, the medical and rescue equipment bags with which they had been practicing the last few days had been carefully stowed into the same nooks and crannies as on the LIFE-STAR aircraft.

While Lawson went over the rules again, the crew was handed flight suits and helmets. Struggling to pull the jumpsuit over her shorts and T-shirt, Angie found the Nomex material clung to her sweaty skin like plastic food wrap; immediately causing beads of perspiration to form streaming tributaries down her back.

"Take up positions as if en route to a call!" Lawson ordered. Howard took the co-pilot's seat, Alex the captain's, while Russ took the backward-facing seat directly behind Bateman and Angie set about strapping herself into the seat across from the stretcher.

Chief instructor Lawson, parading back and forth, poked his head into the business end of the helicopter. He looked first Russ and then Angie straight in the eye. "Are you guys ready?"

Angie was still wrestling with her seat belt. Because the aircraft was resting at a near forty-five degree angle, her chosen seat was positioned half-way up the wall. It wasn't like she'd had much choice, either, since the seat that should have been to Russ' right was missing.

"Just a sec... okay?" she sputtered, clinging to the wall with one hand while desperately trying to clip the obstinate buckle with the other.

"GO!"

Peter's thundering bellow caught her completely off-guard. Losing her grip on the wall, she fell forward and hit the stretcher face-first.

Swearing under his breath, Russ immediately went to Angie's aid. Helping her crawl out of the chopper, he watched as she gingerly extracted what was left of her upper lip from under her radio mouthpiece. Miraculously, her swollen nose had escaped unscathed, but with the skin scraped off all the way to the gum line, she was still checking for possible missing teeth when Peter bellowed again.

"You've just had a dual engine failure and gone down! The fuel tanks are full and smoke is coming from the transmission! The pilot was killed on impact! The co-pilot has been seriously injured!"

Angie scrambled to help Russ assess Howard's injuries. Howie was playing his part to the bloody hilt... hanging limp as a rag doll from his shoulder straps as he sprawled at an impossible angle across the central radio control panel. In order to get to him, Alex would have to be removed first.

Supposedly snuffed on impact by a tree smashing through the canopy, the flaccid, fish-eyed pilot actually did look pretty dead. At 180 pounds, he was difficult to extract from the cramped cockpit. With fear of an explosion mounting with each passing second, Russ and Angie hurriedly dumped the ketchup-splattered fatality onto the trampled grass. This was an emergency and the patient was supposed to be dead anyway, but it still felt very weird to hear the pilot softly cussing them as they stepped over his inert form.

The pilots' seats were equipped with combination shoulder and lap belts, and because of the way Bateman was lying, Russ could not reach the belt's four-way release buckle without risking further injury to Howie's head and neck. The resourceful medic pulled a pair of industrial-strength scissors from his hip pack and pretended to cut through the straps.

Angie meanwhile, was busy removing any equipment they might need. The scoop stretcher, airway management kit and combination IV fluid/drug roll bag were the easiest to drag out. She immediately returned for the KED splint stuffed behind a seat.

With no time to lose, they carefully slid the splint down behind Howard's back. A strange-looking contraption, the KED was a combination C-collar and backboard used mainly to package entrapped trauma victims with potential neck or spinal injuries. Instead of wasting precious minutes fooling with its dozen velcroed straps, Russ slapped together only the essential ones—the head, waist and crotch belts.

He and Angie groaned with the effort as they removed Howie from the wreckage. Quickly securing him to the scoop stretcher, they carried him a hundred feet due south. While Russ stayed behind to begin a more detailed examination of their patient's injuries, Angie ran back to get the medical bags.

"The portside engine is on fire... the air reeks of jet fuel!" Peter yelled.

Angie got the message. "It's going to blow! Get the heck out of here!" Even though her brain was screaming at her to run, she didn't lose her composure. Instead she scanned the interior of the aircraft one final time.

"It's playoff time! What would Gretzky do? Come on girl, think!" Angie spotted a life jacket scrunched behind the radio bulkhead and a large coil of climbing rope lying under a seat. Acting strictly on impulse, she grabbed for the rope. Then, for some inexplicable reason, she found herself reaching back through the door for the life jacket. It seemed unusually heavy for a vest, but she dragged it out anyway, and with the rope slung over one shoulder and heavy equipment bags in both hands, she scurried across the open area as fast as her sturdy legs could move.

"Rusty!" she screamed. "Watch out... she's going to blo...."

A tremendous blast split the air. Instinctively taking a nose dive into the dry grass, for a few heart-stopping seconds, Angie actually believed the chopper had exploded. When she finally looked up, Peter was standing next to the aircraft with an air horn in his hands. He was looking over the top of his half-glasses at her... smiling.

"The helicopter has just exploded. Any remaining gear on board has been destroyed. Good luck, team number nine."

"How would you like that air horn shoved up your lower gastro-intestinal tract?" Angie muttered, gently fingering her puffy honker and blood-caked upper lip.

Howard should have received an Academy Award as he lay on the stretcher. At times it was hard to tell if he was even breathing. "Unconscious with probable head and spinal injuries. Chest and belly seem okay," Russ called out. "Breathing is rapid and shallow."

While Angie pretended to start an IV, Russ took off one of Howard's boots and squeezed his big toenail. Nothing. Howie's hairy leg remained motionless. Russ gave his partner an exasperated glance.

Angie just smiled as she motioned for Russ to check Howard's pupils. Waiting until Russ was directing a distracting penlight into his eyes, Angie carefully attached a pair of forceps to several long black hairs sprouting from Bateman's muscular leg. A flick of the wrist later, it was all over but the screeching. Caught totally by surprise, Howard let out a violent bellow as he instinctively jerked his leg away.

"Well, would you look at that! He's not paralyzed after all," Angie announced loudly enough for all to overhear.

"He's not unconscious either!" Russ cheerfully chimed in.

Bateman collapsed back onto the stretcher. He could not utter a single sound, at least as long as Lawson was within earshot. He had obviously had it all worked out: an unstable neck fracture causing partial paralysis. Nearly impossible to transport, as any movement of the neck could cause a complete transection of the spinal cord, and respiratory arrest. He had blown it now!

"Okay, we have a semi-conscious patient with unknown head injuries who responds appropriately to painful stimuli." Russ called out. "Vital signs stable, but the blood pressure's kind of high. One hundred fifty-six on ninety-five."

"Head injury, nothing. We're talking congenital psychosis here!" Angie whispered.

Howard's ice-blue eyes abruptly narrowed to mere slits.

The medics quickly took stock of their supplies including one hundred feet of climbing rope and one very heavy life vest. Angie reached over and picked it up.

"Geez, what's this thing made out of... cement?" As she flipped it over, a tightly wrapped plastic bundle fell to the ground. Stenciled on one side was, "TWO MAN DINGHY." They looked it over for several seconds trying to decide whether to take it. Angie spoke first.

"We probably won't need it, but who knows... maybe we'll lose points for leaving stuff behind. I vote we take it along."

"Take it if you want, but it sure the heck won't be me carrying it," Russ snorted.

While scrounging through the various equipment bags, Russ discovered that one of the bags converted into a backpack. Stuffing it with gear, Angie helped lift as her partner struggled to shoulder the unwieldy load.

As the temperature was now a sweltering 25 degrees Celsius, they were both soaked with sweat. Russ, the top half of his flight suit peeled off and the sleeves tied loosely around his waist, checked his map and compass heading one final time before setting out. Chivalrously assigning Angie the lighter "foot end" of the stretcher while he grappled with the much heavier "top end," Russ directed his woman to lead the way as they slowly tottered off down the hill.

Their game plan was simple. They would travel in a southeasterly direction until they intersected with a small stream. From there, it was only a matter of following the stream bed down to a larger creek which would eventually pass under a busy two-lane highway. After that, it would be all downhill, so to speak: flag down a car... get to a phone... call for an ambulance. With any luck, he and Angie would be hoisting a brew to their team's triumph by noon. Twelve-thirty at the latest.

The sun climbed higher, and with it, the temperature. The hum of blood-sucking insects serenaded them while Howard moaned and groaned for effect. After a few minutes, Angie was almost wishing he had stayed comatose. It was going to be a very long day if he kept up this crap.

After laboring to carry the unwieldy stretcher another few hundred feet, Angie found something to smile about. On the path just ahead was a black stethoscope.

Russ motioned to set the stretcher down. "Ange," the medic wheezed, "we'd better rest for a bit. I don't want to wear you out."

Angie absentmindedly scratched under her T-shirt as she contemplated her boyfriend's utterly erroneous statement, then bent and picked up the stethoscope. There was a name engraved on the chrome chestpiece. "Holy geez, I can't believe this. It's Martin's. That hot shot. He's going to be just sick when he finds out he's lost it."

Stuffing the expensive instrument into her flight suit, Angie took a long look at the trail ahead. "You know, they must've had the same idea as us... to find the creek."

"Yeah, but there's one big difference," Russ replied.

"And what's that?" Even Howie stopped his moaning long enough to listen in.

Using the tail of his T-shirt to wipe his brow, Russ pointed at the ground to either side of the trail. It was almost completely overgrown with weeds and tall grass, but there was no mistaking it: they were standing in the middle of the dry creek bed they'd been searching for. And yet, strangely, trampled into the grass, two very distinctive tracks could be seen continuing well past the creek and up a steep incline before disappearing from view.

"You know, those two are a pretty observant pair. How could they have missed it?" the medic remarked quietly. "And why the heck did they start going uphill again?"

Russ checked his watch. It was a little after ten. They had been at this for half an hour already and it was time to get moving again.

Even though they were now traversing a relatively gentle slope, every few minutes another moss-covered rock threatened to unhinge Angie's already-wonky left ankle. Her better-half seemed intent on running her over with his end of the stretcher, and her shoulders and back were being strained to the breaking point. "This is absolutely insane!" she grumbled between gasps for breath. "What the heck is Lawson going to learn from all this?"

After a tough, fifteen-minute hike, she and Russ finally intersected with the second creek. Unlike the first, which had been bone-dry, the second stream roared past in front of them. Ten feet wide and a foot and a half deep, the mud-coloured water did not look inviting.

"Are you sure this is the right creek? Angie asked. It looks so small on the map!"

Russ yanked the crumpled map from his leg pocket. "Nah, this is the creek, alright," the former Hanna farm boy replied with authority. "It's just, with all the spring run-off from the mountains, the water level's a lot higher right now, that's all."

"Spring run-off, my ass!" Angie muttered as she unconsciously backed away from the raging torrent.

Bateman lifted his head. He was not supposed to quit role-playing, but he had to observe how his rescuers coped with the various obstacles they faced. Dragging a thirsty tongue across parched, cracked lips, Howie silently continued taking notes.

After a short, intense discussion with her partner, Angie finally caved in, agreeing they should stick with their original plan of following the creek to the highway.

A scant five minutes later, they were forced to halt again. Because of the stretcher, Russ couldn't see where he was stepping, so was constantly stumbling over rocks and debris strewn along the creek bank. Nearly falling twice, he angrily shouted at Angie to stop. It was time to get the map out again.

With trees and dense brush having closed in along the edge of the stream, the medic was ready to turn around and head back to the dry creek bed. Maybe the bizarre uphill route Martin and Brett had taken was the right one after all... though the idea seemed hard to figure.

"I've got it!" Angie shrieked.

A startled Russ nearly tore his map in half.

"Hon, I've got the answer. I know how we can get to the road!" Angie babbled on. "It's so simple, it's positively brilliant!"

"Only if it involves giving me a heart attack!" Russ fumed.

"Will you listen? First, we inflate the raft and strap Howard on it. Then, we tie a rope to each end and with you walking on one bank and me on the other, we float our patient down the creek!"

Russ shook his head in disbelief. Bateman was also frantically shaking his head, a difficult thing to do with his neck immobilized by the KED splint.

Russ wearily gazed at the radiant blue sky. "A beautiful summer day, just made for kicking back and relaxing with a tub full of beer, and what am I, Russell Patrick Andrews, doing on this gorgeous June morning? I'm stranded and dehydrating in the middle of the mosquito-infested wilderness with a brain-damaged girlfriend and a guy who's just pretending he's brain-damaged."

With that, the medic walked over and placed a comforting arm around Angie. "It's okay, hon. You've just been out in the sun too long. Irrational thought is one of the first signs of heat stroke!"

"No... really, this is going to work!" was Angie's angry response as she twisted round to face him. Howard suddenly started groaning real loud. "Rusty, our patient isn't going to last much longer. We have to take the fastest route out of here!"

Struggling to pull free of his restraints, Bateman had had enough. "Okay you two, the game's over and you both flunk! You couldn't even follow a simple map without getting lost. What a pair of bumbling idiots! I bet every other team is back in Calgary by now!"

"Oh my God," Angie cried out. "Look, he's having a seizure! Where the heck did we put the Valium?"

"Andrews!" Howie screamed. "Your little woman here isn't playing with a full deck. The game is over... don't you get it? Now untie me this damned minute!"

"I'll be the one who decides when it's time to quit," Russ shouted back. "And that won't be until our patient has bloody well died of unnatural causes!"

As their mentally deranged patient turned the air blue, a devilish grin spread across Russ' face. "You know something, Howie? I've been thinking, and it looks like you might be doing a little river rafting after all!"

13
RIVER RATS

Angie and Russ blew every ounce of air they had into their inflatable dinghy. Even though they spelled each other off at regular intervals, twenty minutes later they were both dizzy from hyperventilation.

Eventually, the little craft took shape and Russ screwed the air plugs firmly into place. He and Angie sat back to admire their finished product. "This is supposed to be a two-man raft?" Russ asked. "For two twelve-year-old kids maybe, but for two grown men... there's no bloody way!"

Just then, the crisp crack of gunfire echoed across the valley. Every member of team nine watched in silence as a bright red emergency flare arced high across the empty sky before finally burning out on its downward trajectory. Somewhere, one of the other teams had gotten themselves into a whole mess of trouble, trouble that they could not get out of by themselves. The launching of a flare signaled: "SEND OUT A SEARCH PARTY RIGHT AWAY!"

In addition to a small squeeze bottle of insect repellent, Bateman had a flare gun tucked in the right leg pocket of his flight suit. Lawson's instructions had been specific: the flare gun was to be used only if the crew and patient had somehow become so completely incapacitated as to be in dire need of immediate assistance. Simply getting lost was not good enough.

"You know, that thing came from the same direction Brett, Martin and Dale were headed," Angie remarked quietly. Seeing the look of uncertainty in her face, Bateman's eyes very nearly took on a twinkle.

Angie and Russ went to hold an emergency conference just out of earshot of their patient. Howie lifted his head to watch as both participants nonchalantly swatted and scratched various parts of their anatomy and occasionally, those of their partner. After five long minutes, they slowly walked back to where their patient lay waiting.

"Well, Mr. Bateman," Russ said, "I think we've about run out of ideas."

Howard could not help but sneer. "I'm just glad you've finally come to your senses, Andrews. Now if you get me the hell out of this thing, I'll forget about having you both shot!"

Totally dejected, Angie and Russ knelt in unison to loosen his restraints. Instead of unclipping the various buckles, however, they suddenly yanked down hard against the straps.

"What the hell are you people doing? Untie me this instant! There's no way out of this! It's time to throw in the bloody towel!"

"Who said anything about throwing in the bloody towel?" Angie grunted. "With Martin's team out of the running, we'll have a much better chance at winning, and if we lose you in the water, well... at least we won't have to drag this flipping stretcher back to camp!"

Strapping a rabid wolverine into a child's carseat would have been a whole lot easier than getting old Howie into that life vest. Struggling mightily to escape, the livid instructor expressed his feelings both verbally and through primitive hand gestures.

Anchoring the top-heavy stretcher to the unstable raft also created a few tense moments. Looking like a navy blue hot dog in a bright yellow bun, Howard continued to spit venom as Angie and Russ carefully eased the little craft out into the current. As they were stringing a rope across to the other bank, Angie's half-baked idea wasted little time in taking off. Caught in the powerful current, the small dinghy with its wildly protesting cargo immediately headed downstream; Angie and Russ stumbling madly along behind.

At great personal risk of losing an eye to the overhanging tree branches as he raced along the rocky shore, Russ fought to keep the speeding raft as close to his bank as possible. It was the shallow side of the creek, so the current was weaker there, meaning there was less danger of the raft being swept away.

"Hey Rusty," Angie yelled above the roar of the water, "I wonder if Martin's crew is okay!"

"I certainly hope not, 'cause if they aren't near death, they certainly will be when Lawson is through with them. They'll wish they'd stayed where they were... lost in the bush with that crazy Australian," Russ hollered back.

"I thought Lawson just hated us."

"Heck no! He hates everybody."

Angie smiled. Russ seemed to be in much better spirits now as he struggled to keep the flimsy rubber raft under control. Maybe this insane idea was going to work after all. They sure were covering an awful lot of ground.

The tug of the current rapidly grew stronger as it descended toward the valley floor. Fighting to keep her balance on the slimy rocks as the raft brutally yanked her along, Angie was beginning to think it might be time to pull the raft in and reassess. Forced to duck beneath yet another low hanging tree limb to avoid being decapitated, Angie quickly raised her head again. What awaited her very nearly sent her into cardiac arrest.

The animal wasn't that big for a black bear, probably just a yearling, but it was still a bear... and right then, it was standing on the bank ten feet away.

Her sneakers frantically back-peddling in the slick mud as she instinctively fought to avoid a head-on collision with the equally surprised bruin, the nurse momentarily lost both her footing and her grip on the raft's nylon life line... a catastrophically ill-timed combination that wrenched the end of the thin yellow rope from her hands and sent it snaking into the rushing torrent.

Russ, who'd unfortunately picked that exact moment to check the sky for more distress flares, was instantly jerked off his feet and flung into the raging creek by the runaway dinghy. Horrified, Angie watched Russ fight to stay afloat as the roaring current carried him around a bend and out of sight. In a frenzied effort to remove herself from the scene of her second bear encounter in less than twenty-four hours, Angie leaped blindly into the creek.

Screaming hysterically as the bone-chilling water threatened to knock her feet out from under her with each faltering step, she scrambled up the opposite bank and raced off downstream in pursuit of the rapidly receding raft.

"Lord help me! They're going to drown and it'll be all my fault! All my bloody fault!" she cried as she checked downstream for any sign of the tiny craft. What she saw instead was a bridge... and believe it or not... a car was actually driving past on the road above.

They had been on the right route after all. Rusty would be so pleased!

Traveling at a speed she had not possessed since her high school track days, Angie galloped down the rock-strewn creek bank. Even after slipping and stumbling several times, she would not allow herself to slow down. She was wholly responsible for this awful dilemma, and if her teammates were to survive, it was up to her to save them.

By some incredibly merciful act of divine intervention, the dingy's trailing rope eventually snagged on something and Russ was able to come alongside the raft and grab hold of a handle. When Angie finally caught up, Russ ferociously waved her downstream. The raft could break loose at any moment.

Sprinting another 150 feet along the muddy bank, Angie bravely entered the turbulent, knee-deep water. She was fighting to keep her balance as she waded out toward the middle when a wave of dizziness swept over her. Her head spinning as the icy current licked hungrily at her legs, it was all she could do to keep her thoughts focused on the dinghy. If she could only grab hold of one of the ropes and somehow pull it into shore!

The raft broke free. With Russ clinging to the side for dear life, it was now rushing downstream toward her at breath-taking speed.

Unable to get out of the way in time, the dinghy caught Angie just below the hips, pitching her forward. It was all a blur of yellow raft, rushing water and wild cursing, then she felt something grab her arm. It was Rusty!

"Keep Howard's head up!" he yelled, directing her to inch her way to the front of the raft. Easy to say, but rather difficult to do considering she was sprawled eyeballs to toenails atop their homicidal patient.

The swift-flowing stream quickly carried them under the bridge and beyond. A quarter of a mile later, the mighty Bow River swallowed the raft. Ready or not, Russ, Angie and Howard were on their way to Calgary!

A hundred yards across at its narrowest point and bloated to biblical proportions by recent rains and the seasonal melting of the winter snowpack, the Bow was fourteen feet above flood stage. Spread across a much larger channel than the earlier feeder stream, however, the river's frigid waters were amazingly smooth... almost tranquil.

After several failed attempts, Russ was finally able to swing one leg up into the raft. With Angie's help, he carefully hauled himself onto the side wall of the dinghy. Howie, meanwhile, sandwiched snugly between them, was looking older with each passing second.

Watching as the rotting trunk of a 60-foot Cottonwood bobbed past, the shivering medics began to assess their chances for survival. Howard would probably be the only one to live to tell their gruesome tale. After all, he was the only one wearing a life vest. But as he was also still tightly strapped into the KED, which in turn was anchored to the stretcher, the vest was not going to do him much good if the raft suddenly flipped over. As much as they both detested the guy, they couldn't leave him like that, so very cautiously, as if defusing a bomb, they began to loosen his restraints.

A teenager biking on the path beside the river observed the strange blue and yellow craft as it floated by. He immediately took off for help, pedaling as fast as his mountain bike would go. As luck would have it, he nearly mowed down a yuppie jogger who had stopped in the middle of the bike path to answer his Cel phone. After helping the irate lawyer to his feet, the cyclist somehow convinced him not to sue, and instead dial 911 to report a possible double murder/suicide in progress.

"Two people were lying face-down on an inner tube!" he told the dispatcher. "And there was a third guy between them screaming, 'WE'RE GOING TO SHOOT THE WEIR... WE'RE GOING TO SHOOT THE WEIR! AND WE'RE ALL GOING TO DIE... AND I'M TAKING YOU TWO WITH ME!'"

Angie's left hand had a very firm hold on the dinghy while her right hand maintained its death grip on Howie's life vest. She had already decided that if worse came to worst and the dinghy sank, she would stay with Howie. From watching him during the Water Rescue course, she knew he'd be her best bet for making it to shore alive.

Russ was in a strangely similar position, but his left hand was stretched across Howie's muscular upper body and attached firmly to Angie's flight suit. As he later explained, if he was going to drown, then so was the dizzy broad who had got him into this mess in the first place.

After he'd warmed up a bit, Russ' first rational act was to ease himself back into the water and try to guide the craft toward shore. Within seconds, the blue-lipped medic was back in the boat, rethinking his strategy.

Bateman had settled down somewhat following his initial screaming fit. Although he'd done plenty of white-water kayaking in his day, this was totally different. This SOB of a river was at peak flood stage and only by luck had they so far avoided several raft-flipping rapids. Ironically, the single greatest threat to their continuing existence actually lay awaiting them within the apparent sanctity of the Calgary city limits.

Just past the zoo on the east side of town was a submerged concrete weir which spanned the river from shore to shore. A water diversion project for irrigation, the barrier formed a waterfall four feet high. The base of the falls was one giant, elongated whirlpool with an undertow beyond description. Once a boater went over the weir, inflatable rafts, paddles and people—even those wearing life jackets—were instantly pulled under. The Fire Department's River Patrol had even given the weir a morbid nickname. To them, it was simply known as "The Drowning Machine."

Angie and Russ each put an arm into the freezing water and started paddling for shore. It was tricky to do without spinning the dinghy in circles. It would have helped, as well, if both had been paddling for the same bank, which at times they weren't.

Within a few minutes, there were houses passing by on the shore. They were in the city! Their paddling escalated to jet boat speed, while Howard did his part yelping for help. Five minutes later, the increasingly frightened threesome was swept under the Fourteenth Street bridge on their way downtown. A few minutes later, the gray cement belly of the Tenth Street bridge passed overhead.

"Jesus, somebody must see us!" Russ cussed as they began to circumvent Prince's Island. Looking downriver, he could see the Center Street bridge fast approaching. Beyond the bridge lay St. George's Island and the zoo, and just beyond that... The Drowning Machine!

The current lost considerable momentum as it rounded the small island. As a result, a mammoth Cottonwood tree, its denuded foot diameter branches jutting up out of the water like the horns of a beached Triceratops, had run aground near the north bank just under the main span of the bridge. Angie knew there was little danger of slamming into it as they were floating in the middle of the river now, but it provided Russ with an idea.

Fumbling for one of the dingy's ropes, Russ quickly fashioned a slip knot, then coiled it in his hand, checking that the other end was still firmly tethered to the raft.

"I'm going to swim for the tree and tie the rope to it!" he shouted. "The raft will float past and drift in behind it where the current will be a lot weaker. You should be able to push it to shore from there with no problem!"

Angie and Howard stared. For a brief moment, thoughts of the medic bailing out on them filled Angie's head. One look into his frightened eyes, however, told her a vastly different story. Pausing only long enough to blow her a kiss, the medic rolled over the side and disappeared in the murky water.

At first his finely-tuned body sliced through the icy water as if all the demons of Hell were after him, but it was only a matter of seconds before he started showing signs of hypothermia. The intense cold stiffened the rippling muscles in his arms and legs. His smooth strokes became awkward and clumsy. Losing his sense of direction as swirling eddies sadistically spun him around, Russ looked up to find the massive tree suddenly towering over him.

Stunned by the impact, Russ had just enough presence of mind to loop the end of his rope over the closest branch. A split second later, the wayward raft hit the other end of the rope.

Jerked to a violent halt, the rubber dinghy instantly folded lengthwise, pinning Angie helplessly between the sidewalls. With Howie screaming, all but lost from sight beneath her, the powerful current swept the tiny boat in a broad arc in behind the tree. Here the current was, indeed, much weaker and Angie was finally able to peel herself off Howard and take a quick look around. Incredibly, they were only about twenty feet from shore now. But, looking upstream, she could not see Russ anywhere.

Angie eased herself into the dirty water. Clinging to the side of the raft, she began flutter-kicking toward shore. For several agonizing seconds, nothing happened. The dinghy did not move at all. "Move damn it, move!" she cursed as her thrashing legs churned the water to foam.

On the verge of panic, she sensed something in the water beside her. It was Howard. "We're moving!" he shouted. "Ange, the raft's moving... keep going, girl... you're doing great!"

After an eternity, her knee scraped something hard. The river bottom. They had made it.

With legs so numb she couldn't feel them, Angie stumbled clumsily up the river bank and set off for the half-submerged tree.

Searching, screaming, Angie finally spotted Russ among the snarl of broken branches. Her initial thought was that she was too late.

"Russ!" she shrieked over the roar of the current. Getting no response, she waded out into the river until it was just over her knees. Dangerously close to hysteria, she kept shouting Russ' name over and over until the dazed paramedic slowly raised his head and turned toward her. Angie was sickened by what she saw.

His flight suit torn off by the current, Russ had been attempting to swing his leg up and hook it over the tree trunk. He just didn't have enough strength left to do it, and with each successive try, he grew progressively weaker. Finally, he let his leg flop back into the water. The current immediately shoved him back against the Cottonwood.

Pausing to rest his grayish-white cheek against the ragged bark, Rusty was hovering on the very edge of consciousness. The freezing water had caused his body's core temperature to plummet so dramatically that he was losing touch with reality. His drooping eyelids sagging shut, only a solitary distraction kept him from drifting off and slipping peacefully beneath the water. Something, far off in the distance, was demanding his attention. Very faint. Something above the roar of the river. The sound came and went. Sometimes louder, sometimes softer, it was irritating, grating.

Using every bit of energy he had left, Russ forced open a mottled eyelid. Laboring to bring his wavering eyeball into focus, a beautiful angel slowly materialized before him.

She was flapping her arms about and pointing at something in the water... like she was trying to show him something... or maybe it was something she wanted him to do.

"Rusty, follow the rope!" she screamed. "Follow the God damn rope, you idiot! It'll take you to shore!"

As he watched, the angel ran up the shore and out of his line of sight. Staring now at the empty bank, the medic began to wonder if she had ever been there at all.

But no, she was back again. And she had someone with her. Some guy wearing a life vest.

"Rusty, please follow the rope, please, it will take you to shore," Angie pleaded, panic seizing her throat. "'Cause if you don't, Howard is going to have to go in after you! Just follow the rope, please!" She was crying now.

Russ continued to stare blankly at her. As he watched his guardian angel take another hesitant step toward him, it finally clicked. If Angie was on shore, then so was the raft. With fingers so cold they would no longer bend, he reached up to loosen the rope from around the stump. There was no tension on the rope at all now and it came off easily in his hands. Clumsily, he pushed his arm through the loop. Then, clutching his fist with his other hand, he rolled over onto his back and let the powerful current grab hold of him. With no strength left, he went wherever the water took him... like so much flotsam and debris.

As he floated along, something snagged his arm. Weakly attempting to jerk away, Russ heard a familiar voice. "It's okay big guy," Howard said, "I've got you!"

It was all Angie and Howard could do to drag his dead weight out of the water and up onto the river bank. All three collapsed in a heap on the muddy ground. It was 1:10 p.m.

In less than thirty minutes, they had covered nine miles. Having overshot Parkland Hospital by a good twelve dollar taxi fare, they were now only eight short blocks from the other accredited trauma hospital in the city... the Riverside Medical Center.

Even with his team-mates' arms wrapped tightly around him, Russ' teeth were still chattering uncontrollably ten minutes later.

Assessing the situation from a strictly medical point of view, Bateman disengaged himself from the half-frozen medic and got to his feet. "Jackson, if we're ever to get your boyfriend here warmed up, we've got to get him moving. Enough of this cuddling B.S.!" he growled. "It's time we got our butts in gear! There's still a race to be won!"

Angie and Russ nearly stopped breathing.

"According to race rules, you guys can't quit until you're physically exhausted... or until I tell you to... and since you haven't listened to one damned thing I've told you to do so far, I'm ordering you to deliver me to the nearest hospital, which in case you haven't noticed, is the Riverside Medical Center, just down the flipping road. So let's get a move on, shall we?"

"What are you talking about?" Russ mumbled through numb lips. "The race is history. Even a tough old buzzard like you would've croaked after what we've put you through. The only thing to do now is flag down a taxi and hitch a ride back to Parkland... in disgrace."

"This bleeping race ain't over till I say so, Andrews!" Howie barked as he pulled the wobbly medic to his feet. "This is a team effort, remember? And I'm part of this team. And as you can plainly see, I'm not dead, am I? Well, am I?"

"It's just the idea that you're actually going to cover for us... " Angie sputtered. "It's... well, so... so uncharacteristically charitable!"

"Ange, I don't know what he's up to, but I'm game if you are."

"I'm always game!" Angie replied tenderly as she took her boyfriend's outreached hand.

It was only when they returned to the dinghy to retrieve their gear that the threesome realized the race was far from theirs to take. The raft was gone. So was their bagful of medical equipment. The only thing not carried away by the torrential current was the heavy scoop stretcher, lying half-buried in mud.

With no time to waste, Russ and Angie reloaded Howard onto the stretcher and carried him with great effort up the steep river bank. Less than fifty feet beyond lay Memorial Drive... a major thoroughfare pointing like an arrow, straight east to the Riverside Hospital. There was only one problem—they could not get one bleeding vehicle to stop!

To be honest, they did make quite a sight, encrusted with muck, hair tangled and plastered to their heads. And what about their good buddy lying sprawled in the grass beside the road? Obviously drunken or drugged or both!

Suddenly an ambulance and fire truck raced past going east, sirens blaring and lights flashing. They didn't slow down as they shot through the intersection, and they certainly didn't notice the two misfits waving frantically at the side of the road.

"There goes our ride!" Angie cried.

"If you think that's bad, look behind you!" Russ said. The Fire Department's River Patrol jet boat went flying past, also heading east.

Angie had had enough. Stomping to the intersection where several vehicles were waiting for the light to change, she boldly commandeered the first pickup truck she came to. After she explained their situation, she and Russ loaded Howard into the back; five minutes later, they were carting their patient into the Riverside Medical Center.

Hopping off the stretcher, Howard scurried to phone Lord Lawson at Parkland, then returned to give report. "You're not going to believe this, but so far you guys are the first... no, let me rephrase that, you people are the only team to have made it back to civilization in one piece, never mind transporting your critically-injured patient safely to a hospital. Mr. Lawson asked me to pass on his congratulations on your outstanding effort. And on that triumphant, if not thirst quenching note, let me be the first to buy you two half-drowned river rats a well-deserved beer!"

14
THAT FLOATING FEELING

"Ange, if I'm going to teach you to swim, I need two very important things from you, and I don't mean the foam blocks stuffed in your suit," Dale said. It was Monday evening at the pool.

"First, I want one hundred percent effort because I won't accept anything less," the Aussie continued. "And second, you've got to have complete trust in me and my training methods. If you truly believe... I can teach you to swim."

Her heart already starting to pound, Angie studied the gray eyes that were asking so very much from her. Deep down, she knew exactly what he was trying to say—he was asking her to believe, not so much in him, but in herself. She had to take that first courageous step, however, a step she barely achieved with the feeblest of nods.

"Good girl! Now, the next thing I need to know is why you're so afraid of water? What scares you about it?"

"Well," Angie hesitated, "whenever I have to put my face in the water, I feel like I'm going to smother. You know, getting wet doesn't scare me and drowning doesn't scare me... it's that part in between I'm afraid of... you know, the awful suffocating, panicking part before I finally lose consciousness from anoxia and die! I'm sorry Dale. I can't do this. I'll never make...."

The pilot cupped his hands around Angie's trembling shoulders and looked into her frightened eyes. "It's alright, luv. That's exactly what Russ told me over the phone last night, and I won't let that happen to you, okay? After I talked to him, I stayed up until two this morning trying to figure out how to get you around that road block."

Angie found herself gazing, almost mesmerized, into Dale's eyes. She had never seen eyes quite like his before. Bluish-gray with flecks of green, they seemed to reach down into her very soul. At the same time, they were warm and caring and genuinely sincere, reflecting a gentle peacefulness she had never dreamt possible in a man's eyes.

"When I was with the Coast Guard," he was saying, "I had a mate who couldn't swim, either. He was even worse than you—scared to death of water and you know what? It was a diving specialist who finally taught that bloke how to swim. Heck, once the guy caught on, he turned out to be a bloody natural in the water... eventually went on to became a navy frogman!"

The Aussie smiled and handed her a bulging gym bag. "I want you to put this thing on and be back here in five minutes. We've got a lot of stuff to cover tonight."

As Angie trotted off, she unzipped the bag for a sneak peek at its mystical contents. Crammed inside was a pale green wet suit.

Waiting until she was in the change room, the eavesdropping Russ wasted little time expressing his doubts. "Is that story really true or did you just make it up for Angie's benefit?"

"Oh, it's all true. Willard turned out to be one heck of a diver. Darn shame what happened to him, though."

"What happened to him?"

"Well," Dale drawled out his answer, "it seems he and a buddy were diving off an old shipwreck and from what we could piece together, a shark must've got them."

"From what you could piece together? Morgan you're full of it!"

"I swear it's the honest truth, but don't worry, Mate," Dale teased with a lustful grin, "the only man-eating shark that'll be after your girl tonight... is me!"

Hurrying back in her skin-tight wet suit, Angie found Dale and Russ sorting through a tangle of material. She knelt down for a closer inspection. Resting in front of her were two silver air tanks.

"Ange, do you know what SCUBA stands for?" Dale asked.

"It stands for 'Self-Contained Underwater Breathing Apparatus' and it was invented by the legendary Jacques Cousteau," Angie replied as if learning the acronym had been part of her nursing training.

"Uh... pretty smart cookie we have with us tonight, Russ. It's always easier to teach someone who isn't too bright. The smart ones always slow things down by asking a lot of dumb questions."

"Really! Like what?" Angie demanded.

"Oh, stupid stuff like who used this regulator last? I hope to God they didn't have anything contagious like herpes? And these flippers... have they been sanitized? I heard about somebody getting jungle rot that way! Ate his entire foot clean off!"

Dale first had Angie pull on an inflatable vest called a Buoyancy Control Device. Once it was snugly fitted, he slipped one of the pressurized air cylinders into a pocket on the back.

Casually admiring her teacher's lean, muscular physique as he fussed over her, Angie's wandering eyes liked what they saw. "Angela!" Dale interrupted her train of thought. "Are you with me here? Alright, the first thing I'm going to teach you is how to scuba dive. That way, we'll kill two birds with one stone—it will help you get used to being under water, and because you'll be able to breathe with the tank, you won't suffocate. Even if you sink to the very bottom and have to walk back to the shallow end, it'll be impossible for you to drown."

Dale then showed her how to put her face mask on so it formed an airtight seal around her eyes and nose. "Always remember, breathe through your mouth, not your nose and never hold your breath, okay?"

"What kind of idiot does he think I am?" Angie wondered. "Good God, I can barely breathe through my nose as it is!"

"This little gauge measures the amount of air left in your tank. Check it at least every five minutes and never let your tank go completely dry. If that happens, moisture can get sucked inside. Moisture causes rust and rust can be fatal to your tank... and YOU if I see it happen. Next, see this little button? It's called a purge button and when you press it, it blows your mouthpiece free of water. If your regulator ever gets knocked out of your mouth, just pop the thing back in, put your tongue over the hole and press this button. Remember the tongue part because if you don't, you're going to purge your lungs full of water. Understand?"

The look on Angie's face was not one of complete confidence. In fact, had Dale not had a firm hold on her regulator hose, his wild-eyed student would have bolted straight for the parking lot.

"But that's not going to happen to you because you're a smart girl... right? And you're not going to try to breathe through your nose or forget to purge your mouthpiece... are you?" the pilot calmly reiterated the lesson.

Angie nodded meekly.

"The vest you're wearing is connected to your tank by this hose. By adjusting the amount of air in the vest, you affect your buoyancy, allowing you to either float upward or sink to the bottom. You can also balance it until you're actually weightless in the water.

"This pool is only ten feet deep, so if you screw up and suddenly shoot to the surface, you won't hurt yourself. Now, on the other hand, if you were diving in a lake or, heaven forbid, the ocean and you were down forty feet, I don't have to remind you, a licensed medical professional, what happens to a gas under decreasing pressure."

Angie solemnly nodded. "It will expand and if you don't allow enough time during your ascent for the pressurized oxygen and nitrogen molecules to filter out through your lungs, they will expand and form bubbles in your blood vessels, which in turn, will travel to your brain or lungs or heart and you will develop the bends and die a horrifying death!"

"Jackson!" Dale sternly corrected. "You would develop an air embolus... easily treated by a quick trip to Edmonton for some time in a hyperbaric chamber. None of my students die, not unless I feel the need to kill them first. Remember that!"

Reaching for her hand, Dale lead the nurse out into the pool until the water was lapping at their chests. Flashing Russ the "thumbs-up" sign,

Angie announced she was ready to submerge.

Dale asked her to simply sit down on the bottom of the pool. It seemed straightforward enough, but when Angie tried to sit down, she floated with a good two feet between her butt and the bottom. Worse, her regulator didn't seem to be working. Inhaling for all she was worth, she just couldn't suck any air from the blasted thing. Thrashing like a eggbeater, she clawed her way to the surface and yanked out her mouthpiece.

"This bloody thing doesn't work! I can't get any air out of it!" she sputtered.

"Next time, luv, try breathing through your mouth," Dale sighed. "The nose compartment on your mask only holds about an ounce of air and once you've inhaled that, all you're left with is a vacuum."

Furiously, Angie shoved the regulator back in her mouth and took a deep breath. Her stunned look spoke volumes. Feeling like a complete moron, Angie tried once again to sit on the bottom of the pool, but again hovered just under the surface.

Dale tapped her on the shoulder and pointed to her buoyancy control vest. Good God, she had forgotten all about it, too. What was wrong with her? She hadn't remembered a single thing Morgan had just spent ten minutes trying to teach her.

Fighting hard to look like she knew exactly what she was doing, Angie began to play with the control. After letting some air out, she found herself gently drifting downward. Settling on the bottom, she watched as Dale used a magic marker to jot something on his writing board. "Slow your breathing down. You're hyperventilating."

Then, rubbing the slate clean with the back of his arm, he quickly wrote another message. "Now lie flat on your back."

Angie's laughter sent up an effervescent cloud of bubbles. Reaching for the board, she borrowed his marker, and wrote, "In your wildest dreams!"

Dale grabbed his marker back and wrote "TRUST ME" in big red letters. Angie might have trusted her coach a bit more if he had not simultaneously flashed her a wolfish wink through his mask.

As she started to hyperventilate again, Angie slowly let more air out of her vest until she felt her tank grate against the bottom. As she rested awkwardly on her back, Dale held his writing board horizontally over her face so she could read it. "Okay, slowly breathe in for 5 secs, pause, then slowly breathe out for 5 secs."

Angie did exactly as she was told and almost immediately felt herself begin to rise toward the surface. By the time five seconds was up, the astonished nurse found herself floating belly-up on the surface of the pool. Letting her breath out now, she gradually began to sink and within seconds, her air tank was once again scraping on the bottom.

For the next ten minutes, Angie surfaced and submerged like a mini-submarine. It was kind of fun! Every time she came up, she gave Rusty a big grin before vanishing beneath the waves again.

"We'll end the lesson on a high note" Dale announced, "by learning how to clear your mask." First he pulled the bottom of his mask away from his face until both the nose and eye compartments filled with water. Then, tilting his head back, he breathed out through his nose. The escaping air floated up under the mask, forcing all the trapped water out through the bottom.

It looked so easy, but, just in case she panicked, Dale had her practice in the shallow end of the pool. With both hands nervously clutching the sides of her mask, Angie reluctantly sank beneath the surface. Battling to keep her demons in check, nearly a full minute passed before she gathered the courage to pull the mask away from her face.

Cold, chlorinated water immediately flooded her face-piece. Using every ounce of willpower she possessed not to panic, her eyelids welded tightly shut, Angie carefully tilted her head back and breathed out. Anxiously awaiting the feel of air bubbles rushing up past her face to displace the water, she felt nothing. On the verge of kicking hysterically for the surface, she paused just long enough to cautiously crack open an eyelid. Her mask was clear! And her teacher had a big happy face drawn on his board.

Night two, she learned how to tread water.

Night three, she graduated to wearing fins, learned to swim underwater, and ended the evening by proudly doing ten laps of the pool, fully enclosed in her cumbersome scuba gear. While it was true her stroking technique had all the elegance of a harpooned Moby Dick, that didn't faze her growing enthusiasm one bit. For the first time in her life, she was actually having fun in the water.

It was sometime during her fifth class that Angie Jackson learned to swim. Like the first snowflake of winter, it materialized out of nowhere. She had been working so hard, concentrating on each simple task Dale set out for her, that she had not seen it coming.

Suddenly, all those rudimentary exercises just seemed to come together: one minute she was struggling to tread water, the next she was breast stroking across the pool.

Only someone who has repeatedly tried and failed at something could ever hope to imagine the ecstasy Angie felt as her hand touched the far end of the pool.

She had learned something else, too; something far more valuable. She had learned to put some trust in the male of the species again.

15
NEVER TRUST ANYONE OVER FORTY

"What a difference a week can make!" Angie kept thinking during the Water Rescue test. Everything Dale asked her to do now seemed so simple. Treading water, the front crawl, the back stroke, the breast stroke, even saving the drowning victim—played to loving perfection by Rusty.

Dale finally snapped his clipboard shut and told her to climb out of the pool. While there was little danger of her being asked to try out for the U of C swim team, she had performed well enough to legitimately pass the course.

Following the congratulatory round of hugs and kisses from her beaming coach and number one cheerleader, Angie hurried off to shower and change. Returning to the pool ten minutes later with her swim bag slung jauntily over one shoulder, she was surprised to see Russ and Dale, still in their warm-up sweats, in the midst of a vigorous discussion.

When she pulled up alongside her boyfriend to casually slip her hand in his, Russ shot a strange look in the Aussie's direction, almost an apprehensive look.

"Come on, you guys! Get changed so we can get out of here. We have some serious celebrating to do."

"Yep, I'm going right now!" the medic blurted. With head down, he plodded off toward the showers, then abruptly spun around to face Dale. "I just hope the hell you know what you're doing!"

Dale gave him an icy stare. An uneasy feeling crept over Angie as she struggled to make sense of Dale's belligerent body language and Rusty's' bizarre parting comment. Something foul was in the wind; no doubt another juvenile dispute between the two men.

Depositing herself on the floor, she was just about to ask Dale if he knew when the final LIFE-STAR selection results would be posted when the chopper pilot came to life.

"Uh, could I get you to help me for a second?" he asked without making eye contact, then knelt beside an open equipment bag. "If it's no trouble, I'd like you to try something on for me." He fished a cumbersome navy blue bundle from the bottom of the bag. It was a regulation Buoyancy Control vest with several little pockets sewn into each side. The pockets each contained a lead weight, and must have added 20 additional pounds to the vest.

"What's this thing used for?" she asked as Dale helped her put it on. "Burial at sea?"

Dale forced a smile as he zipped it up. "You're close. It's a combination Buoyancy Control vest and weight belt."

Checking that it was properly in place, her instructor stepped back. "I came across it in the dive shop when I was picking up the tanks. I just wanted to make sure it's the correct size before I buy it." All the while skillfully avoiding Angie's inquiring eyes, he added hastily, "I know a girl back home who's about the same size as you and she's been trying to get her hands on one of these for a long time. Trouble is, she can never find one to fit properly."

What a lame duck story! Morgan was up to something, but what? Trying to read his thoughts, Angie failed to notice Rusty standing just outside the change room door, watching.

"Russ... look out!" Dale shouted, suddenly staring at something behind her. Angie spun around, feeling as she did, something grab hold of the back of her vest.

Grinding his teeth with the effort, Dale picked up his trusting student and heaved her into the deep end.

As her scream-distorted face vanished beneath the water, Russ came at a dead run. "You didn't have to throw her in so bloody hard, did you?" Russ spit, his eyes scanning the bottom of the pool.

"What the heck did you want me to do, Andrews? Coo sweetly in her ear and ask her to jump in when she was good and ready? This has to be as real as possible if she's to learn anything from it."

"The whole thing sucks! Good God, you just got her over her fear of water—she trusted you, man! And now you've destroyed it all. For what? She passed the bloody test, couldn't you have left it at that?"

"Look Andrews, she's proved she can swim in a pool, but I've got to know if she can do it when it's going to count... when she's out in the real world. Remember yesterday when I had her fishing hockey pucks out of the shallow end? She thought she was cock-of-the-walk until I slipped that plastic baggy over her snorkel. Bang! Totally lost it. Came completely apart as soon as she couldn't get any air. I've got to know she can save herself... that she can think her way out of a dangerous situation without panicking. I just have to be sure."

The tsunami waves Angie had generated were now ripples. Dale checked his watch. "Thirty seconds gone. I'll give her one minute."

Angie had had a split second to gasp for air before the water closed over her head. As if outfitted by the Mafia, she was dragged straight to the bottom. Landing heavily on one knee, she staggered to her feet. Kicking hard for the surface, she ascended only a few feet before drifting down again.

Lungs screaming for oxygen, her first rational thought involved walking to the shallow end. But after two laborious steps in extreme slow motion, she frantically abandoned it.

"Come on, Jackson!" Dale muttered as he paced the pool's edge. "For Christ's sake woman, settle down and think your way out of it!"

Forty-five seconds had passed. Russ was leaning forward into his dive when Morgan roughly grabbed his arm. "She's still moving around down there! She's okay. She won't learn a damn thing if you go in after her!"

Russ savagely shook himself free. "You jerk! If she ends up in the hospital, you are going to the morgue."

Her oxygen-starved heart felt like it was going to rupture. Angie yanked hard on the vest's zipper. Too hard. Its teeth jammed with fabric... the plastic pull-tab snapped off in her hand.

Hysterical thoughts were now impairing her judgment. Her fumbling fingers clutched at the collar of the vest as she tried to tear the zipper apart. But the tight-fitting vest clung like a funeral shroud.

"Come on, luv! Don't make me come down and get you!" Dale breathed. A minute had now passed.

"She's got ten more seconds!" Morgan lied as Russ once again took up a diver's stance.

Angie was on the verge of blacking out, her struggle nearing an end. With her body's billions of cells running strictly on oxygen fumes now, she sluggishly reached up behind her neck. For a moment she thought she was hallucinating as she felt the vest slide up. She pulled again.

Slowly it moved over her head. Flinging the thing aside with a final convulsive spasm, she kicked for the surface.

A strangled wheeze spilled from her lungs as her head broke the water. Alternately coughing and crying, she splashed wildly, clawing to stay above water.

Gradually the anoxic fog clouding her mind and her vision began to clear. The blurry outlines of two people standing at the pool's edge slowly came into focus. Mechanically obeying their frenzied shouts to swim toward them, three feeble stokes later, she felt her fingertips brush the edge of the pool.

Russ hauled her limp body from the water. Wrapping her in his towel, he half-carried, half-dragged her to a deck chair. Several minutes of retching, gagging and ragged breathing passed before Angie recovered enough strength to raise her head and take a long look at the man kneeling in front of her.

"Why?" was all she managed to croak before succumbing to another coughing fit.

"I'm so sorry." Dale's voice cracked as he reached out to caress her wet tangle of curls.

"I didn't want to do it... but if I'd passed you... I'd have never known... known for sure you could save yourself. I had to know that if Russ or I weren't around, that you could fend for yourself if you got in trouble. And you proved that, luv. I know I promised I would never let something like this happen to you and rather than try to explain my way out of it by saying I did it for your own good, I just hope that someday you will forgive me."

Cocooned in Rusty's arms, Angie eyed the man before her. There was no doubt his hurt was real. It was in his voice... his heart-felt words... his gentle touch.

"I only hope that you can forgive me," she whispered hoarsely. "That vest of yours is still lying on the bottom, and I will be damned if I'm going back down there to get it!"

16
HEY, WHAT ARE FRIENDS FOR?

Russ had been forewarned about the final sink-or-swim test, so he brought along an extra sweatshirt and pair of jeans for Angie. Half an hour later, the trio stepped out into the brilliant sunshine of a gorgeous July day.

His anger still very much evident, a brooding Russ began a quick walk-around of his rusting clunker in search of flat tires just as a downcast Captain Morgan, two rows over, was about to unlock the door of his gleaming white Saab turbo.

Caught in the middle, Angie could feel each man's pain. Slipping a comforting arm around her boyfriend's waist, she swallowed her pride and whispered a face-saving solution.

"Hey Morgan, what are your plans for the rest of the day?"

Dale looked up, surprised. "Oh, I don't know. I thought maybe I'd go home and tease the neighborhood pit bull for awhile... you know... with maybe the tom cat from across the street."

"Well that certainly would bring new meaning to the term 'kitty litter!'" Russ snorted. "If you really want to see fur fly, why don't you come along with us? What with Angie passing her test and me not being able to kill you until you've handed her results to Lawson... we've got some serious Stampeding to do."

Dale looked blank. "Morgan, for crying out loud!" Russ said. "This is Calgary, and it's the second week of July. You don't have any allergies do you? Like to horses, cows, manure, corn dogs, chuckwagons, midway rides, caramel apples, beer, fireworks...."

"I don't think so," the Aussie replied. "But then again, I've never been exposed to that many health hazards all at once. To be quite honest, I've been so busy with this selection business. But I have heard about your celebrated rodeo, though. What did they call it—'The Greatest Outdoor Show On Earth'? Isn't it a bit out of character for you Canadians to boast like that about anything?"

This time it was Angie who let out a snort. "Rusty, did you hear that. I think we should show this sadistically-warped foreigner what he's been missing! Make him eat his words... or twenty-five corn dogs, whichever comes first!"

Dale climbed into the back of Rusty's road-weary roadster. As Angie turned around to chat with her "drowning coach," she had to position her elbow "just so" to avoid several exposed coil springs. "First thing we'll have to do is teach you how to yahoo. I'm sure that after a few tries, everyone will think you were born here."

"Funny you should mention that," Dale replied, distracted as he idly glanced around the back seat as if checking for signs of rodent infestation. "When I landed in Edmonton on the way down here, I got talking to one of the security guards at the airport. When I mentioned I was headed for Calgary, he said, 'Well, you better watch yourself then, 'cause this time of year, that city's just crawling with yahoos.'"

Stampede Park was a magical place for the 120,000 souls reveling in the sun-drenched festivities. The midway with its whirling, shrieking rides was pulsating with the bass beat of rock music. Loud and impudent barkers hawked their games of chance while the greasy-sweet aromas of burgers, pizza, corn on the cob and cotton candy drifted tantalizingly on the breeze. For three starving, fun-loving people, the Stampede was a beckoning oasis of heavenly delights.

Because Russ had worked as a paramedic at the rodeo for several years, it didn't take him long to wrangle up three free passes to the infield. Parked behind the chutes and hidden from the spectators' view was a privately-owned and -operated ambulance which the Stampede Board hired for the ten days of rodeo action.

Perched on a nearby metal fence were two men. Decked out in boots, jeans, western shirts and straw hats, they looked just like the other hundred cowboys milling about. The only give-away was the black walkie-talkie slung on each man's hip like a six shooter.

Russ called up to one of them, "Hey Joey, any good wrecks today?"

The man turned and broke into a grin, revealing a lip-line of wind-blown dirt across his front teeth. He tapped his buddy on the arm to shift over, then motioned Russ and his entourage to climb aboard.

As the medics on duty, Joey and Gord had been instructed to show up in "undercover" cowboy duds. Rodeo was a dangerous sport—no one disputed that. But having medical personnel roosting like vultures on the infield fence in their familiar baby blue shirts and black slacks would have been excessively ghoulish.

The "Novice Bronc Riding" event was underway. Each time an aspiring bronc rider was tossed from his crow-hopping mount, Joey put a big red X next to his name in the rodeo program. Leaning closer for a better look, Angie discovered that some cowboys had two, some three Xs.

"An X is a buck off," Joey explained. "Two X's means it was a real crowd pleaser and three means the guy should've died and we really should go and check him for a pulse once he crawls out of the arena.

"Hey Rusty, remember that wreck about four years ago, in the bull riding? The guy got his hand hung up and the bull dragged him around for a good five minutes."

"How could I forget?" Russ said. "After he was knocked all but senseless, he waved Joey and me away, staggered from the infield under his own power—no damn way he was going to let the audience know he had been hurt.

"That guy had cracked ribs, a dislocated wrist and the only thing holding his busted ankle together was his cowboy boot... and he still wouldn't let us treat him. Said he wanted to wait till his buddy completed his ride first—if he was still hurting after that, he'd stop by a medi-clinic on his way out of town... to the next rodeo!"

"Yessiree Bob," the rodeo commentator was introducing the next event, "some of the finest bull riders in the world today got their start in this here event. The cowboys and cowgirls competing this afternoon are all five and six year olds and they're going to show us just how hard it is to stay on one of God's tastiest critters. That's right, it's MUTTON BUSTIN' TIME AT THE CALGARY STAMPEDE!"

Dale's jaw flopped open. "You people don't actually ride sheep up here... do you?"

The gate to chute number four swung open. With a hockey helmet strapped over her pony-tail and both hands clutching a soft cotton rope hidden in the thick fleece, sheep rider number one stuck out her wee chest and leaned back as her bouncing, elastic-legged mount headed due west at a nominal rate of speed. After her sheep negotiated a sharp left turn which she didn't, the cowgirl briskly dusted the seat of her jeans and ran to pick up her rope... hotly pursued by a colorfully painted rodeo clown in baggy pants.

Mutton Buster number two, a tiny native contestant by the name of Trevor Running Rabbit, was doing well until his sheep, too, made a sudden left-hand turn. But, sticking to his woolly mount as if he were Velcroed, Trevor refused to relinquish his rope. Leaning hard to starboard as his sheep went to port, the balancing act could last only so long before, finally, the sheep over-balanced and flopped onto its woolly side... with Mr. Running Rabbit still perched proudly on top.

Thrusting a jubilant fist into the air, the green-haired, bulbous-nosed clown plucked the beaming five year-old up in his arms as his steed bounded to its cloven hooves and skipped from the arena like a windblown powderpuff.

Following the rodeo performance, Angie, Russ and Dale wandered over to the Roundup Center to challenge Lady Luck. Sipping on an icy cold beer, Angie watched as the men played the various games. Oblivious to everything around them, both amateur card sharks were down about twenty dollars when Angie glanced at her watch and, squeezing between their bar stools, slipped an arm around each of their shoulders.

"Do either of you boys have enough money left to buy me dinner or should I start sniffing around for another couple of sugar daddies?"

"Come on, Morgan," Russ sighed. "We'd better get her fed and watered before she heads off in search of greener pasture."

Struggling to hide a grin as Angie swatted his muscular behind, Russ took her by the hand, and with Dale surgically attached to the other, they headed off in search of an early dinner.

Dale had seen it once on television, but standing next to the fence and feeling the ground actually shudder as horses and wagons rumbled past was something else entirely. Four wagons, thirty-two horses, twenty men. It was chuckwagon racing time!

Reins stretched taut, the four drivers strained to hold their high-strung horses as they eased them into their starting positions in front of the grandstand. The chuckwagons were replicas of the cook wagons which once served up beans, flapjacks and coffee to the hard-working cowboys out on cattle roundups.

A horn sounded. "Aaand theeeey're off!" drawled the announcer. Outriders pitched stoves and tent poles into the back of the chuckwagons. They then scrambled to board their skittish mounts and avoid being run over as the wagon drivers lashed their teams in tight figure-eight patterns before charging out onto the oval racetrack.

Pounding into the first turn, the wagon drivers jockeyed for the coveted rail position, sending a choking cloud of dust billowing into the cool evening air. Thousands of spectators roared as the frenzied maelstrom of horses, wagons and riders covered the half-mile distance in just over a minute and thundered down the homestretch toward the finish line.

Standing at the track-side fence, Angie, Russ and Dale had to hastily shield their plastic beer glasses as hoof-sized chunks of dirt rained down on top of them. As he watched Dale fish a lump of animal by-product from his beer, Russ could not help casting a friendly barb in the Aussie's direction. "Remember the other night in Canmore when you told me our beer tasted like strained cow pee? Well, now you know how we distill it."

As the last of the chucks headed for the barn and twilight cast a golden glow across the park, Russ and Angie set out to show Dale the world-class exhibits of stock and show animals, the Olympic displays, the city police K-9 demonstration, even the horse-shoeing competition and the wonderfully weird and wild pig races.

Pleasantly weary, the three eventually found themselves sitting on the steps of the Saddledome, home of the Calgary Flames hockey team. From their vantage point, the glittering amusement park spread out before them.

Angie gazed up at the sky. Velvety black and studded with stars, the Milky Way spilled across the heavens. Truly at peace with the world, she wished she could put this moment in a bottle, cap it, and keep it forever.

Just then the darkness overhead split into a thousand shards of light. Fireworks! Because the sound traveled more slowly than the light, the whistling crescendos and deafening booms were strangely out of sync with the light show. Reverberating off the Saddledome's mammoth superstructure, the mortar barrage's fading echo rumbled like distant thunder, as the acrid smell of gunpowder wafted slowly down from above.

Dale had climbed the steps to get a better view, and during a lull in the fireworks, glanced down at Angie and Russ. They sat snuggled in one other's arms, her head resting lightly against his broad shoulder. Deep in thought, the pilot leaned heavily against the metal railing and watched the stars awhile before starting down the stairs.

"Uh, sorry to intrude. I probably should've told you earlier, but I've got some news regarding the Medical Crew selections."

The cuddling stopped.

"I got a call last night from Lawson. He'll formally announce his Air Medical Crew selections tomorrow morning. The old fart knew I wouldn't be testing Angie until today, but apparently Bateman told him he'd already seen more than enough of her talents to make a decision."

Angie felt sick. Russ tightened his arm around her waist. All this agony, the written exams, the rope climbing, the bear attacks, nearly drowning in the river, nearly drowning in the pool. It had all been for nothing.

"They had a heck of a job you know," Dale continued with his grim task. "Some very qualified medics and nurses didn't make the final cut. Calgary is so darn lucky... you folks have such a wonderful EMS program here. Peter stuck Alex and me with the lousy job of contacting all the people who didn't make the team. We spent most of last night breaking people's hearts. I really hated doing that."

It was now very dark where they were sitting. Angie and Russ sat holding one another, pretending nothing had happened... that their whole world was not about to collapse.

"Uh, hello? Do I have to repeat myself or what?" Dale asked. "I said we phoned all the ones who didn't make the cut last night."

Still they sat there. The Aussie descended the stairs until he was standing right in front of the deaf-mute couple. "Are you two brain dead? Read my lips. We called every one of those poor suckers LAST NIGHT!"

"You called all of them... LAST NIGHT?" Angie repeated, her voice wavering.

"Every... last... one," Dale said, milking each syllable for maximum effect.

"You mean... " Russ couldn't finish.

"Lord help us!" the Aussie exclaimed. "I hope to heck Stevens is a little faster on the uptake when Lawson phones him in the morning with the good news."

"Kyle made it too?" the medic gasped.

"Stevens made it with flying colors and so did you two, although right now I'm not sure we made the right decision. I think your brains have atrophied from too much necking!"

"Oh, I don't know about that!" Angie squealed as she collapsed on top of Russ, pinning him to the ground, smothering him with kisses.

A blissful minute of smooching later, reality finally set in. Jumping to their feet, the couple descended in unison upon their new co-worker.

"Did you have to torture us first?" Russ blasted, relieving the Aussie of his new Stetson and using it to beat him over the head.

Angie, being female and thus non-violent by nature, elbowed her way between the two men so she could plant a generous, heartfelt kiss on the Australian's weathered cheek. "Dale, I truly couldn't have done it without you. I don't know how I can ever thank you."

"Oh, I can think of a few things you might like to try," the 'copter pilot whispered flirtatiously as he moved in to land a congratulatory kiss of his own.

"NO SHE WOULDN'T, MORGAN!" Russ interjected from the darkness. Thus amid the sounds of someone being whacked and warned to watch his hands, the fireworks eventually resumed... setting the heavens ablaze with chrysanthemum-shaped explosions, bursting rockets and streamers of liquid stardust.

17
SECOND THOUGHTS

Angie met with her Nursing Unit Supervisor the very next morning. Jean Wallace had been aware of Angie's extra-curricular activities from the very beginning; it had been her glowing letter of recommendation that had resulted in Angie's invitation to the training camp in the first place. With the Mountainview Intensive Care Unit already short-staffed, however, and nurses with critical care experience hard to come by, Jean was not exactly "overjoyed" when Angie broke the news to her.

Knowing she was about to leave a secure position behind, Angie shrewdly covered all her bases by asking her employer if there were any openings in the unit's relief pool.

By offering to work relief, the RN hoped her seeming generosity would be viewed in a positive light. The summer months were always a hectic time and Angie knew from past experience that the NUS would be scrambling to replace sick calls and vacationing staff. While relief status would eradicate her many years of seniority and all of her benefits, it would accomplish two very important things: 1..keep her on good terms with her NUS and 2..allow her to keep her ICU nursing certifications up to date.

On a somewhat more realistic note, if the LIFE-STAR program did end up in the dumpster after the Olympics, Angie didn't want to be left treading water financially... without any other source of income. By becoming a relief staffer, she was leaving her bridges intact.

As she finished out her final two weeks, Angie caught herself more than once wondering if she was doing the right thing. Here she was, replacing a secure though stressful job with something even more stressful and with a future suspect at best. For a nurse already suffering from burnout, it did not seem like the wisest of decisions.

Angie's last shift ended with her fellow nurses hauling her off to the nearest lounge for an impromptu farewell party. Amidst tears of joy and sadness, Jean Wallace spoke for everyone when she raised her glass in wishing Angie all the best in her new endeavor.

Though invited, Connie Harrington, the unit's overbearing assistant NUS, never did put in an appearance at the festive sendoff. She would later claim she couldn't get her car to start.

Their new career as flight medics to begin the next day, Russ had planned to celebrate when he invited his favorite female out for dinner. Watching her pensively sip her cocktail, however, he realized that, for Angie, things were no longer so straightforward. As the rum-laced fruit punch released a flood of apprehensive thoughts, he quietly listened.

While he couldn't deny her concerns were valid, Rusty managed to put the whole issue in perspective. "The choice is yours, hon. You can while away your days in a nice, secure job keeping dead people alive and emptying bedpans for the rest of your life, or you can follow your heart and put all those God-given talents of yours to good use."

Angie exhaled and nodded, smiling for the first time all evening. Russ leaned across the table and took her hand. "Want to hear something that'll really make you smile. You remember in the Rescue Race when the team in front of us, Fleming and Harris shot off that distress flare? It was because they encountered, get this, a moose!"

Russ went on to relate how a senile old bull, with a rack of antlers spreading at least as wide as the Trans-Canada Highway, suddenly appeared on the path ahead. Instead of running off like most self-respecting members of the docile deer family, however, this one stood its ground.

Harris, "Mr. Cocky" himself, shouted at the ugly beast to scare it away. To everyone's surprise, especially Harris', the scruffy, long-legged brute refused to budge. Instead, it bellowed a challenge of its own, and charged!

Fleming and Harris bolted. Madly scrambling up a steep embankment, they made straight for the nearest stand of poplar trees. Clawing his way through the foliage, Fleming accidentally lost his grip on the top end of the stretcher. With their freaked-out patient spewing a colorful string of Australian obscenities, Harris shot past his partner, dragging Dale backwards through the bushes just ahead of the rapidly-closing moose.

Having chased his quarry into the dense thicket, the haggard old beast grudgingly abandoned the chase. So as not to appear totally defeated, however, the "bearded horse with antlers" immediately began venting his frustrations by savaging a tree. Bawling angrily, shreds of freshly-peeled bark dangling from his massive rack, the enraged moose then viciously pawed at the ground, tearing out great clumps of sod and heaving them high into the air.

Yanking at the snarl of straps holding him to the stretcher, Dale finally fell free. Fleming meanwhile, checking over his shoulder for the moose as he ran, tripped over the spread-eagled Aussie, and went cartwheeling into the tall grass. Staggering to his feet, the medic found he couldn't put any weight on his left foot. All the while cussing their stunned teammate, Dale threw Fleming's arm around his neck and hopped him further into the thick underbrush.

Harris dragged the empty stretcher another thirty feet before realizing his three-man team had shrank to a single member. Unable to ignore his companions cries for help, Harris raced back to the two men at a dead run... and ran smack into an overhanging tree branch.

Fleming crawled over to his partner's crumpled form. After assessing Brett's general lack of consciousness and the condition of his own rapidly swelling ankle, the flight medic "wannabe" raised his arms in surrender.

His head aching, Dale wearily reached into the leg pocket of his flight suit. Retrieving a small pistol, he fired a single shot into the air. The mighty rescuers were soon to become... the rescued!

Angie burst with laughter as Rusty recounted the unbelievable story.

Leaving Angie's apartment that night, Russ pulled her into his arms one final time. Standing in the dim, stuffy hallway, he brushed his lips ever so softly across her forehead. Following the curve of her face down to the sensitive area just below her ear, it was several minutes before the kiss-starved paramedic came up for air.

"Babe, everybody dies, but few people ever really live! You should greet each day as if it's your last. Cherish every sunrise."

Angie pulled back in astonishment. This was about as philosophical as she had ever heard her boyfriend get.

Drawing her close again, Russ tenderly caressed her strawberry-blond curls, savoring the satiny softness as it slipped through his fingers.

Angie dreamily closed her eyes as she surrendered to his gentle touch. She had long known of Russ' reputation as a lady's man. Because she had never been exposed to that sinfully delicious side of his life until recently, however, she had never understood why. For starters, the living room of his tiny ground-level apartment was a tasteful littering of exercise equipment, dusty house plants, a legless CPR practice mannequin, the occasional orphaned sweat sock and the current copy of Playboy.

There was never any food in his refrigerator except for the staples...

beer, Coke and pizza. His car was a ten year-old beater with terminal metastatic rust, and his choice in clothes had always made Angie suspect he was either color blind or just plain blind.

"Yeah, Rusty will never make the cover of Gentleman's Quarterly, or Better Homes and Gardens," Angie confided to a nursing buddy one evening, "but Lord is he ever good in... well, you know!"

18
THE HANGAR

Angie's new place of employment had all the comfort and charm of an auto repair shop.

While the helicopter enjoyed a spacious, fully-equipped, heated hangar in which to rest its landing skids, the same could not be said for the Flight crew's living quarters. Among the cramped office's appointments were an ancient wooden desk (elaborately etched with termite carvings), two dented metal file cabinets (minus the keys), and a tattered, 1986 calendar entitled "The Hot Men Of Calgary."

Produced by local firefighters as a fund-raising project for Parkland Hospital's burn unit, the calendar immediately caught Angie's eye. Flipping through its dog-eared pages, she quickly located the object of her desires. Clad only in sunglasses and a flirtatious grin, Mr. May was seductively draped across the cab of a lemon-yellow fire truck, as if sunning his well-muscled physique.

Angie giggled. It had been crazy hot that day, forcing the fire hall crew to repeatedly hose down the pumper's hood so their model wouldn't sizzle anything on the scorching metal. Talk about a cool tom cat on a hot tin roof! The prime Alberta beefcake belonged to none other than Rusty Andrews—firefighter turned paramedic extraordinaire!

Reluctantly tearing her eyes from the calendar, Angie hurried to catch up with the tour. A combination kitchen/TV room/lounge led off from the office. While it did boast a fridge and a microwave oven, there was no sink or running water, and the second-hand furnishings were obviously refugees from someone's unsuccessful garage sale.

A small color TV, complete with floppy rabbit ears, was the room's crowning glory, perched proudly on a coffee table in front of the sway-backed couch. A lone red balloon inscribed, "I Dig Doug's Used Cars," was tied to one of the antennas. Floating with the air currents, it waved a breezy "Hello" every time someone entered.

The room to the left of the office had a small, hand-written note stuck to the door: "BEWARE... PILOT GERMS!" This was the LIFE-STAR pilots' domain. Large maps of southern Alberta and British Columbia had been pinned to the walls, showing the 150 mile radius of the helicopter's maximum range and the locations of the numerous fuel depots scattered across the countryside. Several thick binders were neatly arranged in alphabetical order in a bookcase against one wall. Stuffed to overflowing with navigational headings, they also contained the phone numbers and radio frequencies for every rural hospital and EMS user group within LIFE-STAR's vast territory.

Across the hall, two small rooms contained bunkbeds for the night crew to sleep when they could. Further down that hallway, with wire mesh for a door and a massive padlock bolted to the frame, was the single most important room in the entire LIFE-STAR headquarters. Not because it safeguarded the program's narcotic and drug supplies, but because it contained the one thing keeping the helicopter in the air—the LIFE-STAR approved line of Public Relations merchandise.

From floor to ceiling, the broom closet-sized room was bursting with a colorful array of fashionable T-shirts, golf shirts, sweat shirts, sweat pants, coffee mugs, lapel pins and baseball caps... all embossed with the familiar LIFE-STAR logo of a little red helicopter superimposed on an ECG tracing.

Several Air Medical Crew members, chequebooks in hand, had gathered outside the locked room. Eager to buy gifts for family and friends, they were patiently waiting for Howard Bateman to return with the key.

"The government will only fund this program while the helicopter is actually in the air," Howie growled as he unlocked the door. "They won't cover any of our expenses while we're sitting on the ground waiting for a call. Because of that, we have to depend on private donations, corporate sponsors and the clothing business to stay alive. Okay, who's first. I take credit cards, cheques and cash!"

The LIFE-STAR washroom facilities were apparently located somewhere out in the vast recesses of the aircraft maintenance hangar.

Too shy to ask, Angie and her distended bladder instead listened keenly as Peter gave directions to one of the other rookie flight nurses.

"Just go past the supply cupboards, through those doors at the end of the hall and you'll be in the main hangar. Make a right and try to keep along the near wall. They're doing some sanding and refinishing in there so don't touch or step in anything, okay? Keep going till you pass the Caribou and an old yellow Buffalo. When you come to a Grumman Goose without a rudder, turn right."

The petite brunette, not wishing to appear stupid in front of her new boss, quickly expressed her undying gratitude before scurrying off down the hall. Hustling to catch up, Angie burst through the double doors in pursuit, an action that very nearly flattened her knock-kneed nursing colleague who had, for some unknown reason, chosen to pause on the far side.

"Thank God it's you, Ange! You've got to help me! I don't have the faintest idea what a Caribou looks like, never mind a Buffalo, even if it is painted yellow, and just what the heck is a Grumman Goose? I thought this was an airport... not a frigging zoo!"

Their orientation tour completed, Angie, Russ and Kyle visited with the other paramedics and nurses chosen for the new flight program. Michael Brown was there, the luckless medic very nearly delivered into the jaws of a grizzly by Dale's down-drafted helicopter. The instructors must have felt that "dropping in for a quick bite" would be enough to make anyone lose it.

Angie asked about Larry Moyen, the Park Ranger they'd helped rescue. Michael had been a frequent visitor to his bedside. Forty-seven units of blood and 500 sutures had been required to patch Larry's shredded body back together. Then a near-fatal blood-clotting disorder and a potentially lethal infection had kept him attached to a ventilator and hovering near death for almost a month.

He had survived, however, was out of hospital and planning to return to his job as a Forest Ranger, though it would probably be from behind a desk and not the back of a horse. And the grizzly? At Larry's insistence, it was not hunted down and destroyed. Instead, the bear was relocated to a more remote area of the park. It was Larry who had invaded the magnificent creature's domain. Why should it have to pay with its life for his momentary carelessness?

Rubbing his hands together, a beaming Peter Lawson ushered everyone into the TV room. It was time to get this show of his off the ground.Following an impassioned welcoming speech to his troops, he eagerly delved into the bold and exciting world of air ambulance. He started off by regurgitating a mountain of dry, brain numbing statistics with respect to the program's two years of operation to date without full-time Air Medical Crew.

Thirty minutes later, after nearly lulling his captive audience into a coma, Peter recaptured their attention as he announced the agenda for the coming week: classes on mobile radio etiquette culminating with the Ministry of Communication's radio exam, instruction in rapid-sequence intubation, external pacemaker training and finally, lectures on managing critical emergencies occurring during flight and the medically-delegated procedures they would be allowed to perform without a doctor being present.

Eyes glowing, Lawson went on to explain that all LIFE-STAR personnel would automatically become part of the medical services branch of the Calgary Winter Olympic Organizing committee. Their territory would include all the city Olympic venues plus, 65 miles west of the city, the Canmore Nordic Center and nearby Mount Allan, site of the downhill skiing events.

While the LIFE-STAR pilots were to familiarize themselves with landing areas, Medical Crews were to bone-up on the myriad of injuries specific to each winter sport. In addition, the medics would learn Olympic protocol, so they would know who to address as "Your Royal Highness," "Your Majesty," "The Right Honorable," "Your Lordship," or whatever.

Russ nudged Angie. "I can see it all now," he whispered. "I'll be doing CPR on some old geezer and instead of trying to remember what drugs I should be pushing next, I'll be trying to remember what the heck to call him if I luck out and he regains consciousness!"

Drawing his lengthy sermon to a close, Lawson proudly watched as Bateman presented each crew member with a personal pager, a LIFE-STAR ball cap and a crisply pressed royal blue flight suit. Accented with "glow-in-the-dark" silver and red piping on the arms and legs, the garish flight suits reminded Angie of Mork from the old TV series, *Mork and Mindy*. She wasn't alone.

Hearing the snickers, Lawson staunchly defended his choice of colors. "I'll have you people know that these flight suits were scientifically-designed with only one purpose in mind—visibility. The royal blue tint is one of the few colors not found in nature, and is particularly potent when combined with the reflective taping. With on-scene safety our major concern, we wanted our medical crews to be highly visible against any backdrop, not only to the chopper pilots, but to other rescue personnel, as well, and especially to distracted, neck-craning passing motorists. Anyone have a problem with that?"

After curtly instructing his charges to slip into their new duds, Peter ordered everyone outside. Polished and gleaming in the afternoon sun, the program's cherry-red helicopter would serve as the backdrop for the first official LIFE-STAR photograph.

Among other things, the photo would be used to promote the RCMP's provincial "Check Stop" program.

"DON'T DRINK AND DRIVE... " was to grace the top of the poster, while the caption on the bottom read: "OR YOU COULD END UP GOING FOR THE RIDE OF YOUR LIFE... WITH THESE FOLKS!"

While the majority of medics and pilots proudly mailed copies home to their mothers, it was Angie alone who fully grasped the campaign's intent. She sent one off, not only to her parents, but to each of her party-loving siblings, as well.

19
MYSTERIOUS CROP CIRCLES

After a slow start, word of the revitalized LIFE-STAR program spread, and calls trickled in with increasing frequency.

Financially, however, the fledgling flight service was still experiencing turbulence. After the Games were over, if support from the private sector suddenly dried up, the operation could go right back to its previous month-to-month existence. Keeping a helicopter and crew on 24-hour standby was an expensive undertaking. With the provincial government agreeable to picking up only a portion of the cost, LIFE-STAR was going to have to peddle a hangar-full of clothing and trinkets each month in order to stay in the air.

How much was a human life worth? Angie wondered. If she had to choose between an hour-long ambulance ride over a jarring gravel road with a nervous first-aider along for company, or a twenty minute hop by chopper with an emergency doctor, a paramedic and a critical care nurse on board, she knew which one she would pick.

Anxious to get involved, her first few weeks on the job were racked with frustration. After working five 12-hour shifts, she was still a flight nurse virgin. It wasn't that she was praying for a multi car pile-up or a ruptured aneurysm or anything so morbid. It was just that, if an accident were pre-destined to occur anyway, why couldn't it happen on her shift?

Rather than saving lives, she spent her shifts checking equipment, ordering supplies, watching the latest in-service video and learning how to operate the Lifepak 10 ECG monitor—a wondrous "power-packed" gadget capable of both externally pacing and jump-starting a tiring heart.

She had practiced with the Lifepak 10 so many times she was starting to dream about it. Even then, she still had her doubts. How would she do in a real situation... when the patient's heart wouldn't be the only ticker on the verge of stopping?

To counter her fears, the ICU nurse kept reminding herself that she'd never be alone, that there would always be a medic or a doctor close by. Russ was always so confident about himself. "Once you get a couple of missions under your bra, you'll be just fine!" he reassured her.

Nine hours into shift number six, Angie finally got her call. LIFE-STAR 1 was scramble dispatched to the town of Vulcan, 50 nautical miles southeast of Calgary, for a young man who had been critically injured in a motorcycle accident.

It was a brisk autumn afternoon as Angie and Kyle sprinted across the tarmac toward the purring helicopter. Flaxen hair streaming from beneath her white helmet, she could only describe the experience as one tremendous, mind-blowing adrenalin rush.

Once in the air, the pilot made a bee-line for Parkland Memorial where the on-call flight doctor was awaiting pick-up. This, too, had been part of Peter Lawson's plan to save valuable minutes: having designated on-call flight physicians meant he or she was always available rather than having to search for a doctor to go on the flight.

Upon lift-off from Parkland, Kyle told Angie to radio Calgary dispatch and let them know that LIFE-STAR 1 was air-borne and en route to Vulcan. She was also to give the dispatcher an ETA, Estimated Time of Arrival, to the rural hospital.

The dispatcher acknowledged her transmission with crisp professionalism, but before signing off with the usual, "Have a good flight LIFE-STAR," he solemnly added: "May you live long and prosper!"

Glancing over at Kyle, Angie found the medic forming the famous "V" hand salute. Yes, it was true. They were heading to the mystical birth place of *Star Trek*'s Mr. Spock. Fighting back a giggle, Angie responded, "Thank you Calgary Dispatch, Kirk out."

Arriving at the hospital, the LIFE-STAR team was met by a security guard who escorted them to the emergency department. The patient, a gangly, long-haired 16 year-old had slammed his bike into the back of a parked car. Deeply comatose, the boy lay strapped to a wooden spine board. The force of impact with the car's bumper had smashed his face. Both eyes were swollen shut. Blood trickled from his left ear.

Quickly wrapping up his assessment of the patient, the LIFE-STAR doc ordered his crew to aim for as brief a turn-around time as possible. "There's some shadowing around the heart on the chest X-ray. Could be a possible aortic tear. If that's the case, he's going to need immediate surgery!"

While Kyle was busy helping the doctor intubate the patient, Angie began slipping pressure infuser bags onto the various intravenous bags. In hospital, if an infusion was not running fast enough, she would simply have extended the IV pole, increasing the gravitational pull on the fluid. In the helicopter, however, the IV bags were hung directly from the aircraft's ceiling... a mere two and a half feet above the patient. Without pressure bags taking the place of gravity, the IV solutions would either infuse very slowly or not at all.

Seventeen minutes later, with their patient loaded on board, LIFE-STAR 1 and her three-person medical crew lifted off and headed back to Calgary.

Halfway into the return trip, Kyle looked up from suctioning his patient's airway to find Angie staring intently at the wall-mounted Propaq monitor, a nifty multi-use device which displayed not only the patient's heart rhythm and blood pressure, but temperature and oxygen saturation as well.

"I can't seem to get the O2 sat to register anymore. The probe's on his finger alright, but there's no wave form. BP's dropped from one ten over sixty to ninety over seventy and his heart rate's zoomed to one hundred and thirty-five. What the heck is going... I can't find the radial pulse anymore! I'm going to check for... DEAR GOD, THERE'S NO FEMORAL EITHER!"

With her mind scrambling to remember which of a half-dozen complicated medical algorithms she should be following, Angie's nimble fingers hurriedly released the roller clamps on her patient's two IV lines so the saline fluid could infuse wide open.

"How's his airway, Kyle," the flight doctor asked. "Maybe the ET tube's worked its way down into his right main stem somehow?" As Kyle checked his patient's breathing tube for proper position, Angie started doing chest compressions.

Undoing the front of the C-collar, the doctor made a grave discovery. "We're in big trouble here people. Look at this guy's neck veins! They're all the way up to his ears! Angie, I'll take over CPR. Find me a fourteen gauge needle NOW! I've got to decompress his chest. He's developed a tension pneumothorax."

"I don't know... ," Kyle wondered aloud as he continued to force 100% oxygen into the patient's lungs. "If he had a pneumo, I should feel increased resistance. This guy's easy to bag. No resistance at all. Equal chest expansion... good compliance."

Handing a large bore needle to the doc, Angie squeezed her mike button as she simultaneously injected a second amp of Epinephrine into the patient's IV line. "Calgary dispatch, this is LIFE-STAR One. We have a trauma Code in progress on board. Our ETA to the Parkland heli-pad is approximately ten minutes. Please advise both the Emerg department and hospital security of our arrival and tell them we'll need help getting this patient unloaded. As well, we are also requesting a surgeon be standing by... just in case they have to crack this guy's chest and do open heart massage!"

As the doctor inserted the 2-inch long needle between the kid's second and third ribs, no air escaped. Trying the other side, he got the same result. "Damn, if it's not a tension pneumo...." The doctor paused as he bent over his patient. "What's he had so far?"

"I've given him a total of two amps of Epi and dumped a litre of saline into him," Angie answered breathlessly as she resumed chest compressions. "His ECG rhythm has decayed from a narrow sinus tach to a wide complex bradycardia. The heart is still beating, but it's not pumping any blood."

"He's tamponading," the doctor exclaimed as he grabbed for his mike. "Alex, this is Dr. Underwood. I want you to land immediately. This kid's crashing on us and I need to do a medical procedure on him right now or he's going to die. Just put her down, ANYWHERE!"

Alex glanced nervously at his co-pilot. Beneath their skids, and stretching for miles in any direction, was nothing but lush fields of green barley.

As LIFE-STAR 1 began its descent, the doctor had Angie pull out the central line IV kit. With no cardiac needles on board, he was going to have to improvise. Tearing open the package with gloved hands, the doctor felt the 'copter settle onto the ground.

"Stop CPR!" the doc told Angie. Using a 4-inch needle he had scrounged from the central line set-up, he expertly inserted it just below the patient's sternum. Simultaneously drawing back on the plunger as he carefully advanced the needle several inches, a fountain of dark red blood suddenly filled the barrel of the syringe.

As the tremendous pressure in the sac surrounding the heart was released, the chaotic rhythm on the cardiac monitor showed immediate improvement. The young man's heart was struggling to contract. After several brief flings at lethal rhythms ranging from squiggly runs of ventricular fibrillation to flat lines of asystole, it finally kicked into a beautiful sinus tach at 112 beats a minute.

"Do we have a pulse with that?" the doctor called out as blood continued to drain from the distended pericardial sac.

"I've got a femoral," Angie responded as Kyle leaned over to flash his penlight into the teen's eyes.

"Pupils sluggish, but equal."

"I'm getting too old for this stuff," the doctor exhaled. "You boys up front, if you're listening to any of this, we just bought this kid some extra time. You're cleared to throttle up and launch!"

As the chopper's rotorwash blasted the aircraft skyward, a strangely bemused Alex watched as stalks of barley whirled past his window. Turning to his co-pilot, he observed dryly, "I always wondered where crop circles came from."

20
SCRAMBLE!

Sometimes Angie worked with Dale, and sometimes with Russ or Kyle, but the program had been in operation for two months before she, Russ and Dale shared the same night shift. Jan Elliot, a former forestry pilot, was to split the flying duties with Dale this particular evening.

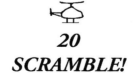

Kyle had flown three busy missions on day shift, and been forced to stay late to finish off the required paper work. With his feet propped on the office desk and a bag of Cheezies balanced on one knee, he was trying to make sense of a statistics form he had incorrectly completed on all three of his flights. Using one of Angie's "letter perfect" stats sheets as a guide, the medic absently crunched and munched as he dabbed correction fluid on one of his many blunders.

The night crew had completed their mandatory equipment checks, and were now relaxing in front of the TV. The airless room was sweltering hot, but following one of Peter's many regulations, they were all duly outfitted in their Nomex flight suits. Made of a flame retardant cloth, the suits would not melt or stick to the wearer in the event of a chopper fire, unlike synthetic materials such as nylon or polyester. Under the suits, white cotton golf shirts, cotton underwear and shorts, and in the women's case, a cotton "wireless" bra, were mandatory.

Sipping on some freshly-brewed decaf, the night crew had settled back to watch an old episode of Star Trek. A die-hard Trekkie, Angie just had to bring up the fact that her very first mission had been to Vulcan. "It was supposed to be a quick, simple hospital transfer. Yeah, right! Things started off so smooth. We had the patient assessed, tubed, packaged and airborne in under twenty minutes. Then, the next thing I know, the kid's Coding on us and we have to ditch in a barley field of all places. A Code inflight! A forced landing! An emergency pericardiocentesis! I'm cursed I tell you. Why couldn't my first call have been a nice, easy NICU baby trip!"

"A nice, easy baby trip!" Russ sputtered, spraying his mouthful of coffee. "I've never known you to do anything the nice, easy wa...."

The ringing of a cellular phone interrupted him.

Snatching it up, Kyle repeated the information as he got it. "Okay, so you're scramble dispatching us to a scene call seven miles northeast of Strathmore on secondary highway six-nineteen... a semi-trailer vs a car... multiple patients involved, several still trapped... one, possibly two will require immediate transport." Kyle covered the receiver and called to Dale who was already in the pilots' room talking with the weather office on another line. "Did you get all that? It's a scene call, northeast of Strathmore, about seven miles. Are we a 'Go' or a 'No?'"

"Tell them it's a go," the chief pilot yelled back, "but just barely. We've got reports of a heavy rain squall in the area. We'll head out, but we could be forced to turn back if the ceiling drops." Jan meanwhile, was examining a map of the area, studying the cluttered maze of side roads, radio beacons and navigational hazards. Stuffing the map into the chest pocket of his flight suit, he threw on his jacket, grabbed his helmet and ran to catch up with the fleet-footed Morgan who was already on his way out the hangar door.

Prior to departing the office, Dale had notified the hangar support staff of the impending mission. Within seconds, the enormous 35-foot hangar doors began to slide open and a tractor moved into position to pull LIFE-STAR 1 out onto the tarmac. The aircraft was still being towed when the pilots jumped aboard to begin their pre-flight checks and coax the twin turbine engines to life.

Kyle scribbled further accident information on a scrap of paper while Russ and Angie ran for the washrooms. It was an unwritten rule that the flight crew visit the can before departing on a mission. There was absolutely nothing worse than flying for an hour with a bursting bladder and a patient who was going down the tubes. Tightly belted in... leaning over a critical patient... in an aircraft that was bouncing all over the flipping sky. It was an experience not unlike airsickness, except from the other end.

Angie slipped on her anti-nausea wrist bracelets and thought briefly about popping a Gravol—the weather didn't sound very good and it would probably be a rough ride. On the 12 missions she had flown so far, she hadn't been sick once, but looking down while monitoring a patient would occasionally make her feel queasy. She wasn't alone. Especially during a night flight when the crew was unable to look outside and focus on the horizon, it was not uncommon to see doctors, nurses, medics and yes, even the lead-stomached pilots covertly slip a hand beneath their seat... just to make sure a leak proof bag was within easy reach.

Airsickness was even worse for the poor patients. Flat on their backs and strapped tightly to a stretcher, the urge to "up-chuck" was a natural response to illness or trauma. As a result, to protect against possible aspiration inflight, it was standard LIFE-STAR operating procedure to intubate all critically injured patients and inject them with an anti-emetic such as Gravol prior to liftoff.

Angie buckled on her waist pack, then hurriedly searched for a small blue nylon bag tucked away in the fridge. Her waist pack contained the medical supplies that she liked to keep close at hand: spare airway, stethoscope, tape, alcohol swabs, heavy duty trauma scissors, penlight, kelly clamps. The blue bag meanwhile, contained specialized IV drugs which required refrigeration—such as potent paralytic muscle relaxants, sedatives and insulin.

Kyle quickly reviewed the mission information with Russ. Fully suited up, the medic listened intently while stuffing a candy bar into his already bulging backpack. His "if I'm lucky enough to survive the crash" kit contained a pair of mitts, toque, hunting knife, hard toffee, water-proof matches and other odds and ends of survival gear.

"Since you seem to know all the facts, Kyle, why don't you come along? We're not taking a doc and from the sounds of it, there'll be plenty of patients for everyone. How about it?" Kyle did not have to be asked twice. He paused only long enough to make a quick call home before grabbing his helmet and racing Russ for the hangar door.

Less than six minutes had passed since the call to scramble had come in and with the last remnants of twilight silhouetting the mountains to the west, Dale brought the 'copter's engines to full power. Slowly pulling up on the collective with his left hand while simultaneously feeding in side pressure on the cyclic with his right, the masterful pilot expertly countered the clockwise torque of the rotors by gently pressing down on the left foot pedal. The delicate dance of hand, eye and foot caused the BK to rise gracefully into the air. LIFE-STAR 1 and her five-person crew were on their way to Strathmore, 37 miles to the east.

21
GOLDEN HOUR

"Thank you Calgary. Please keep us advised. This is med-evac Charlie Gulf Papa Foxtrot Lima, out." Having concluded his conversation with the control tower, Jan glanced over at his flying partner. As if totally unaware that the BK's wiper blades were fighting a losing battle to keep the deluge of rain from obscuring the windshield and thus invalidating Visual Flight Rules, the laid back Aussie casually reached down to extract something from under his seat. It was a bag of cookies.

"Anybody for some munchies back there? Dale said he made them himself," Jan inquired as he handed the bag through the curtain that separated the pilots from the medical crew.

Licking her sugar-crusted lips three cookies later, Angie stared silently out her window at the darkness below. Feeling as the helicopter began its descent into the murky night, she keyed her mike. "Strathmore EMS, this is LIFE-STAR one. How do you read, over?"

"LIFE-STAR one, I read you loud and clear. This is scene commander Dave Connop. We've got a bad MVA down here. An Olds Cutlass T-boned a cattleliner at a railway crossing. Three patients and possibly more are still trapped in the vehicles. Extrication is in progress. Be prepared for a possible two patient transport. Over."

"Has a landing area been set up and secured?"

"The RCMP have set up a landing zone on the highway just west of the accident. They have it marked with red flares, but watch out for powerlines along the south side."

"Strathmore, we copy your transmission. Our ETA to your location is three minutes. This is LIFE-STAR one, out." Pulling on latex gloves as she contemplated the horrific scene that awaited her, Angie suddenly wished she had taken a Gravol.

"Okay people, help us out back there," Jan calmly announced over his headset as Dale began his initial orbit of the landing site.

"We've got a row of powerlines off the port side, but keep your eyes open for any other hazards. It looks like a real mess down there."

Scrutinizing the chaos below, Angie sucked in a breath. Brilliantly illuminated by the headlights of the fire truck, ambulance and RCMP cruiser already on-scene, a massive semi-trailer lay jack-knifed across the road. Tilted crazily over on its side, the trailer's tires jutted awkwardly into the air, giving the truck the hideous appearance of a dying monster. Steam billowed in rolling clouds from its cab. Worse yet, the limp, lifeless head of a cow lolled through a gaping tear in the trailer's metal siding. "I see the truck, but where's the car?" Angie asked.

"It looks like it harpooned the trailer nearly dead-center," Russ replied. "Look just in front of the rear duals. You can see the yellow rear bumper and trunk sticking out."

The helicopter's landing skids settled heavily onto the wet pavement. Receiving the okay to exit the aircraft, the Medical Crew ran, crouched over, toward the police car. Immediately stepping from his vehicle, a rain-soaked Mountie motioned the rescue team to gather around him. "Thank heavens you people could make it! I'm Constable Gagnon and we've got one heck of a...."

The cop paused as a half-ton truck with "Animal Clinic" stenciled on the side, rolled to a stop beside them. "I hate to have to haul you out on such a pissy night, Wade," the French-accented constable called to the driver, "but there's a bunch of cattle on this truck that need to be put down. I've already had to shoot a couple myself. Could you take a look?"

"No problem," the paunchy, middle-aged vet drawled as he climbed out. Picking up a small tackle box lying on the seat beside him, he trudged off through the pouring rain toward the trailer.

"Sorry about that. Anyway, here's the scoop," the constable turned his attention back to the medical team. "From what one of the truckers could tell us, the trailer hydroplaned after hitting a puddle and jack-knifed sideways. An Olds Cutlass traveling in the opposite direction T-boned the trailer broadside and submarined under it. To top it off, the whole frigging mess is resting part-way across the train track. The firefighters believe at least one person in the car is still alive because they can hear somebody moaning in there, but what with the trailer lying right on top of it, it could be coming from one of the dying cows for all we know!"

"Has the truck driver been extricated yet?" Angie asked.

The constable seemed stunned by her question. "When the trailer flipped, part of the railway warning arm went right through the cab. It went right through... everything. The driver and his passenger are still in there. That's where the medics are right now. They took one look inside that cab and called you people."

"Kyle, you assess the people in the car. Angie and I will go check in with the medics," Russ directed, then turned to the constable. "Did you notify the railway to halt all traffic on this track?"

"Yes, we've been in touch with the railway office in Calgary."

Upon hearing that, Angie and Russ scurried off toward the semi-trailer. It was shortly after 9:30 p.m.

A twisted tangle of steel was all that remained of the truck's cab. Resting on its left side with its shattered grill wedged tight against the railway signpost, a single eight-foot section of rusted angle iron had viciously impaled the unit, side to side. The jagged metal rod, all that remained of the red and white striped barrier arm, protruded a good two feet out beyond the passenger door.

Moving to the front of the truck, Angie and Russ found a Strathmore paramedic digging through his equipment bag, while only the rear end of his partner was visible through the shattered windshield.

"Hello there, we're the medical team from LIFE-STAR. What can we do to help?" Russ had to shout to make himself heard above the cows' incessant bellowing.

"You guys don't waste any time," the paramedic replied, his voice strangely monotone. He motioned the LIFE-STAR crew to follow as he stepped away from the truck and up onto the highway. "Just so you know, we're all alone here. Our second ALS unit blew a tire while en route and hit the ditch. Nobody hurt, but that leaves us with just a BLS unit from Rockyford for backup, and they're still thirty minutes out. Not that any of that matters. These poor guys are beyond the help of a mere mortal paramedic. What these guys need is a priest!"

The young man paused to rub his neck with a blood-stained hand. "There's two middle-aged males trapped inside the cab. The swamper's semi-conscious with a fractured right femur and he has a chunk of angle iron two inches wide shoved through the left side of his abdomen... just below the rib cage.

"The other guy is the driver and he's... he was impaled by the same piece of metal... entered through the right side of his lower chest... shattered most of the ribs on that side. He's coughing blood and I haven't been able to find a pulse, never mind a blood pressure since we arrived, and that was thirty minutes ago!

"By the way, I'm Dave Connop and my partner is Rob Hardgrove. We're with Strathmore EMS."

Following the medic back to the truck, Angie dropped to her knees in front of the truck's smashed windshield. The carnage before her was as bad as she expected. But the worst thing about it... the part she would never forget... was the smell. Choking fumes of diesel fuel intermixed with the sickly-sweet aroma of vaporized engine coolant was the bouquet wafting from the cab. The full-strength stench inside, however, was beyond anything she had experienced in either her sixteen year nursing career or growing up on the family farm. Blood, vomit and other unmentionable body fluids had curdled and fried upon contact with the blistering engine block.

Abruptly yanking her head from the cab, Angie dashed into the surrounding darkness where she promptly emptied her stomach of three cookies and everything else she had eaten in the past six hours. Even as she bent double with the dry heaves, a terrible thought raced through her brain. As a LIFE-STAR nurse, her job was to render assistance to the rural EMS medics in whatever way she could. Big help she was going to be, puking herself silly in the ditch.

By the time she staggered back to take her place beside him, Russ had already decided upon a plan of action. "Okay, Dave, let's get a firefighter over here to knock out what's left of the front window. Our first priority will be extrication. We can't transport these gentlemen back to Calgary if we can't get them out of the truck!"

As Jan was to fly the return leg of the mission, he had wisely elected to stay away from the action and remain in the chopper. He could listen in on his portable radio and yet remain focused on the job at hand... that being the safe delivery of his crew and an as yet unknown number of patients back to the Riverside Medical Center.

Dale meanwhile, having performed his co-piloting duties of contacting dispatch of their arrival on-scene, sauntered over to the wreck. It was like nothing he had ever seen in all his years of rescue work.

The local vet, his husky frame perched on the trailer's tailgate, played his flashlight over the terrified animals huddled inside. Forty red blinking eyes reflected back in his light.

"What do you think... can you unload them?" Dale inquired.

"Not a chance!" the vet grunted as he spat out a plug of chewing tobacco. "First, we have to pull the trailer back onto its tires. Then, we're going to need a cutting torch to remove the tail gate. Once that's done, we can start winching the dead heifers out and get a welder inside to cut through the inner partitions. We're also going to need to set up a portable chute and holding pen to corral these frightened beasts once we get them out of there."

The disgruntled animal doctor glanced over at the man he had been chatting with all this time. "You the chopper pilot?"

Dale nodded.

"Well, from what I've heard, this is all-for-not anyway. You probably won't be taking anybody back with you... not alive that is."

"I truly hope our medics can pry some sorry devil out of this mess alive," Dale countered. "Our mandate is to transport the most critically injured patient back to Calgary and to be honest, I don't relish the thought of having to fly home with a cow strapped to our stretcher!"

Kyle hurried over to where several firefighters were working. They had been struggling for nearly half-an-hour to lift the cattleliner off the car. With the trailer section tilted forward, its massive weight had all but flatted the roof of the Cutlass... right down to the door locks. Worse still, the forty-five foot trailer was leaning at such a steep angle that the heifers trapped inside were crowded up against the far left wall. Tufts of brown and white hair poked out through numerous ventilation slats that ran the length of the cattleliner. As well, manure mixed with urine made for treacherous footing both inside and around the trailer as the slurry of animal waste dribbled down the slanted aluminum deck to splatter onto the asphalt roadway.

Having enlisted a firefighter by the name of Tim to cut a small hole in the roof of the car, Kyle was just about to aim his flashlight through it when the trailer directly above his head rocked unsteadily. Its hooves clattering and kicking, a 1200 pound cow lost its footing on the sloping floor, falling heavily against the metal sidewall.

"They don't pay me enough to do this," the visibly rattled medic muttered as he shoved his flashlight back into the hole. Shouting to make himself heard over the bawling cattle, Kyle began calling out his findings to Tim. "I can see a man and woman in the front seat. Both of them motionless. The woman's slumped forward... has the dash embedded in her face and chest. Can't tell if she's alive or not. The man is lying on his right side. Major facial smash. But he's breathing! He's blowing bubbles through the blood."

Switching the flashlight to his opposite hand, Kyle swung the narrow beam toward the rear seat. It took a few seconds for his eyes to adjust to the shadows. When they finally did, what he saw sent a chill knifing through his heart. "We've got two infant-sized car seats buckled in the back seat. One's empty. The other's facing away from me. Tim, hustle around to the back and see if you can shine your flashlight in from the other side."

A few seconds later, there was a screeching howl. "Thank God for car seats!" Tim exclaimed. "We've got a beautiful baby back here. Two, maybe three months old. My light must've scared him. Doesn't appear injured. Moving all four limbs. Don't cry sweetie. We're going to get you out of there."

"That leaves us one kid short," Kyle remarked quietly, directing his flashlight toward the front seat again. His fears were confirmed. Crushed against the dashboard while cradled in its mother's arms, a baby's bloodied foot could be seen poking out from beneath the woman's hip. Twins.

The medic leaned heavily against the side of the car for several seconds before stepping aside. As a pair of firefighters attacked the door with the hydraulic Jaws of Life, Kyle relayed the news to Russ over his chest-mounted radio.

Receiving his partner's update, Russ turned toward the helicopter. A solitary figure peered back at him through the rain streaked Plexiglas. "Jan, did you catch all that? I want you to get a hold of dispatch for me. I need to know the ETA for that unit from Rockyford. If they're more than fifteen minutes away, advise the dispatcher that we've got six critically injured patients to deal with out here and that I'm requesting an additional ALS car be scrambled from Calgary. If they can spare it, ask them to send two!"

As firefighters removed the last of the glass from the truck's windshield and covered the opening with a tarp, Angie again dropped to her knees in front of the cab. Sucking in her empty gut, she squirmed through the window.

Her task was to reassess each man's injuries. The swamper in the passenger seat was sporting a C-collar to support his neck, a high-flow oxygen mask and had a large-bore IV in his right forearm. From the location and direction in which the bar had entered his swollen belly, Angie knew it had most likely perforated every major organ on the left side of his body. As if to rule out any doubt on that diagnosis, an eight inch loop of intestine protruded from the gaping exit wound in the man's lower back.

The plan was to cut off both ends of the metal shaft, leaving it in place inside the patient while they extricated him from the cab and transported him to hospital as fast as possible.

Gently, Angie palpated the area surrounding the metal bar. She could feel only soft tissue beneath her probing fingertips. She thought for a moment. If Plan A didn't work and they couldn't extricate the patient any other way, those last two remaining inches of muscle and skin could be sliced through with a scalpel. Yes, it could be done... but would she have the guts to actually do it?

Turning to the driver, Angie found a ghostly-pale figure tightly wedged between the bent steering column and the seat. Because the other patient was lying partly across him, it was difficult to get a jugular IV line started. Forced to suspend the litre bag of saline from the door handle, Angie was taping the IV to the side of his neck when the middle-aged trucker abruptly roused from his stupor. Opening his eyes, he raised his hand to touch the cold metal rod embedded in his chest. Staring at the blood dripping from his fingers, his dazed look slowly changed to one of horror.

Watching as Angie fussed with his IV, the old trucker suddenly clutched at her wrist. "Don't let me die!" he wheezed. "Please Miss... don't let me die!"

"You're not going to die!" Angie's reply was automatic. "We're going to get you out of here. Now, if you let go of my arm, I'll give you something to help numb the pain, okay."

Very slowly, the driver released his grip. Angie drew up a syringe of Morphine and injected it into the man's IV line. In less than 30 seconds, he had slipped into a narcotic-induced haze.

Unable to do more, Angie exited the cab. Leaving the two truckers in the capable hands of the Strathmore medics, she headed off in search of Russ. He was with Kyle and the other would-be rescuers standing huddled around the squashed Cutlass sedan, heatedly debating what to do next.

"Let's settle down here, people," Russ was saying. "First things first. Constable, the railway has been notified about the track closure... right?"

"They are aware and have a repair crew en route!"

"All right," Russ continued, "this is what we're up against. We can't move the trailer until we extricate the two guys in the cab. We can't get at the people in the car until we winch the trailer off, and the vet says he won't be able to unload the cows from the truck until a welder and a portable chute arrive."

One of the firefighters jumped in. "The angle iron impaling the truckers will have to be cut in at least three places. There's not a lot of room to move around in there, but if we used the Jaws to snip off the outside sections, and a hacksaw for the inside work, we should have both men out of there in twenty minutes. Half-hour tops."

Dale studied the destruction before him. "Thirty frigging minutes before we can do anything else? There has to be a faster way. What if, while you're cutting the angle iron, the rest of us are working to uncouple the trailer from the cab? Once it's apart, maybe we can pull the trailer off the car by using the fire truck. That way, we could be working on two projects at once."

"Do you really think one fire truck can lift that monster?" Russ retorted.

"The trailer's at a hell of an angle now!" Tim interjected. "A slow steady pull just might do it. For God's sake, nothing else has worked!"

LIFE-STAR 1 had been on-scene for seventeen minutes and they were no closer to loading a viable patient into their chopper than when they had first touched down. The critical "Golden Hour" was rapidly ticking away.

22
ROCKS AND HARD PLACES

While Angie and Russ removed the stretcher from the helicopter, Tim and a buddy firefighter were using the Jaws of Life to cut off the outer sections of the metal rod impaling both truckers. A scant minute later, the job was completed and Russ crawled inside the blood-splattered cab to begin sawing on the bar where it protruded from the swamper's back.

Constable Gagnon walked over to where Dale was watching the firefighters battling to pry the trailer's locking bolt free. "I've got a truck full of oil rig workers stopped up the road a ways. They want to know if there's anything they can do to help."

"Sure, send them down," Dale replied. "Maybe they can help us with this blasted thing!"

Moments later, a truck carrying five husky young fellows materialized from the darkness. They quickly pulled tools from the back of their one ton and hurried to the trailer to assess the situation. With the bolt holding the "locking collar" partially sheared off, the firefighters had been struggling to jimmy the trailer's kingpin free using crowbars. Getting nowhere, they were now attempting to utilize a hydraulic spreader to the same end.

With the extra manpower to hold the awkwardly shaped ram in position, the troublesome bolt popped upward with ridiculous ease. A split-second later, the locking mechanism released with a bone-splintering crack. Unable to withstand the added torque, the already-weakened kingpin had snapped off at the base.

No one was more surprised than Russ. Flung forcefully against the back wall as the cab suddenly pivoted to the right, the medic didn't even have time to cuss. Both patients, even though sedated heavily, screamed in agony. The angle iron impaling their bodies had twisted a full quarter-turn.

Angie hastily broke open another Demerol amp as Russ fumbled about on hands and knees, trying to find his hacksaw. Blindly probing the pitch blackness, the medic noticed something odd. He seemed to be throwing a shadow.

Having handed his flashlight to Angie so she could see to draw up the

Demerol, as he glanced in her direction now, Russ noted the downward-pointing flashlight clutched under her arm was causing the curving outline of her face and upper body to glow in silhouetted relief... a seemingly impossible feat.

With more pressing concerns occupying his thoughts right then, Russ located his saw and ran his fingers along the sticky, blood-slicked bar, searching for his old cut marks. He found something else instead. The powerful jolt of the cab breaking free of its trailer had broken the two-inch shaft cleanly in two.

"I'm through!" the medic shouted, turning back to face Angie. "Help me get...." The words froze in his throat as he stared past her into the darkness beyond.

Seeing the look on his face, Angie spun around. Off in the distance, four white lights in a triangular pattern were approaching. They were incredibly brilliant... like aircraft landing lights. Stabbing into the blackness, their beams illuminated the passing wheat fields for a quarter-mile.

"Oh no!" Angie screamed over her radio. "There's a train coming! Dale, Kyle, everybody... did you hear me... we've got a southbound train on the tracks!"

As shouts of chaotic panic filled the night, it was Dale who assumed command. "Tim, we're going to pull the trailer over and drag that car out of there right now! We've got time. No need to run for cover just yet." Dale sounded so calm, so sure. Watching Tim race for the fire truck, the Aussie signaled the remainder of the terrified rescue crew to gather round him.

"Get a second cable on the car!" he ordered the rig workers. "As soon as the trailer is hauled upright, you start winching and you don't stop until you've dragged it well clear of the track. Got it?" The men scurried away like cockroaches exposed to light.

The train's headlights had grown much more intense and, even though only seconds had passed, the entire surrounding area was now bathed in an unearthly white glow.

A bloodcurdling scream exploded from the truck's cab. With time running out and nine inches of angle iron still protruding grotesquely from the man's back, Kyle and Dave abandoned EMS protocol as they forcibly dragged the injured man from the tangle of hissing, steaming metal. Frantically strapping their patient onto a back board, they slung the stretcher between them and bolted for the chopper. As they ran, the ground beneath their feet began to vibrate with the awesome braking action of the unrelenting freight train.

The truck driver, still hopelessly pinned, stared silently at the lights bearing down on him.

Unable to just turn his back and walk away, Russ gently slipped his arms around the man's chest and attempted to lift him up in the feverish hope that the corroded metal rod would slide easily out of his body. "STOP IT! PLEASE STOP!" the burly trucker screamed.

"You can't...." he gasped as he looked up at his distraught rescuer. In those few seconds, as the two men looked into one another's eyes, the unspeakable truth became clear.

"Son, it's not your fault," the man's hoarse voice cracked as he reached for Russ' hand. "The jig's up and you know it. Shoot me if you have to, but please... don't just leave me here to die." Struggling for each breath, the trucker coughed, sending a shower of bloody phlegm down the front of Russ' flight suit.

"For God's sake, boy! I heard them... heard them shooting the cows! Please, I don't want to be awake when that train cuts me in half!"

Angie was kneeling behind Russ. The train's lights were so intense now, they seemed to be burning the back of her neck. She wanted to run away. Away from this truck and away from this freight train... a death train that seemed intent on snuffing out the life of her patient.

Her gloved hands were already reaching for the medication pouch on her belt. It usually contained two ampoules of Morphine and two of Demerol, but she had already used up one of the Morphines and both of the Demerol amps. As she drew up the remaining 10 milligram Morphine vial, she knew it would not be enough. "Russ, give me one of your Morphines!" she yelled over the locomotive's deep-throated throb.

Russ grabbed her by the arm. "What the hell are you doing, woman? We've got to get out of here RIGHT NOW!" Angie shook him loose.

"Give me your God damned Morphine, Andrews!" she screeched, reaching for the black pouch attached to his belt.

The cows were bawling their lungs out. The train's unrelenting warning horn was threatening to rupture eardrums. Rescue workers were shouting orders to one another. A truck engine roared as it strained to pull the trailer off the car. Over his chest radio, Dale was screaming at Russ and Angie to get their asses the hell out of there.

Russ removed the medication pouch from his belt. Fishing out a Morphine amp, he handed it to her. "Angie, it's wrong! Listen to me. We're going to get into a shitload of trouble for doing this. Just because we can't get him out doesn't mean we should euthanize him. For Christ's sake, girl, think about the legalities! What's Peter Lawson going to say? What's the Medical Review Board going to say?"

Though it could mean both their licenses, Russ did not make a move to stop her. Watching Angie's trembling hands draw up the powerful narcotic, he knew it was the only humane thing they could do.

Hand-in-hand as they raced toward the safety of the helicopter, Angie suddenly pulled free of her boyfriend's grasp and turned back. Even with her terrified heart hammering against her ribs, she felt compelled to watch this horror story's final chapter unfold.

Fifty yards away now, the 200 ton locomotive's shrieking steel wheels were spitting a boiling cloud of sparks and fire. Like Satan emerging from Hell, its blazing headlamps reached out to devour the darkness between it and its trapped prey.

Everything was happening in slow motion. Before her eyes, the massive stock trailer slowly began to right itself in response to some imperceptible force. Hesitating briefly at a 45-degree angle, the bottom-heavy trailer abruptly overbalanced, sending its steel-belted radials crashing back to earth. At the same instant, the flattened Cutlass and its entombed occupants lurched backwards down the highway. Using their truck's slender winch cable, the oil rig workers were putting their very lives on the line in a courageous final attempt to somehow drag the car clear of the tracks. It was going to be close!

The train slammed into the truck's white cab with a sound strangely like that of a garbage truck's compactor... instantly slicing it in two. Crushed by the engine cowling, the cab's front section survived the initial assault intact, only to be smashed to pieces as it struck the stationary trailer.

Jolted backwards several feet by the brutal impact of 30 million pounds of onrushing train, the cattle trailer miraculously remained upright as tanker cars filled with propane and liquid natural gas began whipping past, mere inches away.

As it rumbled by, a flatbed railcar carrying two mustard-yellow combines clipped the side of the trailer. The seemingly glancing blow savagely wrenched both combines sideways, snapping like thread the half-inch chains holding them in place. With the tension suddenly released, one of the broken chains exploded outward in a sweeping arc, coiling itself around a nearby power pole. As the hopelessly unbalanced combines were about to vanish into the darkness with the remainder of the freight train in hot pursuit, the snagged chain abruptly jerked the $250,000 worth of farming implements over the side.

After scattering wreckage for a half-mile, what remained of the truck's cab mercifully broke free from the locomotive's cowling, and tumbled down into the ditch.

LIFE-STAR 1 made two flights that night. The first was for the truck's swamper; the second for the father and the surviving twin. While the infant was virtually unharmed, the father would spend the next two months in hospital... followed by another three in rehab.

Just prior to lifting off with the impaled trucker, co-pilot Dale sneaked a clandestine peek at the action taking place in the back of the 'copter. Russ was using both hands to pin their thrashing patient to the stretcher while Angie struggled to inject a medication into his IV line.

"Quit squirming around, damn it!" she finally yelled. "I don't care if you are scared of flying, you're coming with us!"

23
HINDSIGHT IS 20/20

The eastern horizon aglow with fiery pastels, police and railway officials talked quietly among themselves as they surveyed the eerie accident scene. The decapitated cattleliner, its twisted, manure-caked interior still steaming from the welder's cutting torch, lay like a rotting cadaver in the east ditch. Across the road in the opposite ditch, the remains of a two-door Olds Cutlass were visible. Literally cut to pieces, only the frame was recognizable.

The portly county Medical Examiner, having recited his observations into a hand-held tape recorder, told his assistant to put away his camera. With all the angles of the death scene captured on film, it was time to bag and tag the bodies of the mother and child in the car, and start gathering up the truck driver's scattered remains.

Using green garbage bags, two grim-faced police officers and the coroner's apple-munching associate spent the better part of the next two hours combing the tall grass... collecting the bloodied fragments that had once been a loving husband, a caring father, a kind and gentle grandfather.

It was only after a certain number of major body parts had been accounted for that the pathologist could legally pronounce the trucker deceased.

The dreadful accident affected the flight crew in vastly different ways. Morgan, the hardened veteran of the group, had come through the experience with nary a nightmare. Having dealt with Incident Stress Management in the past, the LIFE-STAR chief pilot asked Lawson for permission to debrief each of his crew, to see how they were holding up and ascertain if they would do anything differently if they had the entire thing to do over.

After listening to Kyle agonize over his feelings of helplessness in preventing the trucker's death, Dale confided that several years earlier he had been involved in a comparable incident in Australia. A massive brush fire had sprung up on the outskirts of Melbourne, threatening the city. Piloting a support chopper, Dale's job had been to ferry ground-crews to and from base camp. A million acres of sun-baked forest and grassland had already gone up in smoke, stretching the limited number of firefighters to the breaking point: physically and mentally.

Forced to run for their lives as the shifting wind sent a crackling wall of flame suddenly racing back toward them, one six-man crew had been forced to watch helplessly as a nearby farming community was cremated before their eyes.

"You know, some of those poor blokes honestly believed the town's destruction was their fault. If they'd only moved a little quicker... worked a little harder... maybe cussed a little louder."

Dale rested a steadying hand on Kyle's shoulder. "You did the best you could, son. Heck, you weren't even supposed to be on that flight. Thank God you were! By pulling together, you guys made a difference. You saved three lives. Try to think of it from that perspective and remember this... if we hadn't gone out there the other night, those three people would not be alive today!"

Kyle nodded somberly. "In this business," Dale added, "if you can learn from your mistakes and cherish your successes, you'll do alright. More importantly, you'll be able to sleep at night."

Because of the drastic step she had taken, Angie had naturally been the most deeply affected. The unanswerable question, "Had she done the right thing?" coupled with the frightening possibility she had overreacted to the situation, haunted her every waking moment. During the day, she found herself replaying the dreadful scene over and over in her mind... trying to second guess the final outcome if she had not decided to "play God."

Even sleep provided no release. Angie was jolted awake night after night with a pounding heart and tangled, sweat-soaked sheets. The nightmare was always the same. Peter Lawson was the doomed trucker. She could hear his agonized screams... feel his fingers digging into her flesh as she deliberately injected the overdose of Morphine into his IV line... watched the terror in his eyes slowly fade to blank as the painkiller took hold.

Three nights later, on their next shift together, Dale spotted the deep purple shadows under her eyes. Snagging some Cokes and potato chips from the vending machine, he sat her down on the grass outside the hangar for a little heart-to-heart.

First, he cleared up the mystery of how a freight train had ended up on the tracks that night. Apparently, upon receiving a static-distorted message of an accident blocking the line ahead, the engineer had mistakenly concluded the wreck's location to be the main Trans-Canada Highway crossing... not an isolated level crossing ten miles to the north.

"I heard the engineer's booked off on stress leave... blames himself for what happened," Dale said as he snapped the pull tab on his Coke.

"You know, Ange, when a person experiences a stressful event, it can make you feel real mixed-up inside. You start replaying the situation over and over in your mind... begin second-guessing your actions. That's why I asked to get together with you tonight. If you want to talk, I'm here to listen."

Knees clutched tightly to her chest, Angie stared off into the distance. "You want to know the truth," she murmured, "since the accident, my emotions have been all over the map. One minute I'm angry, the next I'm full of guilt, and then I wallow in remorse and pity for a while. And then it's back to guilt again. The only thing I know for sure is that, if I had left that man to his fate, I would never have forgiven myself. Not ever."

Dale's weather-hardened features softened. "Luv, I don't profess to be a medical expert, but did you really have a choice? You listened to your heart and courageously put mercy and compassion ahead of blindly following protocol. If only more people would do that, the world would be a heck of a lot nicer place to live!"

Russ, too, had been jolted to the core by the dreadful incident. His loony, witless girlfriend had risked not only her career, but also a possible ten to twenty year stretch in a penitentiary.

Deep down, the medic knew only too well why Angie had acted the way she did. Many years earlier, driving home from a rural high school dance, he came across an accident. A farmer had lost control of his pickup, skidded down into the ditch and struck a culvert. Upon hitting the corrugated metal pipe, the truck's engine had exploded through the firewall, leaving the badly-injured farmer pinned between the seat and the steering wheel. A fifty-five gallon slip tank mounted behind the passenger compartment immediately began to vent highly flammable gasoline fumes. Within seconds, the farmer's lit cigarette ignited them.

Across the desolate, windswept stubble fields, the farmer's screams carried on the calm night air; wordless waves of agony rising specter-like above the fire's hushed cracklings.

Desperate to try anything, seventeen year-old Russ approached the blazing wreck only to be repeatedly forced back by the intense heat. Without a fire extinguisher, and with the closest farm house four miles away, the quick-thinking teenager resorted to using his boots to carry water from a slough to throw on the flames. For all the good it did, he might as well have pissed on it.

The fact that someone was trapped in that inferno was horrifying, but being forced to listen helplessly while that person roasted alive was almost beyond human endurance. After an eternity, the screaming faded, consumed by the flames as the truck melted into a smoldering heap of white-hot embers.

Upon arriving home, the distraught teen confessed to his father that if he'd had his rifle with him, he would not have thought twice about taking aim at the writhing, flame-engulfed figure and pulling the trigger.

Remembering how it felt to stand helpless and alone beside that blazing funeral pyre, Russ found himself drawn to rescue work and the fire department following graduation. It was as if he were subconsciously trying to atone for the past.

Yes, with that awful memory for comparison, Russell Andrews knew exactly the torment his girlfriend was suffering.

"You're so much more impulsive than I am," he said quietly after listening to her pour out her tortured thoughts to him one night. "You can see what needs to be done and you take action, without regard for your own safety or personal well-being. You've got to quit doing that, girl. You're making the rest of us cowards look bad!

"Hon," he added with a tender sideways smile, "heck, if I were dying and your sweet face was the last thing I saw before the lights went out, I'd think I was in heaven already."

Angie's muffled sobs instantly edged up to a wail as she reached out her arms for a hug. "Don't ever say that Rusty, not even in fun!"

Caressing her hair as he held her tight, Russ responded by attempting to deliver a reassuring kiss.

Pulling away, Angie was not about to be pacified. "Okay?" she sniffed. "Promise me... okay?"

"Okay," Russ murmured as he gently pressed his cheek against hers. "I was just thinking about you, that's all. I mean, I was the one who got you into this line of work and if anything ever happened to you, I'd never be able to forgive myself. Not ever."

24
FACING THE MUSIC

After discussing the possible medical and legal implications with Howard, Angie was instructed to sit tight for the next couple of days. Bateman explained about how the Medical Examiner's office had already performed an autopsy on the trucker and that the final report was still pending. As there would be little doubt as to what the coroner's toxicology findings would show, however, Angie was to meet with her boss to examine her options.

Sitting across from Peter's battered wooden desk, Angie stoically awaited her fate. After perusing the Patient Care Record one final time, Lawson slowly removed his reading glasses and rubbed his eyes.

"I received a call this morning. It was from a Dr. Melford down at the M.E.'s office. He had some very real concerns regarding the deceased trucker's lab work. Apparently the man's bloodstream was laced with so much Morphine, he probably never knew what hit him!"

Angie remained stone-faced at Peter's news, but the nagging doubt regarding the effectiveness of her action had finally been answered.

"Angela, I think we both know why you're in here this morning. I've already spoken with Russ and Kyle and, to be quite frank, I think you've got a heck of a lot of explaining to do, young lady."

Angie nervously cleared her throat. "Well sir, the train was less than a hundred yards away and there was just no way we were going to get him... the truck driver... out of there in time. As a last resort, Russ even tried to pull him free, but the poor guy was screaming for him to stop. The piece of angle iron went right through his chest and out his back. Half of his insides were coming out. I can't begin to describe it. It was... geez, unless you were there, you can't possibly imagine what it was like.

"The guy could hear the cop shooting the cattle. He could see the train coming. He was crying. Pleading for us to give him something, anything, to knock him out. It was awful. I couldn't just turn and walk away. I kept thinking... what if it'd been me or Russ or Kyle trapped in there. It felt like the train was right on top of us.

"Sir, I honestly didn't know what else to do. I pushed twenty milligrams of Morphine into the man's jugular line. Opened the control clamps wide open, so it would flush in real fast. He was already in deep shock. Lost consciousness almost immediately...."

Her throat squeezing shut, Angie's faltering, disjointed statement abruptly halted in mid-sentence. Pausing to inhale several deep breaths, she valiantly attempted to finish her story. "Sir, we could've reversed the effects of the Morphine. I had the Narcan already drawn up."

Forced to stop because she didn't know what else to say, the rookie fight nurse had the sickening feeling she had said too much already.

His face etched with deep lines, Peter remained silent for a long time. Finally he looked at her. "Ms. Jackson, what we're dealing with here is an extremely complex situation, raising a lot of very difficult medical and ethical questions. Questions I don't think even the Surgeon General would have answers for. Apparently the local M.E. doesn't have the answers either, because he's contacted the Chief Medical Examiner up in Edmonton. The Fatality Inquiry Board has become involved and they've called a hearing for Tuesday of next week.

"Trust me, Angela, the last thing you want to do is come across like some teary-eyed, emotional basketcase while you're trying to defend your actions. If you do that, those boys will eat you alive! This is strictly off the record, but I believe you did what you thought to be morally right. Under those same circumstances, I'm not sure what I would've done.

"One thing I am certain of, however," Peter's fatherly tone abruptly soured as he tossed the PCR form into a manila file folder, "is the fact that I do not want people in my organization who deliberately ignore protocol and think they can get away with murder!"

Lawson sprang up from his chair to jab red plastic pins into the wall-mounted map behind his desk. Clear in the knowledge that her once stellar nursing career was over, Angie looked around for something to throw up in. Instead of a Valium, she should have popped a couple of Gravol before the meeting.

Having run out of pins, a sober-faced Lawson slowly turned around. "I spoke with Morgan yesterday. He assured me you were riddled with remorse, drowning in guilt and that you swore you'd never practice freelance euthanasia again... except maybe on him. Angela, you didn't kill that trucker, the train did. All you did was try to ease his pain and suffering and under the circumstances it was probably the most merciful thing anyone could've done."

Her eyes brimming with tears, Angie stared at the scuffed tile floor.

"Look," Peter added softly, "I know we've had our differences, but I'm not about to throw you to the wolves. The last thing I need is for you to be served up as a sacrificial offering to smooth the ruffled feathers of the medical community. In their eyes, only a physician is allowed to play God. As senior representatives of the LIFE-STAR organization, Howard and I are going with you to that review hearing and we're both willing to testify in your defense, that is, if you want us to."

With tears blurring her vision, Angie did something she never thought she'd ever want to do. She reached out and gave her grumpy old bear of an employer a great big hug.

Peter had been dead-on in his predictions. The medical hierarchy had, indeed, wanted Angie's head served on a platter. It was only Peter's and Howard's indisputable reputations as no-nonsense medical administrators that ultimately won her a stay of execution. Grateful to have escaped the harrowing inquisition with her nursing license intact, Angie accepted her punishment with head held high: two weeks suspension from work without pay, six months probation, mandatory retesting of her medication knowledge and prohibited from administering narcotics of any kind without direct medical supervision for a period of one year.

While the determined RN fought hard to put both the nightmarish accident and its legal repercussions behind her, every time she heard the mournful cry of a train whistle, the memories would come flooding back... of a rain-soaked stretch of highway... a cattleliner tipped on its side... and a man who knew he was about to die, and who bravely made one last request.

25
BACK IN THE SADDLE AGAIN

September was a busy month for LIFE-STAR 1. The program was averaging two calls a shift, and each time the cellular phone rang, Angie's heart skipped a beat. Would it be an acute MI patient in cardiogenic shock, a suicidal drug overdose, the fire department asking for an air search of the Bow River for a possible drowning victim, the city police requesting the helicopter's three million candlepower spotlight to help track down a murder suspect, or the usual, another grisly multi-vehicle accident.

Head-on collisions, T-bones, rollovers. More than once, Angie had arrived on-scene only to find her prospective patient in full cardiac arrest and the ground medics frantically working to restore a pulse. Trauma arrest victims rarely survived. It was a documented fact. Knowing that grim statistic, however, did not make it any easier when she had to stare at an empty stretcher on the sombre flight back to base.

In addition to the regular trauma and medical fare, Parkland Memorial also depended upon LIFE-STAR to transport its Pediatric and Neonatal ICU teams. While the PICU team dealt mostly with infants and young children, the NICU team was called upon whenever a critically-ill newborn was delivered at one of the far-flung rural centers. Arriving months too soon, the neonates, some weighing as little as a pound and a half, were often born with severely underdeveloped lungs. More than once, members of the transport team found their way to a country hospital's nursery simply by zeroing in on the desperate sounds of a struggling baby's grunting cries echoing down the hall.

Angie liked baby flights. The paperwork was minimal, the tiny infants were fascinating, and the only real labor involved was loading the team's cumbersome isolette into the back of the helicopter. Three hundred pounds. Lifted three and a half back-breaking feet. Straight up!

It required at least three strong people and had to be done ever-so-gently so as not to disturb the fragile newborn clinging to life inside. It was enough to rupture a disc.

As the NICU team usually consisted of two women, the pilots, even through they were not supposed to, would often help lift. Because the helicopter's departure always drew a crowd of curious onlookers, however, the pilots usually had little trouble persuading a husky spectator or two to lend a hand. It was a male thing. For some reason, the fly-boys just could not stand idly by while their all-female medical crew struggled to lift the incubator off the ground.

To Angie's way of thinking, it didn't hurt to play the weak, helpless female once in a while.

One rainy October evening, Peter called his group together for an update on the Olympic game plan. With in-depth security checks, ID pictures, orientation lectures and clothing fittings to be completed within the next two months, Peter announced that McMahon Stadium's Volunteer Centre would become a second home to his loyal employees for the next little while.

Happily munching on hot buttered popcorn which a gracious Howard tastefully dispensed in disposable barf bags, Peter's team then sat back to watch the highlight of the meeting: the infamous videotape of Canadian National Team downhill skier Todd Brooker's horrific crash in Kitzbuhel, Austria.

It had occurred several years before, but was still considered among the worst non-fatality skiing accidents ever captured on tape. Peter was using the video to demonstrate how Brooker had been quickly airlifted off the mountain using a Bauman bag and a sling. Because Angie and Howie were the only ones present who could personally relate to this form of rapid transport, Angie hoped Lawson would not call upon her to describe how it felt to be dragged behind a 'copter screaming through the air. Good God, riding a Brahma bull at the Calgary Stampede would be less frightening!

Poor Todd meanwhile, was shown carving a real nice, clean fall line at

60 miles an hour when suddenly, he caught an edge. His skis exploded in different directions as he pancaked the rock-hard course. Mercifully knocked unconscious, his body, bending in places no human being had ever bent before, began to tumble wildly, end over end, down the nearly vertical slope.

A totally relaxed body can absorb a tremendous amount of punishment. Just ask any drunk driver who has ever staggered away from a car crash, while his stone-sober victims were being airlifted to the nearest organ donor facility. It was this fact which probably saved Todd's life.

His flaccid body continued to windmill down the mountainside for another five or six horrifying seconds before finally slamming, head-first, into a wooden snow fence.

No one touched their popcorn as Peter replayed the ghastly video. Several of the nurses, Angie included, ended up closing their eyes so they wouldn't have to view the awful spectacle. Even some of the paramedics, Kyle and Russ included, averted their eyes.

Sensing he was losing his audience, Peter decided it was time to spring his surprise. "I'm extremely proud of the way you people have jelled together as a team in the last few months. Everyone in this room has worked hard to make this program a success. As our schedules will grow more cluttered as we move closer to the Games in February, I can't think of a better time to begin the venue tours than right now. I've posted a sign-up sheet in my office, so please check off which ones you can attend. These tours are free, and your significant others are welcome to come along."

Peter looked around the room. Yes, by golly, he had their attention now. Several were even picking at their popcorn again.

"In addition to the tours, Canada Olympic Park has kindly invited all LIFE-STAR personnel to visit the park this Friday evening. They'll have a ski jumping demonstration going on, and for all you weekend warriors, for a measly twenty bucks, you can try sliding down the track in either a bobsleigh or a luge. Sounds like a lot of fun!"

"A lot of fun!" Kyle grunted as he and Russ went to sign up. "I nearly killed myself the last time you and Angie dragged me out there. Jen was ready to divorce me. My body was so black and blue from that damn luging, she said I could have passed for a member of the Jamaican bobsled team."

Russ laughed, "Come on, Kyle, it wasn't that bad. Why don't you bring Jennifer along? We could strap her on a sled and send her down as her very own doubles team!"

Kyle's handsome face beamed. "Doubles is right! That pinballing experience would put her into premature labor for sure!"

"When's the big day again?" Angie asked.

"Just two more weeks!"

"Well, I guess we'll let you off the hook this time, but only if you name the baby after me. Angie if it's a girl and Jackson if it's a boy."

"And Rusty," Kyle added, "if we're not quite sure!"

They were still laughing when Dale sauntered over to add his name to the venue tour list. "This sports night sounds kind of interesting," the Aussie grinned. "I've always wanted to ride in a bobsleigh. But tell me, what the heck is a luge?"

26

LIFE IN THE FAST LANE

By the time Dale put in an appearance, Angie and Russ had been cooling their heels in the Canada Olympic Park Sport Centre for half an hour.

"Sorry I'm late," the Aussie explained, "but it was my night to register at the Volunteer Centre. Had to fill out a bunch of forms and get my ID picture taken. Then I had to be measured for my clothing package. You should've seen the lineup. Must've been two hundred people ahead of me!"

Giving his name to the desk clerk, Dale was handed a lengthy insurance/injury waver to complete. Pausing to read over the form, the cocky pilot never got past the first paragraph. "Ah, excuse me people, but what's this part about not suing for damages if I die or suffer dismemberment during my luge run? What kind of sport is this?"

"A suicidal one if you ask me!" Russ spouted.

The furrows creasing Dale's brow abruptly deepened. "Don't listen to him," Angie retorted, shooting Russ a steely glare. "Rusty's just trying to rattle your chain. Luge is a safe sport. You must've got a... uh, no, you probably never got a sled for Christmas when you were a kid, did you? Come to think of it, does it even snow where you come from?"

"It used to!" Dale replied. "Why I can remember my grand-dad telling us kids they had to close the schools in Melbourne once because of blizzard conditions!"

"And, like, when the heck was that?" Russ yipped.

"I think it was during the Mesozoic era... lost a whole pile of Sheepasaurus that winter!"

As they walked toward the loading dock, Dale kept gazing at the immense structure they were about to tackle. Built at a cost of fifty million dollars, the combination bobsleigh and luge run was considered to be one of the finest ever built. Listed among the fastest tracks in the world, its 14 magnificent curves glowed with an eerie incandescence... their massive, steeply-banked walls of ice rising up like ghostly sentinels on the treeless hillside.

"Where's Stevens?" Dale asked. "I thought he was coming out, too."

"He and the Mrs. are over at the ski jump," Angie replied. "They're just killing some time until the bobsleigh rides start."

Returning from his car with a bulging equipment bag slung over his shoulder, Russ joined Angie and Dale and ten other rookie sliders for the short truck ride up to the Tourist's Start.

Once inside the small, heated Start House, Angie immediately opened the bag: three helmets, three dark blue speed suits, several oddly-shaped foam pads, an old cotton tea towel, bottle of shampoo, a fat roll of silver duct tape and three clear plastic bubble face shields carefully wrapped in pillowcases were soon sorted into neat piles on the floor.

First, she and Russ helped Dale on with his ankle and elbow pads. Once they were duct taped into position, Russ handed the pilot one of the speed suits to try on. Even with the medic helping, it was a struggle to force Dale's lanky frame into the airtight suit. With the space-age fabric clinging to him like a second skin, Angie instructed him to breathe out as she yanked the two sides of the back zipper together.

"It's too bloody small!" the pilot wheezed.

"No it's not!" Angie fired back. "It has to fit tight if you want to go fast." Upon finally getting him zipped up, the RN then poured a dab of shampoo onto one of the face visors and showed her ungrateful student how to buff it with the cotton cloth.

"Why the shampoo?" he asked.

"Keeps the plastic from fogging up when you're breathing on it."

Angie seemed to know exactly what she was doing and it made Dale wonder—either she was one heck of an actress, which he already knew was not true, or Angie and the bizarre sport of luge were not total strangers.

Her left ankle heavily taped and padded, a seemingly antsy Angie slipped her jacket over her speed suit and escaped outside to watch as the last member of the Italian luge team shot past the Tourist Start. A streak of pale blue, with his skateboard-shaped sled hidden beneath his powerful upper body, it looked as if he were magically floating on a cushion of air. Gliding from curve to curve with a minimum of runner chatter, the world class athlete held a near perfect line as he plunged feet-first down into the labyrinth. Vanishing from sight, the Italian reappeared seconds later, spat out like a giant watermelon seed as the finish curve's 4 G centrifugal force hurled him down the track toward the final timing light.

Fully suited up, Dale went outside and found Angie kneeling beside one of the sleds. Nothing more than two slender wooden runners connected with steel bridges, it looked like it could fall apart at any second. "So this is an Olympic luge?" the Aussie exclaimed. "I have a floor mat in my car bigger than that!"

"This is just a training sled. It's not meant for racing," Angie explained. "Trust me, it might not look like much, but this little beauty can get the job done."

"Only if the job is to do me in!" Dale winced. "Where the heck are the handles to hang on to... and where are the brakes on this bloody contraption?"

Angie exhaled audibly. "Just slip your hands under your butt and sit on them. That way, you won't bang them on the walls. As far as braking is concerned, real lugers don't need them. We drive till we die!"

"WE DRIVE TILL WE DIE? Uh, tell me something, Miss Jackson. You seem to be the only person out here tonight who's not scared spitless. Why is that?"

Angie continued to examine the little sled. "I used to slide. Long time ago. Even made the provincial team, but I got too old. Couldn't get enough time off to train so I... uh, had to give it up."

She was lying. Feeling Dale's questioning eyes upon her, she abruptly turned her attention to a second sled leaning against the track railing. Tugging fitfully at the crotch of his speed suit, Russ chose that exact moment to join them. "What about him?" Dale asked.

"I got the boys out sliding a couple of times last year," Angie replied. "Rusty, well... he wasn't too bad."

"What do you mean... 'wasn't too bad?'" the medic shot back. "Heck, everybody told me I had awesome form!"

"Let's just say you showed a lot of potential," Angie giggled, fighting off her boyfriend's attempt to shove a fistful of ice shavings down her back. "As for your buddy, Kyle, now that was a show and a half! You know what that guy's biggest problem was? He didn't trust himself. He'd be cruising along just fine in the straightaway, then every time he felt his sled start climbing a wall, he'd plop those size twelves of his down on the ice."

Catching a spooked expression floating across Dale's face, Angie back-peddled. "It's like this, Morgan. Once you put your feet down, you are no longer in control of the sled... it is in control of you. In Kyle's case, as soon as he put his feet down, the sled started to skid sideways. That scared the heck out of him so he tried to sit up. That was mistake number two, because once you sit up, it's all over but the ambulance ride."

"Just lie flat," Russ calmly reassured, "look at the sky, the sled knows the way down. If you race from Ladies' or Men's Start, then you have to do some actual driving, but not from here at the Tourist Start. Just pretend you're lying on the couch at home and watching TV through your toes."

"How come you're supposed to put your head back and look at the sky?" Dale asked. "Aerodynamics?"

Before his nemesis could answer, a rookie slider out enjoying a last minute smoke, spoke up. "It always helps to look God straight in the eye when you're praying to Him to keep you alive!"

"TWO MINUTE WARNING TO THE TOURIST START," the PA suddenly announced. "RUSS ANDREWS TO THE TOURIST START POSITION."

Angie held the sled steady while he positioned his muscular behind on it. Russ then stretched out on his back and placed his legs gently against the sled's runners. Extending his neck until his helmet touched the ice, the medic slowly brought it back up until he could just see over his chest. With a slight bend at the knee and his toes pointed forward, he looked up at Angie for her approval.

His form was textbook perfect and Angie smiled as she flashed him the "thumbs-up." She particularly liked the way he filled out his speed suit. His rock-hard physique was very easy on the eyes. And to think she got to take him home afterwards.

Russ had been just as nervous as Dale before his first run. But as he had later confided to Angie, once he'd made it safely to the bottom, he was hooked. Luge was such an incredible rush. He liked the speed, he liked the challenge and he particularly like the fact that once you started your run, you were committed to finishing it. If you got into trouble and started losing control, there was none of this "stopping to analyze your mistake" crap. You just had to bite the bullet and try to drive your way out as best you could. It was, he decided, a lot like riding a bar of soap.

Angie smacked her lips in lustful delight. "You never looked better. You've been practicing your position, haven't you?"

"Nope, I just had a good teacher that's all," the medic replied with a cheeky grin, "and I always remember what you taught me: that lugers love to do it on their backs at eighty miles an hour!"

As all the male sliders within earshot turned to see who Russ was referring to, the overhead PA mercifully interrupted.

"THE TRACK IS CLEAR FOR RUSS ANDREWS FROM TOURIST START."

"Honey, are you sure you've mentally prepared yourself for this run?" Angie fretted.

"I'm mentally and physically prepared at all times. Now about tonight...."

Angie pulled the visor down over his face. "Andrews, you remind me of a pheasant during mating season. You know, when the males are driven so crazy with lust that they just plain forget to look both ways before they cross the road and end up a mess of tail feathers and legs poking out of a car radiator? You won't be able to do anything later tonight if you break your leg, so please get your brain back on sliding... okay?"

Rusty lifted his visor. "You'd be amazed at what I can do with a leg cast on." With that, he slid his visor down and pulled off.

"LUGE IN TRACK... DALE MORGAN TO THE TOURIST START POSITION."

Forty-seven seconds later, the PA clicked back on: "THE TRACK IS CLEAR FOR DALE MORGAN FROM TOURIST START."

"Okay, Dale. That means Rusty made it down without crashing. Now it's your turn. Are you ready?" Angie asked.

The Aussie gave a feeble nod.

Watching as he disappeared down the track, Angie's heart started to thump.

"LUGE IN TRACK... A.Y. JACKSON TO THE TOURIST START POSITION."

A tidal wave of feelings surged through her. It was just like the old days as a promising provincial racer... back when the track announcers would call her by her initials because they thought it sounded classy. But just as the good memories came rushing back, so did the bad ones.

With a heart pounding so violently it seemed her chest shuddered with each beat, Angie positioned herself on the sled, took a deep cleansing breath and closed her eyes. Allowing her body to totally relax as she slowly counted to ten, Angie drifted into a trance-like state.

The slider on deck watched in fascination as she'd tighten a calf muscle or push down slightly with a shoulder or tilt her head one way or the other. Just by watching her, he was able to tell what curve she was mentally driving through.

In many ways, a luger needed all the skills of a jet fighter pilot—top physical conditioning with laser-crisp reflexes to handle the crushing G forces, split-second decision making and probably most important: an unquenchable thirst for speed. It was not a sport for risk-takers or linebacker types. A momentary loss of concentration was all it took to reduce a careless slider to a plasticized sack of splintered bones.

High above the track in the timing tower, the PA announcer turned to his assistant. "I was in Placid when she crashed. Helped load her into the ambulance. For a while there, people were saying she might never walk again!"

"Yeah," his assistant yawned, "but that kind of thing happens to every slider eventually. The good ones bounce back from a crash. She never did. Lost her nerve. But in this crazy sport, I don't guess that's such a great sin."

"A FORMER CANADIAN CHAMPION, THE TRACK IS CLEAR FOR A.Y. JACKSON."

Angie gulped down several deep breaths; blowing each out forcefully. So focused on what lay ahead she had not picked up on the announcer's glowing acknowledgment. All she'd heard was the important part... "THE TRACK IS CLEAR...."

Pulling the visor down over her face, the sweet smell of shampoo instantly jogged another memory—of a visor exploding as it smashed against the ice. Fighting to remain focused, she stretched forward to grasp the metal start handles. Her heart pounded in her ears.

To spectators watching as she gracefully slipped from one curve to another, Angie looked for all the world like she was asleep. Gliding with an effortless, fluid motion, it was as if she and the sled were of one body, one spirit, one soul. A picture perfect run, to the slider involved, however, it was just another futile attempt to relive the past.

Coasting to a stop at the finish dock, Angie picked up her sled and hustled over to where Russ and Dale were waiting for the truck. "Well boys, how'd it go?"

"The ice is so slow tonight," Russ groaned. "I thought I was going to stop in curve thirteen."

Not to be outdone, Dale let out a heavy sigh. "I thought this was supposed to be a thrilling, chilling, death-defying sport. Good heavens, woman, the escalator at Eaton's is faster than that!"

Angie's sweet smile instantly switched to a smirk. "Well, we'd better haul that skinny butt of yours up to the Junior Start then. We let the twelve year-olds race from there. I can arrange it if you think you're man enough to give it a go?"

Pompously gathering up his sled, Dale marched to the truck. "If this is all there is to this wussy-assed sport, I just might have to let my name stand as a member of the Australian Olympic Luge Team!"

Knowing his cargo of Italians were at the top of the training order, the driver slammed the truck into gear as he high-tailed it up the hill toward the Ladies Start. As the panel truck swayed precariously from one hairpin curve to the next, it was all Angie could do to hold onto her awkwardly-shaped sled and keep her rear end in contact with the narrow wooden bench. Hunched slightly forward, her eyes closed, she had just begun the process of mentally dissecting her run when she felt a toasty pair of lips nuzzle the nape of her neck.

Swinging around, she was about to elbow the juiced-up Romeo a good one when the suave Italian popped his visor up. Even in the shadows, she recognized the dreamy, heavy-lidded eyes.

"Surprise!" he hollered over the truck's rumble. Squealing with pure delight, Angie gave the kissing bandit a one-armed squeeze which he returned as only an Italian male could.

Klaus Stockner was a dear friend from her competition days. A former world champion, Herr Stockner had won the European Championship more times than either he or his wife could remember. Two Olympic gold medals had dangled from his neck. Without a doubt, Klaus was the Wayne Gretzky of the luge world. Now nearing the end of a spectacular career, Calgary's Winter Games would be his final competition. After excitedly introducing the living legend to Russ and Dale, Angie fell to chattering with her old friend, eager to catch up on all the latest World Cup gossip.

Their conversation lasted nine seconds. Traveling way too fast, the truck driver brainlessly hammered on the brakes to make the sharp turnoff to Ladies' Start. The lurching deceleration hurled everyone to the floor in a tangled heap of sleds and cursing sliders. Unaware that his infuriated passengers were now desperately scrambling over one another to regain their seats, the witless teen poured on the power as he continued the steep climb up the hill.

Angie and her Italian stallion had been in the humanitarian act of helping others to their feet when the truck's sudden jerk forward knocked them flying. It was as if they'd been launched from a catapult—one second they were there, the next, they were sailing out the rear of the truck and into the night.

As horrified sliders screamed for the driver to stop, Dale and Russ stared into the blackness. "Dear Jesus, she's probably dead and she had to take one of Italy's national treasures with her!" Russ wailed. "For crying out loud, can't somebody stop this damn truck?"

Unable to wait any longer, the paramedic leaped to the ground and sprinted off down the road, with Dale right on his heels. Running blindly along the dark strip of asphalt, the nearly hysterical medic tripped over something lying on the road. It was a sled. Hobbling painfully about on one leg, cussing that he'd broken his frigging foot, Russ nearly stepped on a motionless human form lying in the dirt by the side of the road.

It was Angie.

Flat on her back with her glazed eyes wide open, she seemed to be staring up at the Big Dipper. "Angie... Honey... are you okay? It's Russ. Speak to me, babe?" Even with her medically-trained boyfriend jabbering non-stop to rouse her, Angie only came around after an agonizing minute had dragged past.

"Did you see it?"

"See what?" Russ repeated as he completed his primary paramedical survey. Satisfied that the important parts of her anatomy were still intact and functioning, he carefully sat her up to cradle her in his arms.

"My time. Did you see my run... how was my form?"

"You weren't making a run, Honey. You fell out of the truck. Don't you remember?" Her unblinking eyeballs wavering about, Angie struggled to focus on the pair of identical faces swimming before her.

Dale meanwhile, had located Stockner twenty feet further down the road, hunched over the mangled remains of his best racing sled. Swearing wildly in German, English and Italian, he was holding his sled's broken runners in his trembling hands. Even with Dale's limited knowledge of luge sleds, it was obvious that, had Klaus' sled been a horse, they would have had to shoot it.

Considering how fast the truck had been moving when they had fallen out, it was a miracle neither Angie nor Klaus were killed. They would be sore for a few days, but their helmets had spared them a possibly catastrophic head injury.

As the driver backed up his truck, the rest of the sliders piled out to help load Angie and the sleds into the back. Stockner staggered directly toward the truck driver. Forced to grab hold of the door's side mirror to keep himself upright as he windmilled his other arm about, Klaus cursed the driver in every language he knew.

By the time the truck finally arrived at Ladies' Start, it was an incensed Italian team that shouldered their heavy sleds. With a sense of balance only a certain tower in Pisa could be proud of, a stubborn Klaus Stockner refused assistance as he crawled from step to step, dragging his battered sled behind him.

Angie's double vision had been replaced by a pounding headache, but she, too, was determined to wobble off the truck under her own power. She was trying to make sense of the conversation she'd overheard while riding up to the start. Her limited understanding of German was just enough to ascertain that Klaus was also suffering from an aching head and that his teammates didn't think he should make any more runs.

Upon relaying this bit of covert spying to her boyfriend, Angie found him in complete agreement. In Russ' expert opinion, there was no doubt that the legendary luger was suffering from a mild concussion. Sliding in his present condition would be suicidal.

Reaching out to take Klaus' muscular arm as he paused on the steps, Angie suggested that maybe they should both hang their sleds up for the evening.

"Nein fraulein, Ich... I'm... do dopples run... uh now." Weaving slightly as if fighting a strong wind, the great Italian continued, "Das ist... mein team's... now time to practice here... auf Calgary's rodel bahn before Olympics. Manfred's dopples partner ist kranken... ist sick... kann no practice. Manfred be weltmeister many times, but like win one more race for Italia, Olympic gold!"

Setting his sled down on the deck, the Italian thrust out his thickly furred chest. "Angela, bitte. I do one more run. I be okay."

"You can't make another run tonight, Klaus! Look at you. You can barely stand up, for heaven's sake!"

Klaus held the door for her as they entered the start house, then collapsed onto the nearest bench. He sat there for a few seconds, jumped to his feet and bolted for the washroom. Like most people with a fresh concussion, he had to throw up.

Klaus' teammate, Manfred Burghart paced about the room like a caged polar bear. Angie felt sorry for the guy. This would be the Italians' last trip to Calgary prior to the Games. Every training run was vital when a slider was preparing for a race and this was not just any old race... this one was for all the Olympic marbles.

As Klaus staggered from the washroom and plopped down beside her, Angie was struck by an absolutely brilliant idea. "Klaus, what if Manfred found himself another partner? From what I've heard from other doubles teams, the back man doesn't have to do very much of anything except lie real still. What do you think?"

Klaus looked over at his partner. They exchanged heated German, then Klaus came back with an answer. "Manfred say ja... but who slide mit him? Nein sliders hier... all gone to hotel."

"Nein... nein Klaus!" she said, pointing toward herself. "Ich know someone!"

A tender smile crept across Klaus' classically-sculptured features. "I know you like to help Manfred but your head ist, how you say... nicht good? Ist damaged, too, ja."

Russ and Dale cracked up.

"Not me, Klaus! Nein me!" Angie waved her finger at Dale. "Das guy can do it!"

Captain Morgan's pupils dilated to "brain dead" proportions.

After much German discussion, Klaus replied, "Okay, Manfred say ja. But ist das man a gutte slider?"

"Dale very gutte slider... he like go fast... schnell!"

As Klaus began peeling off his training suit and Manfred went outside to prepare the sled, Russ and Dale hauled Angie into the men's washroom and closed the door. "Are you nuts?" they screeched in unison.

"Why did you say Morgan could do it?" Russ grilled her. "Good God, woman, he's been on a sled once in his entire frigging life! If you think it's that easy, why not send me?"

"Because Dale's a pilot and pilots are supposed to have excellent reflexes, that's why! He's also about the same size as Klaus so he'll fit the sled better. Your shoulders would be dragging on the ice. I truly hate to say this, Hon, but of all the guys I've ever slid with, you have the reflexes of a three-legged porcupine with arthritis. Look, I feel responsible, okay?

None of this would've happened if I'd... if I'd just stayed home."

Angie abruptly turned to stare the apprehensive Aussie straight in the eye. "Dale, trust me on this. Manfred is one of the best sliders in the world. You told me you wanted to go faster, right? Well, just think of this as your contribution to helping an athlete prepare for the Winter Olympics. I'd kill to have this chance!

"I've slid this track as a back man at least a dozen times, so I know what I'm talking about, okay? All you have to do is lie very still and let Manfred do all the driving. Just go along for the ride and have some fun. It'll be something to tell your grandkids!"

Stockner, clad only in his lycra underwear, braved the brisk night air to confer with his partner again. They had a problem. Their technologically secretive coach would never agree to a non-Italian partner swap. "Mein coach will think you ist me," Klaus grunted as he helped the pilot pull on the colors of the Italian national luge team.

"TWO MINUTE WARNING TO THE LADIES' START. BURGHART AND STOCKNER TO THE DOUBLES START POSITION."

Manfred carried his sled to the start ramp. Klaus, still deathly pale, knelt down to hold the sled in position as his partner ritualistically performed several last minute hops and stretches to align the weight vest and cup support he was wearing.

Thoroughly psyched, Burghart straddled the sled. Placing his butt on the raised front seat, he gingerly pulled two nylon straps up between his legs and across each groin. Fastened to a hook behind the seat, with the driver balancing on top of his back man, the straps were needed to hold the two men together.

Klaus directed Dale to take a seat directly behind Manfred. With the spooked Aussie's chest now pressed up tight against the Italian's broad back, Klaus wedged Dale's sneakers into the tiny space framed by Manfred's knees and the top of the sled's runner.

Manfred then abruptly leaned backward, flattening his slightly-built passenger under 180 pounds of solid muscle. Dale vanished from sight.

"Uh, Dale? You still alive down there?" Angie inquired, crouching beside the sled. "Don't worry. You're looking real good. Now pull your head up until your visor just touches the back of Manfred's helmet. Perfect!"

As she stepped off the platform, Angie silently mouthed a last bit of advice to her student: "Don't move!"

"THE TRACK IS CLEAR FOR BURGHART AND STOCKNER."

Angie gazed up solemnly at the moon. "Be gentle with him, Lord. That's a three hundred and fifty dollar, Italian-designed speed suit he's wearing!"

47.024 bone-rattling seconds later, Dale felt Manfred slowly rise into a sitting position. Cracking open an eyelid, the Aussie found himself sailing down the out-run toward the finish dock.

Riding the truck up again, Manfred grinned. "Herr Morgan, you do gutte, but you must... how you say it...." the big Italian labored to find just the right words. "It be like this. You need think of dopples sled as beautiful fraulein. You and fraulein move as one. You move... she move. You see... ja?"

Dale immediately relayed the advice to his coach. "So Manfred says a good run is like fabulous sex, eh?" Angie lamented. "Guess that explains why we Canadians can't seem to get the hang of this blasted sport!"

"I bought you a book, for crying out loud!" Russ interjected. "If you'd only try a few of the ideas from chapter four, you wouldn't have anything to complain about!"

Angie's reaction was immediate. Chasing her boyfriend's rippling derriere down the stairs to the landing, her high-pitched squeals contradicted her earlier statement.

Hearing her laughter abruptly stop, and knowing the reason was that Russ no doubt had her in full lip lock, the Aussie politely turned away to walk back inside the Start House. That's when he discovered Manfred wanted to make a second run.

Fifteen minutes later, the PA announced: "TWO MINUTE WARNING TO THE LADIES' START. BURGHART AND STOCKNER TO THE DOUBLES START POSITION!"

Dale and Manfred strapped themselves into the sled.

"THE TRACK IS CLEAR FOR BURGHART AND STOCKNER!"

Manfred launched the sled down the narrow start ramp. As Dale would later recount to his grandkids, their run was less that three seconds old when his right leg started cramping up. The reason? His foot had somehow slipped out of position on the runner. As a result, Dale's calf was being unmercifully squashed between Manfred's muscular leg and the slender fiberglass runner. With Angie's words still ringing in his ears, however, the Aussie gritted his teeth and didn't move.

Accelerating down the short straightaway toward curve seven, gravitational forces pulled the sled up onto the wall. With the steel edged runners chattering noisily against the ice, Dale became acutely aware that Manfred's body was growing heavier with each passing nanosecond. In addition, it was also becoming increasing difficult to hold his head up.

The pilot's sinewy calf muscle meanwhile, with the added force of gravity now crushing it against the runner, abruptly contracted into one horrific toe curling spasm. Unaware of the possible consequences, Dale instinctively flexed his toes back to stretch out the cramp. This pressed his heel down on the sled's runner, an action that sent the highly-responsive sled darting sharply to the left and straight up the wall.

Manfred reefed against the left runner with every ounce of strength he possessed, while simultaneously dropping his right heel onto the ice. The friction generated by his dragging bootie immediately caused the port yawing sled to pivot back to the right... effectively canceling out his back man's unexpected seizure activity... and returning the sled to its prior course.

Unable to relieve the cramp, Dale once again flexed his ankle back and forth. In doing so, however, this time his foot slipped completely off the runner.

All the while mentally cursing the woman who'd talked him into this mess, the Aussie frantically tried to cram his sneaker back into position. Manfred's main steering appendage, having lost its underlying support, however, had dropped down onto the runner and was now blocking the way. Unable to hold his runner aloft any longer, an exhausted Dale finally had to let it flop onto the ice.

With both sliders now trailing a foot, the sled responded by skidding sideways... past the curve's downward-sloping exit. As the Italian slammed his leg against the left runner in a valiant attempt to pull the sled's nose down, Dale labored to do his part by once again launching skyward with his aching right leg

Club sliders waiting at Junior Start watched in awe as the famed doubles team of Burghart and Stockner shot past them. They would later talk for weeks about how the always-experimental Italians had aced curve seven with two feet on the runners, one foot on the ice and one leg waving about in the air like a rabid tentacle.

Hopelessly out-of-control, the sled abruptly fell off the wall out of curve seven. Immediately drifting to the right, they entered curve eight way too early. A split second later, they were rocketing up the nearly vertical wall. They were now within an eyelash of the paint-scuffed deflector boards bolted to the top of the 30 foot high curve.

The deflector boards had only one purpose: to prevent hopelessly out-of-control sliders and bobbers from being flung out of the track and into Intensive Care.

Even though he was firmly belted in, Manfred could feel himself being hauled upward by the tremendous tug of centrifugal force. Lying out of sight beneath the Italian, a bug-eyed Dale could only watch as his partner's broad shoulders began to lift away from him.

Knowing they were headed for a face-plant of surgical proportions, the Italian abruptly switched feet, dropping his left bootie to the ice and pressing his other leg hard against the right runner.

On the very verge of seeing his life pass before him, a primitive survival instinct deep in Dale's brain suddenly took charge. Making one last desperate kick with his right leg, the pilot reached up to grab Manfred around the neck. Straining to haul the Italian's shoulders back toward him, he felt the sled's nose grudgingly begin to change direction.

With his back man's arm wrapped tightly around his throat and the Aussie's bony right leg spurring out an 80 point ride on his mid-section, it was only Manfred Wolfgang Burghart's world-class driving skills which kept them from spending the next month at Parkland Memorial.

If luge was, indeed, like making love, Dale had a heck of a lot to learn about partner satisfaction.

Miraculously escaping the bone splintering terrors of curve eight with all their flailing limbs intact, the remainder of their run was almost anticlimactic. It was only after they had drifted to a stop half-way down the out-run that Dale felt safe enough to relax his grip on the anoxic Italian.

While poor Manfred didn't appear to be hurt, his glazed, unblinking eyeballs clearly reflected his mental status. Staring into the night sky, his fists clutched the sled's metal handles as if they had been soldered into place.

At the other end of the emotional scale, Dale's reaction to their near visit with a mortician was one of total body collapse. His arms and legs spayed limply to either side of the sled, his head had fallen back until it too was resting on the rock hard ice.

Under the diffuse track lighting and against the white glare of the ice, the two sliders resembled a huge two-headed, eight-legged spider that had just been washed down the proverbial drainpipe and unfortunately, not lived to tell the tale.

The track announcer, having viewed the electrifying run on his monitor, had seen the Canadians make similar runs before, but never the masterful, never-make-a-mistake Italians. Not wanting to believe what he'd just witnessed, the announcer kept waiting for a signal that they were okay. Until then, he could not clear the track for the next slider. Staring at the motionless figures far below, the increasingly worried announcer had his binoculars out now... scanning for possible signs of life. Unable to detect any and unable to stand the ghastly suspense any longer, he finally keyed his mike. "82 IN THE OUT-RUN!"

All the time feverishly hoping the announcer had overreacted and that his services were not required, it was Kyle who scrambled over the track railing and hurried toward the downed sliders. Returning from the ski jump, the medic and his pregnant wife had been watching the action from the finish curve when they heard the secret luge lingo for "urgent medical assistance" paged overhead.

Kyle bent over the glassy-eyed Italian. After calling him by name and getting no response, he reached down to touch Manfred's chest. Mr. Burghart's reaction was not what you would call typical as he abruptly let loose with a curdling yelp.

As if realizing that yes, he was still alive, the seemingly demonically possessed slider leapt to his feet. Forgetting the fact he was still attached to the sled, however, he immediately let out another wail, this time several octaves higher in pitch. In order to undo the tight crotch straps that were now threatening to put an end to any future Burgharts, Kyle had to first get the unhinged Italian to sit back down on the sled again.

With Manfred finally out of the picture, Stevens had fully expected another Italian to emerge from under the first. The medic nearly wet himself when a stuporous Dale flipped up his visor.

"Morgan! What the heck are you doing down there?!" Pulling the rubbery-kneed Aussie to his feet, a thoroughly confused Kyle waved up at the tower.

"I'm sure glad these suits are water proof... " Dale babbled as he feebly attempted to help the paramedic carry the 55 pound sled back to the truck, "'cause I've just had the living crap scared...."

The PA system mercifully drowned him out. "THE SLIDERS ARE UP AND OKAY. CLEAR THE TRACK TO THE LADIES' START POSITION."

27
IS THERE LIFE AFTER LUGE?

"So Dale... like... tell us again what happened on that second run?" Russ laughed as the five friends plunked themselves down around a table at Ringo's, the local country and western hangout they'd fled to after their wild night of luge.

As the grinning Aussie retold his story for the umpteenth time, it was growing wilder with each telling and each beer he consumed.

Angie meanwhile, idly picking at the label on her wine cooler, seemed a million light years removed from the conversation.

"I hope I didn't ruin things between you and that hot-blooded Italian?" Dale asked.

Angie's detached persona instantly changed to a shy smile as she shook her head. "You think this was wild? Heavens, this was nothing compared to the time Manfred went down the Lake Placid luge course wearing only his helmet, his speed booties and a sock."

Jennifer was the only one who had to ask the obvious.

Mindful of Mrs. Stevens' delicate condition, Angie was forced to think long and hard before delivering her reply. "Well, it was like this, the only reason he was wearing the sock was to ward off frostbite and he wasn't exactly wearing it on his foot... if you know what I mean!"

Immediately blushing a deep shade of scarlet as everyone at the table hooted with laughter, the exasperated look on Jenny Stevens' face said it all.

Munching on pretzels as his buddy Kyle gleefully set about relating his bobsleigh run, Russ were just about to order another round when the four-man country band finally swaggered back on stage and launched into a snappy Two-Step. The medic reached for Angie's hand. "Come on, girl... they're playing our song."

Several couples were already out on the floor dancing the Texas Two-Step, or variations of it, but after a minute or so, all eyes were focused on only one couple... Russ and Angie.

With timing and coordination that bordered on perfection, Angie and Russ magically combined into a single entity as they put on a display of spins, intricate two-handed cross-overs and sparkling footwork. Totally in his element on the dance floor, Russ had moves that would have impressed John Travolta.

"Where on earth did you guys learn to move like that?" Jennifer exclaimed when they sat down.

Russ and Angie grinned. "Let's tell them," Angie begged. "They're going to find out, anyway."

Receiving a nod from her partner, Angie motioned everyone into a huddle. "You can't tell a soul, okay? But Rusty and I have been chosen to dance in the Olympics' Opening Ceremonies!"

"I just knew you two would find a way to get in for free!" Kyle snorted. "The eyes of the world will be upon us and how does Calgary respond? With the funky chicken Two-Step!"

"Funky chicken my ass!" Russ retorted. "I'll have you know we'll have three hundred stone-sober yahoos performing some of the finest bar room strutting you'll ever see in your entire life. It'll make you proud to be a Canadian. Make you want to rush out and buy a case of Labatts or a toque or some antifreeze or something!"

Around 11 p.m., Jennifer and Kyle called it a night. Kyle had to work in the morning and Jennifer, who had been quietly sipping ginger ale all evening, had developed a nagging back ache that just would not go away.

With the clean-living Mrs. Stevens now out of the picture, Russ set his beer glass down and gazed across the table at Dale. "Okay, first things first, Morgan. We've got to find you a woman. It can get pretty damn cold around here at night!"

The pilot casually leaned back in his chair as if to check out the bevy of buckle bunnies pressed up against the railing surrounding the dance floor. "What do I do after I've snared one?" he smiled.

"You ask her to dance, you fool!"

"I'm really not much of a dancer... especially compared to you two."

Angie pushed back her chair and walked around the table. "Step into my office, Big Boy, and I'll show you how it's done. Trust me, it's real easy!"

Morgan hesitated. "I've already heard that 'Trust Me!' speech once tonight." But it was Russ he was looking at.

The medic read his thoughts. "Hon, get him up there and try to teach him something. I've got to see a man about a horse." With that, he got to his feet and headed for the washroom.

As Angie dragged the Aussie out onto the floor, the band slowed it down a bit with a mournful ballad of love gone wrong, just perfect for teaching the Two-Step.

A quick learner, Dale picked up the fundamentals right away. Once Angie taught him the trademark "slow slow, quick quick" moves, and had whirled him through two practice dances, Captain Morgan was ready to strike out on his own.

As the evening wore on, and the more beer he drank, the better Dale seemed to dance. "I think we've created a monster," Angie whispered into her boyfriend's ear as they held each other close during a clutch and grope waltz. Hardly moving, the young couple just slowly turned in a circle.

Dale was leaning against the bar... no doubt telling one of his many stories to a mesmerized cluster of bright-eyed vixens gathered around him.

"I wonder if he'll get lucky tonight?" Angie pondered aloud. Knowing the answer would likely be yes, she suddenly felt a tinge of sadness.

"I hope he's not the only one!" Russ interrupted her train of thought by tenderly nuzzling her neck.

"I know how this is going to sound," the woman of his dreams replied, "but I've had a pounding headache ever since I fell out of the truck tonight."

Russ just shook his head and smiled like he always did when he looked down and saw her happily nestled in his arms. "I know the perfect prescription for that, young lady," he purred. "Bedrest. Lots and lots of bedrest!"

28

RACING AGAINST THE DEVIL

The LIFE-STAR program had always welcomed medically-trained personnel from outlying EMS services to ride along on flights so they could witness the benefits of the organization first hand. Having gotten wind of this, a local Youth Court judge telephoned Peter Lawson one overcast autumn morning with a special request.

A juvenile convicted of "Refusal to Take a Breathalyzer" was to come before the judge for sentencing. A cocky little brat, seventeen year-old Ryne Sommerville's latest brush with the law had involved a high-speed crash in which an elderly couple had barely escaped with their lives.

The CEO and majority shareholder of a local drilling company, his father had spared no expense to retain the finest legal minds for his son's defense. With a dangerous driving charge staring his young client in the face, Ryne's high-priced attorney gave the performance of his career as he convinced the jury that his client had been momentarily blinded by the setting sun and thus not seen the car ahead of him stop for a red light.

As brilliant as the defense was, it was not enough to beat the Breathalyzer Refusal rap, however. Feeling the need to extract some measure of justice as he was about to pass sentence, the judge began his summation by re-reading the on-scene paramedic's testimony: "Upon my initial assessment, it was noted that Mr. Sommerville's breath smelled of alcohol. As well, several empty beer cans were found scattered in and around the patient's vehicle."

Scowling down at the smug-faced teen standing before him, Judge Muzeric hoped to observe some show of remorse. Instead, he saw only vile contempt in the boy's cold-blooded glare.

"When people refuse the breathalyzer, they are, in an indirect sense, admitting to their guilt. Mr. Sommerville, as you stated that you were unable to remember any details of the accident, I feel it would be in your best interest to experience first-hand the senseless tragedy of an accident caused by alcohol. Therefore, you are to report to the LIFE-STAR hangar every morning starting tomorrow until you have ridden along on five motor vehicle accident calls. If anything is to change your cavalier attitude toward drinking and driving, perhaps having to stare into the face of a dead or dying fellow party animal will do the trick!"

At 8 a.m. the next day, Ryne had a friend drop him off at the hangar. Acknowledging his buddy's tire-squealing departure with a middle-fingered salute, the smirking teen dutifully reported in for his shift. Ten minutes later, he was stretched out on the couch in the TV room, lazily flipping from channel to channel.

Sitting next door in the nurse's room as she helped Kyle input mission statistics into Howard's second-hand computer, Angie overheard Ryne talking to someone on the phone.

"What a joke. All I've done so far this morning is watch TV! I sure hope I get the same asshole judge next time around 'cause this ambulance duty shit is a God damn breeze!"

Ryne's brooding dark eyes and chiseled features were of GQ calibre, but Angie could feel the foul-mouthed little creep mentally undress her when she walked into the TV room to get a coffee. Trying to appear nonchalant as she leaned against the corner waiting for the kettle to boil, she began to understand how a sexual assault victim must feel.

Even though it was the weekend, Peter Lawson stopped by at noon to drop off another shipment of the latest in LIFE-STAR apparel. Business was booming with ER departments, rural EMS services and benefit organizations from across southern Alberta placing orders for the trendy scrubs, T-shirts and baseball caps.

Just off the phone from speaking with Jennifer, Kyle was attempting to rescue his over-nuked pizza from the microwave when the workaholic administrator wandered in to fetch a coffee refill. "Mr. Stevens," Peter asked, "how's that baby watch of yours going?"

The medic groaned, "Oh, just wonderful, sir. Jennifer cleaned our entire house last night. I was flaked out on the sofa from doing the supper dishes and she was still buzzing around... cleaning the closets, mopping the kitchen floor, disinfecting the bathroom, vacuuming the living room and all the bedrooms. When she ran out of carpet, it was all I could do to keep her from vacuuming our driveway!"

Lawson smiled. "That's a real good sign. Should be anytime now."

"That's what everyone keeps telling me, but she's been like this for an entire flipping week now. It's driving me nuts. I can't sleep... I can't eat...."

"My foot, Stevens! You're the only man I know who's actually gotten freezer burn from having his head in the refrigerator so much!" Angie interrupted as she, Dale and co-pilot Alex Davis strolled into the room.

"Good Lord... Stevens! Jackson! Morgan! Don't tell me Bateman still lets you people work together?" Lawson sputtered as the foursome descended upon the Hawaiian with extra cheese. "I'm going to have a talk with that boy."

"Howie says we're good for business," Angie laughed.

Ryne's lanky frame materialized in the doorway. Shaking his head when Alex offered him a piece, the teen sneered, "Keep it. I got a date lined up for later tonight. My baby knows what I'm hungry for."

A scant four minutes later, LIFE-STAR 1 was being towed from the hangar and readied for emergency launch. Lunch would have to wait.

Robbie Bretton, a teenager from Okotoks, a small town south of Calgary, had been chauffeuring two of his buddies into the city to help him look for a new stereo system. It was to be a fateful outing that would alter all of their lives.

Traveling way too fast in his sister's never-to-be borrowed sports car, a friend in the back seat accidentally burned Robbie's neck while passing him a marijuana joint. Losing control of the vehicle as he instinctively jerked his head away, Robbie suddenly felt the car skidding sideways toward the divided highway's center median. Its speedometer frozen forever at 130 kilometers per hour, the Sunbird gouged a deep rut through the grass, rebounded up into the oncoming lane and into the path of a pickup truck.

Harris Smitke was returning from Calgary with a load of bricks for a long-anticipated fireplace. Swerving wildly, Harris missed the car, but not without catastrophically shifting his ponderous load. Clinging desperately to the steering wheel to brace himself as his truck started to roll, the farmer later told paramedics the last thing he saw through his open window was a black blur of asphalt rushing up to greet him.

By some miracle, the dazed farmer awoke to find himself still alive; shaken but unscathed. The same could not be said for the car filled with teenagers. After dropping down into the far ditch, the baby blue sports car had flipped violently end-over-end before coming to rest upside down.

On the flight out, Kyle went over the situation very carefully with their resident juvenile delinquent. Ryne was informed that he would be a "gopher" on this trip; that is, if extra medical supplies were needed from the helicopter, it would be Ryne's job to go fetch them. Dale, piloting the return leg of the mission, would remain in the chopper and be available to help locate supplies.

As the medic was finishing his lecture with a warning about tail rotor safety, Ryne rolled his eyes ever-so-slightly and turned away to stare out the window. "Look, Smart Ass!" Stevens shouted as he jerked the kid around to face him. "You can walk into that rotor if you want to, but you're going to make one hell of a mess when you do and I'll be the one who'll have to mop you up! Have you got that, Sommerville?"

Angie meanwhile, was on the radio. "Calgary EMS, this is LIFE-STAR One. How do you read, over?"

"LIFE-STAR, this is High River EMS scene commander. I copy you loud and clear, over." To Angie's ears, the ground medic had a very familiar, very sexy sounding voice.

"High River EMS, our ETA to your location is approximately five minutes. Has a landing area been set up and secured, over?"

Angie's radio chatter was crisp, professional. The dazed look on her face, however, was in dramatic contrast. What the heck was Rusty doing down there—her Rusty—amidst wrecked cars, splattered blood and leaking fuel? He was supposed to be working a relief shift in the quiet burb of High River; soaking up the rays and polishing his ambulance. Chewing her lip, the RN listened intently for his reply.

"LIFE-STAR One, this is High River EMS, that is affirmative. You can tell Dale or whoever is on the stick to set that big beautiful bird down on the highway just south of the accident. The RCMP have secured the area. Over." Russ sounded as composed and unruffled as ever.

"High River, can you give us a patient update? Over."

"We have one green and one yellow ready for ground transport and a red still to be extricated. A fourth patient was Code 32 on-scene prior to our arrival. Not to worry though, I'm being good and I'm being careful. This is High River EMS... clear."

Kyle grinned at his partner. "Ange, it's okay. Jennifer says she feels the same way whenever she calls the hangar and finds out I'm on a scene call. What is it about you females? Don't you think your men can look after themselves?" Angie smiled like a robot and nodded, all the time searching out her window.

With traffic in the southbound lanes backed up for nearly three miles, the LIFE-STAR pilots had little difficulty finding the scene. Alex did the usual circuit of the area checking for wires and other rotor hazards before gently settling his multi-million dollar ambulance onto the hot pavement.

Fighting to stay focused as one of the ground medics hurried over to give them report, Angie found herself scanning the immediate area for any sign of her wayward boyfriend. There was none.

"Calgary EMS just left with the green and yellow patients!" the EMT breathlessly rattled off. "We're currently trying to extricate a red patient still trapped in the car. He's the one we want you guys to take. We also have a Code 32 on-scene who can't be moved until the Medical Examiner arrives."

A Code 32 meant that a patient had been found dead at the scene. The young man in question, had paid the ultimate price for his friend's momentary carelessness. A budding hockey star with a major junior team, unbelted Jason Westfall had been hurled face-first through the car's windshield as it rolled. With his lower torso now crushed beneath the 2000 pound vehicle, the tremendous weight had compressed his abdominal contents up into the chest and neck area, bulging the teen's lifeless eyes almost out of their sockets. The once boyishly handsome face was now so grossly distorted by the unrelenting pressure that it seemed about to burst. After going through the needless preliminaries of checking for a pulse, the police had covered the corpse with a waterproof tarpaulin.

Hockey scouts had expected Jason to go high in the NHL entry draft next spring. Apparently this time round, God had the number one draft pick.

Angie and Kyle started their search for Russ in the one place they were sure he would be. Leaving their stretcher on the roadside as they hopped down into the ditch, they both exhaled with relief when they saw a familiar figure worming his way out through the car's crumpled passenger door as firefighters descended upon the vehicle with their extrication equipment.

"Brad and I were tooling back to High River after dropping a sick little tyke off at the Mountainview when we came across this mess. I think it'll be a race between us, the organ donor program and the Medical Examiner as to who gets first dibs on this kid!"

Wedged behind the wheel of the inverted car, Robbie Bretton had only one thing going for him—he was still able to breathe on his own. His swollen face had obviously collided with something very hard. A huge purple bruise, a near-perfect imprint of the car's steering wheel, stood out in sharp relief across the kid's hairless upper chest. A lap seatbelt dangled unused beside him.

Removing the unconscious teenager from the car was going to be tough. Hitting the ditch had buckled the floor boards upward, and Robbie's right foot was caught between the clutch and the brake pedal. Suspended upside-down with the steering column shoved up against his taut, distended belly, long strings of blood and saliva drooled from Rob's shattered mouth, trickling into his jet black hair before collecting in a thick pool on the ceiling.

Despite the awkward position, Russ and his EMT partner, Brad, had somehow managed to strap a KED neck and back splint onto their patient. Robbie's head-down position had made the veins in his neck puff out so dramatically, that three short minutes after arriving on-scene, Russ had a jugular IV up and running. Heck, a blind man could have threaded a catheter into one of those blood-engorged vessels!

The firefighters finished cutting off the doors with their hydraulic Jaws, then waited as Kyle and Russ carefully wriggled their husky frames into the car. Mindful of the shattered glass and razor-sharp metal surrounding them, the medics sheltered the teen's head and chest with a tarp while one of the firefighters gingerly eased a metal bar between the floor pedals, taking great care to avoid the unlaced Nike hightop squashed behind them.

As Kyle was cradling the kid's upper body in his arms, a weird sucking, grating sound suddenly leaked out from beneath his patient's bloodied oxygen mask. The teen was still very much unconscious, yet a primitive brainstem reflex was causing him to chew on his oral airway. As a medic, Kyle knew it was a better sign than no movement at all, but it depressed him all the same. As he would later confide to his wife, it reminded him of a baby sucking, and for the first time in his life, he began to think like a parent.

Somewhere out there were two people who had conceived this child and brought him into the world. They had loved him and nurtured him and tried to keep him safe from harm, and if he were to die today, a part of his parents would die as well. Kyle could not help but think about his own expected child. What would his or her future hold? Would that new life realize its promise, or would it be brutally snuffed out like this?

"We need some more muscle in here!" Russ had his head thrust out the side window, shouting. It was crowded inside the crumpled Sunbird as the three rescue workers once again took up their positions. A second firefighter squeezed in beside the first to grab hold of the crowbar. With a kid's life hanging in the balance, the two men reefed back with all their might. Grimacing with satisfaction, they watched the pedals slowly begin to separate.

Angie, Brad and Ryne had everything ready for Robbie once he was extricated. Stretcher, spine board, Propaq vital signs monitor, head roll, spare oxygen tank and intubation equipment had all been laid out and double-checked.

Impatient to do her part, Angie decided to utilize her down-time by examining the Code 32 victim, just to make sure he was really dead. The police, she knew from Russ' many stories, had occasionally been wrong in this regard.

Ryne was standing next to her when she lifted the tarpaulin from the bloated face. He quickly turned away. Even so, Mr. Sommerville sprayed vomit everywhere... including all down Angie's pantleg.

"There's some sterile water under the number three seat in the helicopter," Angie muttered with disgust as she felt the warm puke soak through to her bare leg. "And ask Dale to find you a towel!"

Still heaving, the chalk-faced adolescent's reply was inaudible as he scurried away.

Stuck in traffic a quarter mile to the north, a Ford Ranger sat idling, its elderly driver silent behind the wheel. Drenched in a cold sweat, his face drained of all color, the man was struggling for every breath. Seated next to him, his equally frail wife was digging through her purse. In desperation, she finally dumped it upside down onto the seat. "Dear God... where is it?"

Her husband remained motionless with one hand pressed tightly against his chest. "Don't worry, Alma. It's just an angina attack. One Nitro and I'll be fine!" Helge Sorensen mumbled as the pressure in his chest threatened to squeeze the very life out of him.

Long-time area farmers, they had been returning home after picking up some combine parts when Helge had spotted the traffic snarl ahead. As he down-shifted, the elderly man felt a heavy ache under his breast bone, the same pain that had seized him two years earlier when he'd suffered a near-fatal heart attack.

Fumbling to remove the screw top on the little brown bottle she finally located, Alma dropped several of the tiny white pills before managing to get one under his tongue.

Five minutes later, Helge asked for another Nitro. The pain had gotten worse, and as the next five minutes crept past with excruciating slowness, Alma had to feed him still another.

Stroking his damp forehead with a trembling hand, Alma coaxed him to lay his head back against the seat and close his eyes. "You'll be fine, dear," she cooed in a tremulous voice. "The pills will take the pain away. They always do. It just takes them a few minutes, that's all."

Her ailing husband suddenly let out a deep, rumbling snort.

"Helge!" Alma shouted, but her husband of fifty-two years did not respond. Instead, his body slowly began to slump sideways. His weathered hand fell away from the steering wheel.

Back in Calgary meanwhile, Jennifer Stevens was busy making phone calls. Her first call had been to her family doctor; her contractions were now a nice steady five minutes apart. Then, upon receiving no answer on the private office line at the LIFE-STAR hangar, she phoned her sister to come pick her up. As they were about to leave for the hospital, Jennifer tried the hangar one final time. Five rings later, she hung up and dialed 911.

The EMS dispatcher assured her that he would contact LIFE-STAR 1, inform Kyle she was en route to Mountainview Hospital, that her sister was driving her and not to worry, everything was okay.

Her attractive features contorted with pain, Jennifer hung up the phone and doubled over. The intense muscle contraction very nearly dropped her to her knees. Glancing at her watch as she waited for the awful cramping to subside, Jen noted that it had been only three minutes since the last contraction. Suddenly she was fighting a deep-seated urge to push.

As Darlene helped her sister waddle down the sidewalk toward her car, it seemed like Jen's hips were out of joint or something. Thinking back to her own pre-natal lectures, Darlene immediately realized it was because the baby's head had dropped down into the pelvis and was now totally committed to finding a way out. As Jennifer was settling into the front seat, her membranes ruptured.

Weaving through traffic as they sped up Fourteenth Street toward Mountainview Hospital, Jen was either apologizing for the mess she was making or clawing at the vinyl arm rests and shrieking at her sister to drive faster.

Forced to stop at yet another red light, Darlene switched on the radio. Tuning in to the raunchiest heavy metal station she could find, Darlene was desperately hoping that the music might drown out her sibling's screams and maybe take their minds off what they were both fearing: that Jennifer was about to give birth to this flipping baby right on the frigging front seat!

Twenty miles due south, Robbie Bretton's hundred dollar running shoe flopped limply out from between the floor pedals. Within seconds, Russ, Kyle and the two firefighters had carefully extracted him from the overturned car and gently placed him on the waiting stretcher.

With his flying colleague off talking to one of the cops, Dale copied the message from dispatch regarding the imminent arrival of the Stevens' stork. "I copy you dispatch. Just to let you know, we should be lifting off here in about five minutes. Once we finish up at Parkland Memorial,

I'll pass on the info and then make a quick hop over to the Mountainview to drop Kyle off. No point in telling the poor guy now. He'll just worry himself sick."

With pre-liftoff "check list" in hand as he glanced out the window in search of Alex, Dale's eyes were meet with a truly unbelievable sight. A beige pickup truck was racing straight toward the helicopter. Having bypassed the traffic jam by recklessly straddling the very inside edge of the pavement, the truck dropped down into the center median. Flinging grass and muck, the vehicle then clawed its way up the opposite embankment. Still southbound, but in the northbound lanes now, the driver seemed intent on suicide.

As oncoming motorists swerved to avoid a head-on collision, the truck just seemed to speed up. The crazed driver was even brazenly flashing his headlights and waving his arm out the window... like he was just dying for attention... or just dying to die!

The RCMP also saw the truck and at first thought it was just some smartass incensed at having to wait in line. Instead of blowing by, however, the truck bounced back across the ditch and squealed to a stop right under the chopper's stationary blades.

The RCMP immediately converged on the vehicle. The driver was a frail, elderly woman. Jerking open the door, the stunned constables took one look inside and started waving for help.

"Stevens, get the hell over here! I've got a cardiac arrest going down right in front of me!" Dale called over the radio. The three AMC stared at each other. Russ and Kyle were still busy with their patient; Angie was it.

Mrs. Sorensen watched tearfully as the police began two-man cardio-pulmonary resuscitation on her beloved husband. As she herself seemed on the verge of collapse, a third constable gently settled her into the back seat of his squad car. The kind-hearted cop took the time to sit down and reassure her that her husband had some of the very best medics in Alberta working on him, and she had done everything she could.

"It's now up to a flight nurse with a history of practicing freelance euthanasia to save his life," an eavesdropping Angie thought grimly as she hustled past on her way to the truck.

Brad had run back and grabbed a spare cardiac monitor out of the ground ambulance. Once Angie had the patient hooked up to it, she found him to be in complete heart block. Unconscious with a heart rate of 30 beats per minute, this luckless fellow had no pulses to speak of and was only breathing at four breaths a minute.

As the EMT quickly set out her equipment, Angie intubated the patient by slipping an endotrachial tube down into his windpipe. By golly, all those valuable lessons she had learned while resuscitating pigs at "selection camp" were finally paying off.

Anchoring the ET tube with her fingers as she instructed Brad to start bagging, she listened to her patient's cold, clammy chest with her stethoscope. Detecting equal air entry to both lungs, she quickly taped the tube to her patient's top lip.

Choosing not to waste valuable time by attempting to start an IV, Angie instead squirted a milligram of diluted Atropine down the breathing tube, directly into the man's lungs. With any luck, the powerful drug would rapidly absorb into the lung mucosa, and from there into the blood stream where it would hopefully speed up the man's barely-existent heartbeat.

The medication worked like magic. Within seconds, the man's heart rate had picked up to 68 beats per minute. After a minute, however, his rate just as rapidly began to slow down again.

After a very thorough search, the only pulse Brad was able to palpate with any certainty was the carotid pulse in the side of Helge's neck. Angie knew that with a blood pressure that low, the old farmer's brain and kidneys would be starving for oxygen. If she didn't do something pretty damn fast, her patient was going to end up with irreversible brain damage or hooked up to a dialysis machine... that is, if he lived to make it to the hospital at all!

As Brad continued to squeeze oxygen into the man's lungs, Angie followed standard ACLS procedure and repeated the atropine. After watching again as the man's heart rate momentarily accelerated, only to revert back to third degree block again, she knew what she had to do.

"Dale!" she called over her radio. "Patch me through to Parkland. I need some covering orders stat and I'm sending Ryne over to pick up the Lifepak 10 pacer-monitor."

"No problem, luv. Consider it done."

As she waited for Ryne to return with the pacer, Angie feverishly tried to remember all the times she had played with it... all the times she had practiced with it... all the times she had prayed she would never have to use it.

Ryne came running with the Lifepak 10. Angie grabbed the monitor and tore open the nylon pouch velcroed to the back. Quickly attaching the large monitor discs to her patient's chest, she carefully connected the two monitor cables from the portable generator to each of the plastic discs. She had already explained to Brad that all she needed was a covering order from a doctor to turn the power on. With her patient all set to go, Angie once again called over her portable radio, "Dale, have you gotten hold of a doc yet?"

"I've been trying, luv, but they have a Code or something going on in their emerg department and I can't get a doctor to come to the radio. I'll see if I can get hold of Riverside's emerg if you want."

Russ and Kyle, in the process of loading their patient into the back of the helicopter, overheard the words firing between Dale and Angie. "Use it anyway, Ange! You can get a covering order once you're in the air," Russ shouted.

"We're here to save lives, Jackson! To hell with protocol... just do it!" The voice was Kyle's, but it didn't really matter as she had already begun adjusting the MA knob on the external pacemaker. She was in the Medical Review Board's bad books already and if they ever found out about this, well, what was the worst they could do? Have her taken out and defibrillated?

As she slowly increased the amount of voltage the machine was sending through her patient's chest wall, tiny little spikes began to march across the monitor screen. Unfortunately, no corresponding heartbeat followed them. The patient's underlying rhythm remained that of a future funeral home occupant—28 measly beats per minute.

Angie immediately retaliated by cranking the power higher and higher. Helge's chest muscles began to twitch at 70 contractions per minute, but his palpable heart rate stubbornly remained fixed at 28. "Work, damn it!" she cussed.

Just as she was about to admit defeat and call Rusty for help, Brad suddenly cried out, "Look...."

There, prancing across the monitor in perfect formation, were paced heart beats... at a rate of 70 per minute! "Can you get a radial with that?" she blurted.

Brad's fingers probed the patient's wrist. "Yes," he shouted, "it's weak, but I can feel it!"

Slowly Angie started to breathe again. "Okay, a radial pulse means we probably have a blood pressure around eighty systolic. We're not out of the woods yet, but I'll take any kind of pressure over no pressure at all!"

From the moment Angie had first taken charge, the entire heart-starting episode had lasted less than four minutes.

As they were sliding their patient into the back of the helicopter, Helge raised an unsteady hand in a feeble attempt to pull out his plastic breathing tube. It was a very good sign.

Watching as Brad hustled back to their ambulance, Russ stayed behind just long enough to secure the chopper's rear doors and blow his flight nurse girlfriend a much-deserved kiss.

While they waited for the chopper to fire up, Angie and Kyle were busy doing their pre-lift off checks... making sure they had all their equipment with them... both stretchers anchored to the floor... back and side doors closed tight... patients' headsets on so they wouldn't suffer hearing loss during the flight... all IVs and monitors hooked up to their appropriate patients and functioning properly, themselves buckled in with helmets on.

There was no room for him, so Ryne was left behind to hitch a ride to the hangar with the RCMP. Angie had a funny feeling that Mr. Sommerville had seen enough today to keep him on the straight-and-narrow for some time to come. And to think he still had four more flights to make!

The helicopter was slow to launch. Angie and Kyle exchanged looks of growing concern as they felt the aircraft's powerful engines strain to pull the chopper into the air. They were at maximum torque and yet... nothing was happening.

Co-pilot Alex finally keyed his intercom button. "Uh, hello back there. As you've probably noticed, we don't appear to be going anywhere. It seems we... uh... I inadvertently parked our red dustdevil on a solar-heated asphalt highway and... uh, I won't bore you with the physics involved, but we don't have enough power to lift off. What we're going to try instead is dump all the equipment you people aren't using right now. Hopefully, if we can download enough, we should be able to get airborne and get the heck out of here!"

Alex climbed out and opened the rear doors. After pulling out several bags of equipment, the pilot figured he had removed enough to get the chopper back in the sky. He was wrong.

Dale could not make LIFE-STAR 1 fly. Even with both engines thundering, all he could muster was ten feet of forward progress; a distance made clearly visible as the steel landing skids etched deep furrows across the hot asphalt.

With the Bretton kid's Golden Hour ticking toward zero hour, it was time for Captain Morgan to go to Plan B. This time, instead of medical equipment, it was Alex Davis himself who got the boot. Angie and Kyle could not believe their eyes as they watched the dejected co-pilot give them a feeble wave before jogging away.

One hundred and eighty pounds lighter now, the BK still was not overly keen to take to the air, but with an increasingly furious Aussie at the controls, it really didn't have much choice in the matter.

"Alright men... oh, and you, too, Ms. Jackson, I've got rid of all the deadwood on this here machine and I'm going to make this sucker fly if it kills me! Make sure everything is strapped down real tight back there. Our take-off may be a little bumpier than normal."

Easing the cyclic stick ever so slightly forward while simultaneously pulling up on the collective control, Dale skipped the helicopter along the pavement at about twenty knots. With some forward momentum now, he got some undisturbed air under the chopper's blades. Undisturbed air meant more lift, and one hundred skid-scraping, vision-blurring feet later, the veteran pilot got the screaming red machine into the air.

A mere five minute hop by air, the trip to Parkland Memorial would have taken half an hour by ground transport; a half hour too long for a teenager from Okotoks to have survived without surgical intervention.

Russ was still at the accident scene packing up his equipment when a tow truck operator got the go-ahead to winch the crumpled car over onto its flattened tires. One of the RCMP constables standing nearby then directed a balding, heavy-set gentleman down into the ditch. It was the county coroner.

Brushing his beefy hand at the cloud of flies attracted by the pool of reddish-black blood, the rural doctor lifted a corner of the yellow tarp covering the bloated body so his camera-toting assistant could snap a few shots of the death scene.

The police were busy taking measurements of the car's skid marks and trajectory for their accident report. A driver's license found in the dead kid's wallet had already been run through the squad car's on board computer. As a result, two Okotoks RCMP constables were at that very moment rolling to a stop in front of the Westfall residence.

Having just finished raking the back yard, an attractive, fit-looking woman of about forty was lugging several bulging garbage bags out to the curb when she spotted the uniformed officers coming up the walk toward her. They were walking too slowly, their faces drawn too tightly.

In unison, both men reached up to remove their caps.

Abandoning her bags of lawn clippings, Mrs. Westfall instinctively began backing away. "No... " her trembling voice rose to a wail. "No!

"Not Jay!"

29
SPECIAL DELIVERY

As members of the emerg team at Parkland Memorial Hospital went to work cutting away Robbie's remaining clothing, Kyle gave a quick history to the attending doc. In less than thirty seconds, the young man lay totally exposed... his shirt, jeans and underwear hanging in bloodied tatters from the sides of the stainless steel examining table.

Kyle had saved precious minutes by radioing ahead to have a surgeon, a cardiologist and the trauma team standing by in the emergency department, rather than running from all corners of the hospital.

The physician seemed to be only half-listening to Kyle's report as he simultaneously barked out orders to his staff. As the medic began gathering up his equipment, the doctor stopped him with a quick question.

"You said this accident happened when?"

Kyle's reply was not what he wanted to hear. "About fifty-five minutes ago."

"Okay," the doctor said, pausing to gather his thoughts. "Have somebody call medical records. Find out if this kid's ever been treated here before. Until we know for sure, I'm going to assume he isn't Jehovah Witness. Is there anyone here who objects to that?"

Except for a slurping, sucking sound as the respiratory techs suctioned a marshmallow-sized bloodclot from the kid's mouth, the room was silent.

"Alright then. Let's get him grouped and cross-matched. Debbie, I want you to contact the Okotoks Mounties and see if they've been able to get a hold of the parents yet. Oh, and Deb, have the unit clerk notify the O.R. Tell them I want to reserve a table and have her page the neuro resident again. We need him down here NOW!"

Stepping aside to let the nurse scurry from the room, a tall, lanky third year surgical resident pushed through the double swinging doors.

"Greg. How nice of you to drop by," the emerg doctor said as he motioned his colleague to the head of the table.

"We have a multi-trauma for you... male, eighteen years old, head injury, belly full of blood. We're just waiting for the neurologist to give us his opinion before I let you cart him off to the O.R."

His role in the medical drama completed, Kyle slipped from the crowded room. Wandering the maze of connecting corridors in search of his partner, he eventually found her leaning against the front admitting desk, laboring over her patient care form.

When it came to giving report, nobody was faster than the great A.Y. Jackson. Her reports came with no added frills or preservatives. An abbreviated rehash of the events leading up to LIFE-STAR's arrival, a brief blurb as to treatment given on-scene, followed by a bare bones update of her patient's condition inflight.

Turn-around time after a mission had to be kept as short as possible. Knowing the cellular phone could ring at any moment with another call, both Kyle and Angie had already packed up their equipment, sponged the blood off the stretcher, remade it with a fresh sheet and blanket and were busily finishing up their paperwork when Dale strolled up to the desk. "We've just been dispatched on another call. You'll have to fax them all this stuff from the hangar!"

As the pilots were never to interfere with the medical end of things; Kyle nearly went ballistic. "Another one? Well you just phone the Trauma Hot Line back and tell them we can't possibly accept it. You seem to be forgetting that most of our supplies and your dyslexic sidekick got left behind on a highway somewhere between here and Okotoks. The gophers have probably made off with most of the stuff already, including, hopefully, Captain Davis, so give us a break, okay? Plus I'm not leaving here until I've had a chance to call home and see how Jen's doing!"

"Oh yes you are, Stevens!" the Aussie commanded. "You people never use half the junk you carry on board anyway, so quit your whining. And it wasn't the Trauma Hot Line that called. It was the city EMS dispatcher. Our medical presence has been urgently requested to a area just east of the Glenmore reservoir so I want you people packed up and ready to lift off in five minutes. Got that?"

As Dale stormed off to fire up his machine, Kyle tore the back copy from his patient care report and slammed it down on the desk. "Who the hell does that jerk think he is?"

Captain Morgan paid little heed as his infuriated flight medic stomped past his window and climbed into the back. Keeping an eye on his instrument panel, the pilot waited until the door closure light went off. Then... he pulled pitch—an abrupt maneuver that caused the chopper to rocket straight up into the air. Flying due south across the city for what seemed like all of fifteen seconds, Dale smoothly brought the chopper around to begin his descent.

"Morgan? Where in heck are you taking us? I just radioed Riverside Medical Center and they haven't heard anything about the city dispatching us to a call east of the reservoir!" Kyle shouted over his helmet radio.

"I should hope not!" Dale spit back. "This mission is of a highly personal nature. A highly personal nature of your own doing, I might add. At least I hope it was. I only pray that we're not too late!"

Kyle yanked the black curtain partition to one side. Staring out through the front canopy window, all he could see was the massive outline of the Mountainview Hospital looming ahead. Suddenly, it all came together.

"Too late... for what?" the medic choked.

Dale twisted around to face the tongue-tied paramedic. "Good Heavens, man, the baby is supposed to arrive by stork, not the father. Didn't you learn anything in pre-natal class?"

Twenty-four minutes later, Jennifer and Kyle became the proud parents of a beautiful 7 pound 14 ounce baby girl... Amanda Lynn.

30
AN OLYMPIC VOLUNTEER

"You're never going to believe this!" Russ' voice shouted from the answering machine.

As if it weren't enough that he and Angie were going to flaunt their fancy footwork in the Games' Opening Ceremonies, now Russ' own personal Olympic goal had been realized. After having spent hours and hours sending in nearly 150 entry forms, he had just received word that he'd been selected, along with seven thousand others, to carry the Olympic torch across Canada.

Rusty's designated kilometer was on the Salmo-Creston Skyway in southeastern British Columbia. Steep didn't even begin to describe it. The highway en route to the mountain summit had a mind-boggling 8% grade, which meant that for every hundred feet of distance, the roadway climbed eight feet. Scheduled for late January, that particular segment was considered by many to be the most difficult stretch on the entire relay. Russ could not have been happier.

One evening, a few days after finding out the news, Russ was at Angie's apartment watching the Edmonton Eskimos annihilate his beloved Stampeder football team yet again. With the score already hopelessly lopsided in favor of the awesome Eskies, the game paused for half-time and Russ turned the volume down.

Angie was stretched out next to him on the couch with her head comfortably nestled in the crook between his shoulder and his muscular chest. She had just finished her second beer, and with inhibitions numbed by alcohol, had become very philosophical.

"Hon, have you ever wondered... you know... if everyone who has ever been born was as smart as you or I... where would the world be right now? You know, like would we still be living in caves or would we have invented electricity? Would there have been any wars?

"Or have you ever stopped and asked yourself where seedless grapes come from? I mean, how do they reproduce and make little grapes if they don't have any seeds? And what about lint? Every time you dry a load of clothes, you have to clean out the lint trap, right? So if you just kept washing and drying that same load of clothes over and over again, would they eventually disappear altogether?"

"Where do you come up with stuff like that, Ange?" Russ rolled his eyes. "God, with insanity running rampant in your half of the gene pool, our kids won't stand a chance!"

"Insanity in my half of the gene pool?" the agile flight nurse quickly straddled his narrow hips. "And just whose crazy idea was it to run the torch up the steepest highway in North America?"

"It wasn't a crazy idea. It was very carefully thought out," Russ replied, pulling her down toward him. "I've driven that stretch of highway and figured that nobody in their right mind would want to run there... except for maybe some of the local jocks. It only made sense to concentrate my limited number of entries in an area with the least amount of competition."

Angie let out a theatrical sigh. "Well I'm just glad that all the time we spent running around to all those gas stations picking up entry forms paid off."

Russ sat up and, with his woman wrapped tightly in his arms, twisted around until he was now on top. Able to snuggle a whole lot closer now, he began his ritualistic foreplay by brushing his lips hungrily across her forehead.

"It was worth it, don't you think?" he whispered, kissing the sensitive area under her ear.

"I'm just thankful that it's you that has to run it... not me," Angie murmured as she nibbled on his earlobe.

"Oh, but you can always pull on those hot pink exercise tights of yours and Two-Step up the road in front of me... you know, to give me some incentive to make it to the top!" Russ replied as his lips and hands slowly started to migrate south.

"And we're going to have to drive all the way out there... and all the way back... in the middle of winter... with all those icy hairpin curves," Angie sighed as she slipped her hands under his pullover.

An unrelenting body shirt blocking his way, Russ was forced to move north again. Lovingly exploring every female nook and cranny that crossed his path with a delicate kiss and warm caress, it was as he tenderly nuzzled Angie's satiny-soft cheek with his nose that he finally found time to respond. "In that case, my dear, we could always book into a motel. I mean, you wouldn't want me driving home through all those mountains at night, would you?"

Her fingers delicately teasing her lover's mane of thick brown curls, Angie paused her lustful massaging just long enough to reach for the remote control. She had never been one for making love by the flickering light of a television set.

"Honey," she moaned, "the Stamps are on the Eskimo's five yard line... looks like they're threatening to score."

"They're not the only ones!" came Russ' muffled reply.

Fumbling with the buttons on his shirt, Angie whispered breathlessly into his ear, "How would you like to start training for the big event right now?"

The medic slowly raised himself up on his elbow to gaze at her. Seeing the puzzled look in his eyes, Angie pulled him back down and gave him a very sensuous, very delicious-tasting kiss. Upon resurfacing for air, she softly concluded, "You can start jogging tomorrow, Mr. Andrews, but tonight I thought you might like to practice the motel part."

31
SOMEONE'S IN LOVE

A four thousand square foot mansion on Lake Chestermere was to be the site for LIFE-STAR'S first annual Christmas party. In an effort to keep the financially-strapped organization's costs to a minimum, one of the more affluent Riverside Medical Center's emerg docs had graciously donated the use of his home for the bash.

Fully aware they were missing the best party of the year, the med-evac crew on duty that night was not a happy lot. With arms folded grumpily and their scuffed leather boots jostling for position atop the rickety coffee table, Dale, Alex, Russ and Kyle had spent the evening stuffing themselves sick with popcorn and complaining about how Bateman always seemed to plan these lavish little soirees whenever they were on shift.

To make matters even more depressing, Angie, the RN scheduled to be on with them, had been grounded indefinitely with a nasty inner ear infection. As none of the other fun-loving flight princesses wanted to pick up the shift, Kyle had selflessly volunteered as a last minute replacement. With Jen and Amanda off visiting her folks in Regina, he was missing his family something awful. Rather than sitting at home and feeling miserable, what with the new baby and all, he really could use the extra money.

Shoveling in another handful of buttered popcorn, Russ lamented, "Angie wouldn't have gone to the party tonight even if I'd had the shift off. Said she was worried somebody might've nominated her for the WIENIE award."

"I thought that honor went to the fly-boy who committed the worst screw-up during the year," Kyle said.

"Stevens!" the usually soft-spoken Alex erupted, "I'll have you know that LIFE-STAR pilots never screw up and this 'TURKEY OF THE YEAR' crap they have for the pilots is just another of Lawson's scheming ploys to keep us underpaid and under-appreciated!"

"I'm behind you all the way, Captain Davis," Dale grinned, mischief lighting his eyes, "but considering I nominated you twice myself, I'd be working on an acceptance speech if I were you! And as for Angie, I wouldn't worry about her. She's a tough cookie. A little teasing won't kill her. Might even do her some good. Make her a bit more humble."

"A tough cookie? God, how I wish that was true," a strangely subdued Russ replied. "That girl is so damn talented. She's the best nurse I've ever worked with. Good head. Cool under pressure. But she's so much more than that. You should hear her play Mozart. Not on piano, but on her guitar... and she plays it by ear. She's twice the computer hacker that Bateman is... and he was the one who taught her. She can do anything she puts her mind to, but only if someone pushes her.

"She never used to be like that. You guys probably don't know this, but two years ago, she was down in Lake Placid for the Canadian Luge Championships. Crashed big time. Damn near sliced her achilles tendon in half. But it wasn't just her ankle that got messed up. You could see it in her eyes... hear it in her voice. The fire was gone... the intensity... the desire. She was suddenly afraid to try anything new, afraid to take a chance, afraid of failing.

"This was a woman who'd once talked me into taking skydiving lessons for Pete's sake. The old Angie was a cocky, balls-to-the-wall speed junkie and her dream... her big all-encompassing dream... was to march into McMahon stadium as a member of the Canadian Olympic team. And it wasn't just a case of wishful thinking. Even after crashing and riding her butt through the finish light at the championships, she ended up taking the bronze medal away from a girl who'd competed for Canada at the Sarajevo Games!"

As if lost in a world of his own, Russ aimlessly wandered about the tiny room as he rambled on. "Emotionally, she'd pretty well hit rock bottom. Not only had she lost her chance of making the Olympic squad, but it was right about then that she got dumped by that Jefferson Logan creep. It was awful what she went through.

"Night after night, bawling her eyes out, babbling on and on that all men... except for me, of course... were nothing but scum-sucking bottom-dwellers and how she was planning on moving to Edmonton for the entire two weeks of the Olympics. That last part really got to me. Calgary will probably never get to host the Games again... not in our lifetime anyway... and for her to miss out on that... well... it would be such a crime.

"That's why I talked her into taking dance lessons with me and trying out for a part in the Opening Ceremonies. You know, she tried hard not to let on, but when we were selected, I think she was more excited than I was. I've even sweet talked her into running the torch relay with me. All the woman needed was someone to help her through the rough spots. Someone she could lean on. Someone she could trust. Someone who could keep her out of trouble!"

Russ' three friends were speechless. Their good buddy had never talked this glowingly about anything, much less about a woman. This could not be the lone wolf, stud-muffin party animal they all loved and, until now, thought they knew.

It was Kyle who finally clued in. "Uh, Andrews, just what are you trying to tell us here, anyway? You've never spoken so highly of a woman before, except maybe your mother. Are you trying to tell us that this girl just might be the one?"

Everyone stopped chewing as they awaited Russ' reply.

The boyish former firefighter replied softly, "The one and only one!" His dark brown eyes welled up with emotion. "I'm taking her out for dinner tomorrow night. I know she can't cook and her homemaking skills are limited to hemming her jeans with a stapler, but sometime between the appetizer and the main course, I'm going to ask that squirrelly, sassy, sexy little ex-luger if she'd like to marry me."

Alex and Kyle were pounding him on the back in congratulations when the phone in Lawson's office rang. A forced smile masking his true emotions, Dale went to answer it.

It was Lord Lawson himself. "Why don't you boys crank up that big red beast of yours and fly on over here?" he said. "If we get a call, you can launch from here just as easy as from the hangar. And you'd better hurry if you want any food, 'cause it's going fast."

As Alex was radioing to have the helicopter pulled out, Kyle suddenly turned to Russ. "It's a shame Angie won't be at the party tonight. You know, the longer she puts this Wienie Award thing off, the worse it'll be when she finally does show her face."

The love-sick medic nodded energetically and speed-dialed her number. The answer, however, was still the same. It was snowing and the roads were icy and she was tired and she'd have to wash her hair and she'd just gone out and rented a video.

Russ cupped his hand over the receiver and relayed her endless excuses to his waiting pals. Dale had the answer. "You just tell that sassy, sexy little ex-luger of yours to get her buns ready and hurry up about it because we're going to be picking her up in five minutes!"

"But, how...." Russ asked.

"Isn't there a playground across the street from her apartment? For an experienced IFR pilot like Captain Marvel here, it should be a piece of cake to set down on... unless he starts drifting sideways in the hover and gets the tail rotor tangled in the jungle gym or something."

As outbound pilot, Alex was not exactly crazy about the idea. What if Lawson found out about their imaginative, not to mention highly illegal night-time "touch and go" in a residential area?

Morgan let out a deep sigh. "You're probably right. It would've been a tricky approach anyway."

"Excuse me, but are you saying it might be too much for me?" Alex demanded. "Get your helmet, cowboy!"

After passing on Dale's plan, Russ quietly set the receiver down. "Men, we've got to depart immediately," he hissed, tiptoeing toward the hangar door, "before she realizes she's arguing with herself!"

Angie immediately called back on a different line, but as she listened to the phone ring, she knew exactly what her weasel of a boyfriend and his nefarious buddies were up to.

There was no time to lose.

Thrusting her legs into a pair of sleek black satin slacks, she began digging like a terrier through her dresser drawer, searching for the pale pink angora sweater that was her honey's all time favorite. Balancing on the edge of the sink in the bathroom now, she looked like a movie on fast-forward as she brushed on eyeliner, blush and lipstick.

With all the fashion flair of a bulimic shark caught in a feeding frenzy, she jabbed a pick through her tangle of blond curls as she hunted through the closet for her camel hair coat.

Exploding from her apartment with a patent leather purse flapping over one shoulder, Angie was still struggling to cram an arm into a coat sleeve as she dashed for the elevator. Inside, she punched the button and fought to catch her breath while hopping about pulling on her knee-high boots. All the while fantasizing about the evening ahead, Angie couldn't wait for the doors to open. Bolting from the elevator, she nearly trampled a middle-aged couple quietly sorting through their mail in the lobby.

Once the smartly dressed husband and wife recovered from their initial fright, their unnerved expressions soon turned to smiles. "Why Angela, darling, we haven't heard... uh... seen you for quite awhile. We were wondering if maybe you'd moved."

"Oh, it's nothing like that, Mrs. Cooper," Angie replied, knowing full well what her nosy neighbor was after. "I've been off work with an ear infection for the last two weeks, that's all. Went out to my parents' farm for a few days of TLC."

"That boyfriend of yours isn't working the night shift again... is he?"

Angie smiled. "Can't fool you, can I, Mrs. Cooper? I really am sick... honest, but yes, Russ has been working nights. You're looking at a very deprived female here, but we're going to a Christmas party tonight, so who knows, maybe all that mistletoe will get things back on track again?"

"Young lady," Mr. Cooper chimed in, "it's not a very good night to be out on the roads. The side streets are glare ice. Our Jag just wasn't meant for this kind of weather. Slipping and sliding everywhere. I do hope this fellow of yours is a careful driver and has a dependable vehicle?" Having many times before requested that the building manager tow Russ' rust-encrusted vehicle from his parking stall, Mr. Cooper was just about to comment further when something stole his attention. The velvety blanket of snow in the parking lot was suddenly swirling angrily... as if a tornado were about to touch down.

Knowing it was the wrong time of year for such meteorological phenomena, Angie faked a big, disinterested yawn as a helicopter dropped out of the night sky and landed in the vacant park across the road.

Watching as a helmeted figure sprang from the BK and sprinted toward them, Angie couldn't help but grin. "You don't have to worry about Rusty, Mr. Cooper, he's always extra-careful when his folks let him borrow the family helicopter."

32
THE PARTY

Displaying all the finesse of an airborne snowblower, the BK's twin spotlights hungrily searched the estate's vast front lawn for a suitable landing site as its powerful rotors viciously whipped the foot-deep snow into a boiling white cloud.

With Angie on his arm, Russ proudly led his little troop up the cobbled walkway to the modest abode. The place was huge. Three stories high, it was a castle overlooking Chestermere Lake.

The crew stripped off their flight suits and set their helmets in an orderly row atop a bookcase, then passed through french doors to the living room. Turning en mass, the revelers enthusiastically greeted their on-duty counterparts with the joyous news that the awards were about to be presented.

Emcee Howie Bateman tapped his microphone. "Ladies and Gentlemen, it gives me great pleasure to present to you tonight... the winner of the Wienie award! This beautiful trophy goes to the AMC who committed the most embarrassing blooper of the year.

"There is one amazing candidate who lead all the others with not one, not two, but three separate nominations. She garnered votes for attacking an unarmed barbecue, attempting to raft down the Bow River during peak flood season without a paddle, and blatantly endangering Dale Morgan's life by strapping him to a crazed Italian and sending him down the luge run.

"Is she here tonight? She's just arrived? Great. Without further ado, the winner of the first annual Wienie award goes to... Ms. Angela Jackson, RN." Hoots of laughter erupted as Howard held up the wall plaque uniquely crafted in the shape of a truly pornographic wiener. Angie fled.

As Russ ran after his mortified sweetie, Dale pushed Alex forward to accept the award. It was while he was being presented with Angie's trophy, that the grinning Bateman handed him a second plaque... a plaque bearing a proudly strutting turkey.

Alex Davis was actually very good at his job, but like his medical co-hort, seemed cursed with bad luck. As such, his understanding pilot brethren had submitted his name a record four times.

His first blunder occurred on a day of back-to-back missions. Upon transporting a "donor" patient to the Riverside Med Center for multi-organ removal, Alex and his crew were immediately dispatched to fly a second patient to Edmonton for heart transplant surgery. It was while en route with the second patient, that the apparently "brain dead" Captain Davis inquired over the chopper's intercom system: "Jodi, I can't remember... is this guy getting the heart or are they going to divvy up his parts like that last poor devil?"

The critically-ill young man, wearing a headset so he would not go deaf during the hour-long flight, fortunately chose to make light of Alex's faux pas and replied, "I'm kind of hoping I'll receive an organ... not donate one!"

Alex had also been solely responsible for the total annihilation of a Christmas display complete with Santa, prancing reindeer and impish elves erected on the roof of a small rural hospital. Setting up for one of his infamous, "never the same twice," approaches, Davis had blasted the entire works off the roof and into a neighboring cow pasture. Twenty minutes later, hospital security were still combing the wreckage for possible bovine casualties as the red-faced pilot and his crew beat a hasty retreat with their patient.

Then there was the time, on a flight to Rapid Creek with the NICU team, he had managed to overshoot the hospital and land at the local nursing home instead. The janitor who met them at the door was mighty surprised to learn that LIFE-STAR was there to pick up a premature baby that one of the home's residents had just given birth to.

Alex's crowning achievement, however, was for single-handedly creating a crop-circle wave of hysteria in Vulcan, Alberta.

With the awards over, the teenaged DJ wasted little time cranking up his sound system. As all his musical selections tended toward heavy metal, the living room floor remained empty until someone shouted, "ENOUGH OF THIS CRAP... PUT ON SOME STONES!" In seconds, Jumping Jack Flash had them all on their feet.

Angie walked over to a middle-aged gentleman standing off by himself. "Could I interest you in a dance?" As his couch-bound wife radiated ill-will, a beaming Peter Lawson accepted his Wienie-winning flight nurse's kind offer.

For a big man, Lawson was surprisingly light on his feet and as he and Angie shared a lovely little ballad with the unlikely title of Wild Horses, they talked about some of the crazier things that had happened over the past six months. Angie was soon relating to her employer a bizarre idea she had heard regarding edible underwear and its possible use as survival food.

"I didn't know Chatelaine carried such thought-provoking articles," Peter remarked with a chuckle.

"I didn't read it in a magazine. Dale told me about it."

"I hope he sticks around long enough to implement it."

"What do you mean?"

"Well, his work visa isn't forever, you know. He's got to make up his mind pretty soon about staying in Canada or going back to Australia. You know how 'flighty' helicopter pilots are... here one day, gone the next. Morgan's got no family here. No ties. What he needs is a good reason to stick around... you know, like maybe finding the right girl, preferably one with Canadian citizenship papers. He's a good man. Even darns his own socks. You wouldn't happen to have any single sisters on the prowl, would you?"

"No, but I have two brothers," was Angie's ridiculous answer.

"I really think Dale would prefer a girl... at least I think he would, but then you never can be too sure about those kind of things. I mean look at Forbes standing over there next to the punch bowl. He looks manly enough, but I've always had a funny feeling his dip stick is a little low in the testosterone department, if you know what I mean."

Angie couldn't help laughing out loud as she nodded her head in complete agreement of Peter's lighter than air depiction of his chief mechanic.

When the music ended, Angie thanked her boss for a delightful twirl on the dance floor and headed for the buffet table. She was about to sample some vegetable dip when a familiar face eased into line beside her. It was the womanless Captain Morgan.

"Reminds me of a guy I used to date," Angie remarked as she held up for inspection a rather limp stalk of broccoli.

"That's cruel, Ange. Real cruel," Dale said, bending to take a look at it. "Anyone I know?"

"Nope!" the RN chirped as she reached up to dangle the shriveled vegetable playfully above his head.

"What in blazes are you doing, luv?" the startled Aussie laughed as he instinctively tried to brush her hand away.

"Quit your fussing, will you, Morgan? I've been all over this damn house and haven't spotted a spray of mistletoe anywhere, so I guess we'll just have to use this." Angie repositioned the broccoli over his head.

The pilot was just about to gallantly surrender his lips to the festive cause, when he stopped. "Pardon me for asking, Ms. Jackson, but won't Russ get upset if he catches you necking with another man?"

"Naw, Rusty and I have an understanding," Angie grinned, slipping her arms around her favorite pilot's neck. "He doesn't care where I get my appetite... just as long as I come home to eat!"

Heading for the dining room so they could chat as they shared a plate of cheese and crackers, Angie got the withdrawn pilot talking about his snowless hometown of Cairns, how they celebrated Christmas Down Under, and about the painful fact that he had not been home to see his son in nearly five years.

"I'd love to see a picture of him," Angie gently coaxed.

Dale immediately fished a small, tattered photo from his wallet. It was a much younger Captain Morgan sitting at the controls of a giant Pelican Coast Guard helicopter. The boy on his lap looked about five or six years old. He was almost out of sight beneath his father's white flight helmet, but only a blind man could have missed the big grin on his chubby face.

"His name's Brian. Brian James Morgan. He turns eleven next month," the pilot stated matter-of-factly as he quickly tucked the faded picture back into his wallet.

"He's a fine looking boy," Angie replied softly. "Looks just like his dad. You must miss him a lot."

Dale nodded. "My Grandma used to have a saying. If a child is conceived under the Southern Cross... during a new moon... while its parents are waiting for a tow truck to arrive to extract their car from a muck hole, that child will grow up to become a great man someday."

"Really! And just what happens if this so-called wonder kidlet inherits two X chromosomes instead of an XY?" Angie laughingly demanded.

"Like I said, she'll grow up and become a great man someday!"

"Where the heck did you and your wife get stuck? Downwind of a nuclear power plant?"

Unable to come up with a witty reply, Dale instead asked a favor. "Could I have this dance?"

Holding her close as they swayed to the music, Dale pushed back the dense curls from around her face. "How long has your ear looked like this?" he whispered.

"All my life, sir."

Their dance over far too soon, Dale, showing the kind of gentleman he was, escorted her over to Russ who was deep in conversation with another LIFE-STAR medic.

"Mr. Andrews, I've brought your woman back safe and sound. Try and keep her that way." Turning to leave, Dale flashed Angie a sly wink as he wandered back toward the buffet table.

Russ gazed down at the smiling woman standing before him. "You've danced with the rest. Now, how about dancing with the best!" He waved his hand to get the disc jockey's attention.

"Now?" the teenager said.

"Now!"

A "Stones" classic began to drift from the speakers.

"Angie," Russ' improvised off-key singing all but drowned out Mick and the boys as he tenderly held his woman. "I pledge to you my heart and soul forever."

The seductive song ended just soon enough in Russ' hormone stimulated opinion. Hurriedly departed the dance floor with his girl in tow, it did not take him long to find an empty room on the mansion's second level.

Russ was in the act of removing Angie's bra when there was a sharp rap on the door. It was Kyle.

"Russ... zip yourself up and get the heck out here. We've been scramble-dispatched to an MVA. Morgan says the weather's iffy, but we should be okay if we launch right away. Andrews... are you getting any of this?"

"Sweet Jesus, why can't people stay home and watch TV like the rest of us?" Russ muttered bitterly as he pulled Angie close.

"I wouldn't call what you two are doing, watching TV." Kyle hollered as he ran off to suit up.

"Here's some money for cab fare," Russ instructed as he forced a twenty into Angie's hand. "I don't want you having to catch a ride back to town with some drunk. Now don't forget to take your antibiotic when you get home and remember, tomorrow night at the Owl's Nest. I'll pick you up at five."

Frantically fumbling to look presentable again, Angie paused to wrap her arms around his trim waist. "Don't worry about me, Big Guy. Have a good flight... and be careful, okay."

"I'm always careful," the medic laughed as he tucked in his shirt. "Heck, that's the only reason you and I haven't become parents yet!"

Delaying at the door to pull on his heavy snow boots and parka, Russ was just about to head into the swirling snow beyond when he suddenly did something he never did. He abruptly turned back and gave Angie one last, passionate hug and kiss... not just a peck on the lips like she usually got when there were other people around.

Shivering in the open doorway as her man jogged toward the waiting helicopter, Angie saw Dale angrily wave at him to hurry it up.

It was 11:45 p.m.

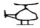

33
THE ROAD LESS TRAVELED

The weather had been beautiful earlier in the evening with a slight wind out of the northwest and temperatures hovering in the -5 Celsius range, but it was not like that now.

Prior to accepting the mission, Dale had checked in with the local Flight Service Station. "You boys are going to earn your money tonight!" the weather observer prophesied.

"The Arctic air mass that was stalled over Edmonton has started to move," he continued. "We're already receiving reports of blizzard conditions in the Red Deer area and have halted all north and eastbound air traffic. Chinook conditions are strengthening as well, so there's a chance the storm could miss Calgary. That's not a definite, however.

"At this time, air travel to the west is still a go, but just barely. The Banff-Calgary corridor is experiencing severe wind gusts, and if night visibility minimums deteriorate further, you could find yourselves spending the night in Canmore. Let us know how you make out. This is Calgary Flight Service Station, out."

Leaving the soft amber glow of the city's street lights behind, Alex Davis had his hands full as the turbulent Chinook headwind kicked LIFE-STAR 1 square in the teeth. Buffeted by 60 knot gusts which were making a mockery of his attempts to maintain level flight, Alex muttered, "If this crap doesn't let up pretty damn soon, I'm all for following Standard Operating Procedures and turning for home! Traffic down on the Trans-Canada is making better time than we are!"

Standard Operating Procedures clearly stated that no mission was worth risking the lives of an entire crew. If there was the slightest possibility of not making it back to base safely, they were not to lift off.

As the pilot with the most flight-hours on staff, Dale agreed with Alex. During his stint in the arctic, the steely-eyed Aussie had done an enormous amount of winter flying. It was while dodging tracer bullets in Vietnam, however, that he had learned his most valuable lesson: there were old pilots and there were bold pilots... but there were no old, bold pilots.

In the back of the lurching chopper, Kyle and Russ were clinging to their seats and discussing the fine art of child rearing. "I know Amanda's a girl, but maybe she'll like monster truck rallies and camping and going to Flames home games. Jen learned to love all those things. Why not my beautiful daughter?"

The chopper suddenly yawed to the right and pitched nose down. "For God's sake, how much longer is Morgan going to let Davis have the stick?" Kyle added through clenched teeth as he grabbed for a fresh barf bag. "I don't have anything left to woof!"

Struggling to keep his own lunch down, Russ unzipped his flight jacket and cracked open his window vent. The numbing breeze against his face felt surprisingly good.

Kyle turned to his partner. "I just don't want to make a mistake. I want Amanda to grow up with pride and respect for her old man."

Russ couldn't help but smile. "She's only three weeks old, for crying out loud! All she wants right now is a full bottle and a dry diaper. Just be yourself. Be fair, admit when you're wrong. Tell her you love her and make sure she knows she can come to you when she needs help, no matter what the problem."

"I have Canmore EMS standing by on provincial," Dale announced.

Kyle squeezed his mike button. "Canmore EMS, this is LIFE-STAR One, how do you read, over?"

"LIFE-STAR One, we copy you loud and clear. We're at an MVA on Highway Forty, about five miles south of the Ribbon Creek turn-off," a female voice replied. "A pickup truck and a car collided head-on about an hour ago. Three patients involved... two yellows and a red. Both yellows have already been transported to Canmore. The red patient is trapped in the wreckage. Condition critical with hypothermia, fractured pelvis, bilateral femur fractures, and a closed head injury. We'll hopefully have her extricated by the time you people touch down. Just to let you know, it's snowing like crazy here and the wind is really howling out of the west so I think we should aim for as short a turnaround time as possible. Do you require further information? Over."

"Ask her if a landing area has been set up and secured?" Russ prompted his absent-minded partner. Kyle quickly relayed the question.

"LIFE-STAR One, that is affirmative. The RCMP have the highway south of the accident marked with flares. The area is free of hazards, but blowing snow could make visibility a problem. Over."

"We copy you, Canmore. Our ETA is five minutes. See you on the ground. This is LIFE-STAR One, out."

Forced to crab into the wind as he set the helicopter down on the narrow snow-swept highway, Alex deliberately landed so the tail of the aircraft pointed away from the accident.

Dale hopped out to guard the tailrotor, pulling his parka's fur-lined collar up to shield his face from the biting cold. His back to the wind as he stood with gloved hands tucked under his armpits, the craggy-faced pilot shivered in silence as he watched Russ and Kyle scurry off toward a lone medic waving at them from the warm confines of one of the Canmore ambulances.

"Man, we were afraid the weather would force you to turn back!" the medic shouted over the wind as he jumped out to greet them. "I don't mean to rush, but in the interests of self-preservation... both ours and the patient's, I'll give you the story as we go, okay? My name's Darrel, by the way." Tugging his frosted neck warmer over his nose, the medic started toward the snow covered wreckage.

"For the past twenty minutes, our firefighters have been trying to extricate your patient, but she's wedged head-down under the dash and every time we try to move her, she dumps her pressure! The Park Ranger who came across the accident had wrote her off as a Code thirty-two. He couldn't find a pulse and stated she had no discernible respiratory effort. I was about to write her off too, when I first assessed her. Severe hypothermia had her so peripherally shut down that it was only after we had her hooked up to our cardiac monitor that we discovered she had a rhythm!"

Both front and rear door posts of the compact sedan had been cut through using the hydraulic jaws. As the medics watched, four firefighters removed the crumpled roof and heaved it into the ditch. With the vehicle's bloodied interior now clearly visible, an EMT could be seen huddled down in the front seat talking to a motionless mound of white thermal blankets piled behind the steering wheel.

A moderately obese, middle-aged female, was buried under those blankets. After 20 minutes of aggressive warming and three litres of IV fluid, she was now semi-conscious, and had a BP of 80 systolic. With a swollen belly and broken pelvis, however, her blood pressure was as high as it was likely ever to get.

She had escaped the crash without a visible scratch, yet she was on the verge of bleeding to death. The force of impact with the steering wheel had ruptured something inside her abdomen, and while blankets and IV fluid were buying her time, her only real hope for survival lay in transportation to Calgary where a surgical team was standing by.

"Why don't you guys get set up," Darrel said. "I'll see if... " "Darrel, it's Tracy," a breathless female voice erupted from his hip-mounted radio. "The RCMP just found another adult male lying in the east ditch. Patient is unconscious with marginal resps and pulses. Major areas of frostbite covering the face and head. I sure could use a second set of hands over here."

"The east ditch?" A cloud of frozen mist billowed from the medic's nose-warmer. "Okay, look, get a secondary assessment done and I'll...."

"You've got your plate full here," the rapidly-chilling Kyle interrupted. "Russ and I can go help her out until you get this patient extricated and packaged."

Guided by the frenzied waving of an RCMP constable, the LIFE-STAR medics were directed to a spot further up the highway. Side-slipping down the steep embankment, both men cursed themselves for not bringing a flashlight.

Stumbling through the darkness, his face stung by ice pellets, Kyle finally saw a flicker of light ahead. A lone EMT was kneeling over something in the snow.

Tracy quickly brought her medical cavalry up to speed. "Hi, you guys must be Russ and Kyle. Darrel radioed you were coming. I'm Tracy. You know, I feel just awful about this. I did a walk-around of the scene checking for patients, but this guy must've been thrown at least a hundred feet. It was a Mountie setting out road flares who spotted him."

Swaddled beneath numerous thermal blankets, only the face of the mystery patient was visible. His frostbitten cheeks the texture of candle wax, a green oxygen mask sat perched atop his gaping mouth. As she slipped a C-collar around his neck, the EMT began her report.

"No ID or MEDIC ALERT on him. Pupils equal and brisk to react. Glasgow coma scale is only six, but his BP's a solid one hundred and forty systolic and his heart rate is eighty a minute. The cold has him pretty much shut down, but aside from the fact he reeks of alcohol, I can't seem to find anything wrong with him. He doesn't appear to have any injuries... no scrapes... no bruising... no fractures... nothing!"

Seasoned BTLS instructors, Kyle and Russ exchanged weary looks as they knelt to examine the patient. However, after several minutes of playing medical detective, they grudgingly admitted defeat as well.

"You know, if I didn't know the circumstances, I'd say this guy just plain and simple curled up in the snow and passed out!" Kyle muttered as he slowly got to his feet.

Gently squeezing a fingernail, Russ had not been able to elicit even the slightest twitch of purposeful movement. Nearly crushing the ultrasensitive nailbed on his second attempt, the medic watched with grim satisfaction as the patient made a feeble attempt to pull his hand away. Bending forward to sniff the guy's breath, Russ asked, "Did you do a dextrose level? He smells a bit like acetone. Could be a diabetic."

Tracy nodded and shook her head all at the same time. "I thought of that too, but I figured it could wait till we had him packaged and into the ambulance. As cold as he is, I doubt if I'll even be able to get an IV into him."

Appearing for all the world as if he were enjoying a peaceful afternoon nap, the stranger suddenly sighed, made a half-hearted attempt to yank his oxygen mask off, then smacked his lips together several times before snuggling under his blanket again.

"It's possible," Kyle theorized aloud as he positioned a wooden spine board next to the patient, "that maybe being drunk and all, this guy was so relaxed when he was thrown from the car... like maybe all the snow cushioned the landing and...."

Tracy and Russ carefully log-rolled the patient onto his side while Kyle slid the spine board underneath him.

"How long did you say since this happened?" Russ asked.

"We've been out here for a half-hour now and the accident probably took place an hour before that. These people are just damn lucky the Park Ranger happened by when he did. With a minus fifty wind-chill, another thirty minutes and they would've frozen to death!"

Russ checked his watch. Ten precious minutes had passed since their arrival. "Okay, this is how we're going to proceed. Tracy and I will get this guy packaged and moved to the ground ambulance. Kyle, you go back to see how the firefighters and that other medic are making out. Give me a shout on the radio when you have her extricated so I can tell the pilots to start up the helicopter."

Regardless of their suspicions, Russ and Tracy treated their patient as if he had a possible spinal injury. Russ called two of the Mounties for assistance. Even then, it was a struggle to lug the patient up the steep embankment and down the roadway to the waiting ambulance

"No you don't, pal. Just settle down. You've been in a little accident, but you're going to be fine," Russ gruffly reassured the increasingly combative patient as he pinned the uncooperative fellow's flailing arms against the stretcher so Tracy could tie them to the side rails.

"His primary assessment doesn't indicate a need to transport him by air. Get him on the cardiac monitor and set up an IV. While you're doing that, I'll go pack up your gear. You be okay?"

"I'll be fine," Tracy replied. "You know, we really appreciate you guys flying out here tonight. What with the weather and multiple patients and all, it's nice to know we have backup if we need it."

Russ, his helmet visor pulled part-way down to shield his watering eyes from the wind, followed the feeble beam of Tracy's fading flashlight as he hurried back toward the ditch. Anxious to find out how his partner was faring, Rusty's numb fingers fumbled for the send button on his chest-mounted radio. "Kyle, you got that patient extricated yet?"

"Almost! Give us five more minutes," Kyle replied.

"Good! I'll notify the pilots to get their bird fired up." All the while dreaming of his nice, warm bed, a chilled-to-the-marrow Russ knelt in the snow to begin gathering up Tracy's equipment.

Using a wooden backboard, Kyle and Darrel carefully removed the woman from her smashed car. Ever-so-gently placing her on the LIFE-STAR stretcher draped with two blankets and a pair of unfolded MAST pants, the medics snugly velcroed the trousers on. Busy with that, Kyle directed one of the firefighters to take a post-extrication BP.

"What? Sixty! You can only get a pressure of sixty on her?" the medic echoed, his frosty breath puffing like a steam engine. "Okay, let's not panic. She just didn't like being moved. Keep the blankets on and let's get her into the helicopter. The secondary assessment can wait until we've got her out of the cold."

Deftly slipping the woman's IV into a pressure infuser bag, Kyle wedged a small disposable hot pack down alongside. The hot pack would hopefully keep the saline solution from freezing up, while the infuser would pump the IV fluid in faster.

Hard at work inflating the MAST pants, Darrel reached over with his free hand to crank up the oxygen flow to the woman's non-rebreather face mask. A patient in shock could never be given too much oxygen, and this babe was definitely air-hungry.

As soon as the MAST pants were inflated, Kyle took another blood pressure. "Alright! We're back up to ninety systolic again. At least we haven't lost any ground," he shouted. "Okay, let's get moving!"

With several firefighters assisting, Darrel and Kyle were carting their patient to the chopper when an unexpected flash of light suddenly washed over them. Glancing back over their shoulders, the rescue workers stopped dead.

A canary yellow sports car was fishtailing wildly from side to side, careening down the hill directly toward them.

Ian McLennon would later tell police that "it all happened so fast." The teenager and his buddy had chosen the seldom-travelled Park roadway to check how well Ian's new Camaro could perform.

Because the RCMP had been unable to drive around the accident site to block-off traffic, a lone constable had walked up the hill to set up emergency flares. Half-frozen, he had been standing guard for over an hour now, and his flashlight was dimming.

Blinded by the driving snowfall, the teens had just narrowly missed running the cop over. As the frantically waving officer streaked past in Ian's peripheral vision, the inexperienced driver reacted in the worst way possible... slamming the brake peddle all the way to the floor.

Black ice, the result of snowflakes melting upon contact with the asphalt, then refreezing, sent the car's rear end into a sideways skid to the right. With all four tires locked up and sliding, the 17 year-old instantly realized his mistake. Easing up on the brake, he reefed the steering wheel hard in the direction of the skid.

The response was immediate. The vehicle quit fishtailing and incredibly, the terrified teen had actually regained control of the car as he crested the top of the hill... at 117 km/hr.

Ian's heart was hammering against his ribs. His birthday present wasn't even a week old. What would his old man say if he totaled it before he'd even made the first payment? The mentally distracted teen nervously squinted at the swirling blizzard of fat wet snowflakes stuccoing the car's windshield. As the wipers swept the slush to one side, what the kid saw next very nearly made his adrenalin-laced ticker stop beating totally.

"At the bottom of the hill were all these flashing lights... cars and fire trucks everywhere. I had to take the ditch or I would've creamed the guys carrying the stretcher. If there'd only been enough room to pass!" the teen whimpered as a stone-faced constable handed him a statement form to complete.

Thirty-five agonizing minutes later, the tearful adolescent was still struggling to get his side of the story down on paper. His hands were trembling so badly he was having difficulty just holding onto the pen. The last sentence was giving him the most trouble. The words on the page swam before his eyes. The cold reality of what he had done eventually proved too much for the Grade 11 student. His muffled sobs echoed in the stark isolation of the interrogation room. Still unfinished, that last line began: "I didn't see the guy in the ditch until we were right on top of him...."

34
ALL THE KING'S HORSES

Sitting at the controls of the revved-up chopper, Dale had seen it all. Now he could only watch as everyone began rushing toward the ditch. Unable to take his eyes from the horrific scene, he prayed. First he prayed that what he'd just seen had been an apparition. But as he was forced to listen to the frenzied chatter spilling out of the BK's radio, he began to pray for a miracle.

Kyle Stevens nearly went to pieces. This was no nameless stranger lying face-down in the snow. It was his best friend. His buddy. Rusty had been closer than a brother.

For several long seconds, Kyle forgot every paramedic skill he had ever been taught. Kneeling beside his unconscious friend, he tried to assess his injuries using the ABC method. The only trouble was... he could not remember what A, B or C stood for.

Darrel finally had to step forward and take charge. "Kyle, I want you to get the airway bag and the extra stretcher from our ambulance. Tracy and I will start the initial assessment."

Alex rushed over to see if he could help. Darrel saw him coming and jumped to his feet. Gripping the hood of Alex's parka, the Canmore medic forced him to turn away from the dreadful scene. After a tense exchange, the sickened pilot hurried off in search of an RCMP constable.

"That was our flight paramedic who went down!" Alex's voice cracked as he relayed Darrel's message to the cop. "We have a medical emergency here and we've got a blizzard bearing down on us from the northeast. Our other pilot is on the chopper radio to Calgary Flight Service right now so I need you to call the Canmore hospital on your mobile. Tell them to package up as much O negative blood as they can spare. We'll be bringing in two major traumas and the medic is requesting that a surgeon be standing by at the pad to accompany us on the flight back to Parkland Memorial."

As the constable vanished into the darkness, Alex looked back once more toward the cluster of bobbing flashlight beams illuminating Russ' crumpled form. For a distance of three feet to either side, the snow was red. Blood red.

Darrel and Tracy carefully rolled Russ onto his back. A reflex action caused his blood-caked eyelids to momentarily flicker open... exposing white eyes. As they watched, the medic's shattered mouth suddenly made a convulsive, fish-out-of-water gasp. While an untrained bystander might have thought Russ was attempting to breathe, one look at his motionless chest told the real story.

Gently probing the side of his muscular neck, Tracy thought she could detect a feeble pulsation beneath her gloved fingers. While feeble wasn't good, it did mean the heart was still pumping... and where there was a heart beat... there was life. Breathing or not, Russ was alive.

The area beneath him actually began to steam as his blood poured out onto the snow. As Tracy cut his flight suit away, a lacerated pelvic artery spurted blood into the night sky. Quickly stuffing a thick wad of gauze into the gaping wound, she felt Russ' shattered left hip collapse beneath her hands. Both feeling and hearing as the fragments of bone grated past each other, Tracy's stomach nearly heaved.

Darrel carefully removed Russ' helmet. The thousand dollar helmet was relatively unmarred, except in the front where a jagged piece of visor had broken away.

Holding Russ' head and neck steady while her partner checked for skull fractures, Tracy stared down at the bluish discoloration already evident under Rusty's eyes. Gently brushing his dark curls aside, the EMT noted a fist-sized bruise behind the left ear as well. Known in the medical business as Raccoon Eyes and Battle's Sign, the bruising most likely indicated a fracture at the base of the skull.

Kyle meanwhile, had returned with the equipment and immediately set up for intubation. Pausing only long enough to suction the throat clear of blood, Darrel slid the endotracheal tube into position and began bagging his patient with high flow oxygen while Kyle taped the tube to Russ' swollen face.

Seven minutes later, LIFE-STAR 1 was airborne and on its way to the Canmore hospital. Even with Darrel suctioning like a mad man to keep Russ' airway clear, dark red blood mixed with clear yellowish cerebral spinal fluid continued to ooze from everywhere. Nose. Mouth. Even from his ears... streaming down the sides of Russ' neck to form a jellied pool under his head. With his bruised eyelids now a ghastly shade of purple and his handsome features rapidly swelling completely out of proportion, Russell Patrick Andrews was mercifully no longer recognizable.

At 500 feet, the relentless Chinook winds battered the aircraft. Even with the Aussie's steadying hands at the controls, the 6,500 pound aircraft seemed bent on yawing to the left and flying sideways.

In preparation for the two-patient flight, Alex had stripped the back of the helicopter of all unnecessary equipment. Even with the spare seats folded up, it was a tight fit sliding the patients in, side by side. With the stretchers butted up against their knees, Kyle and Darrel could barely move as they did a quick reassessment their patients. The woman, adrift in a chemical haze, had stabilized for the time being. The same could not be said of the young man.

With Darrel in charge of Russ' care, Kyle had plenty of other worries to occupy his thoughts. He had four IVs to regulate, a multitude of blood-soaked dressings to reinforce, MAST pants and infuser bags to keep inflated, woefully unstable blood pressures to monitor, and ECG tracings and oxygen saturation readings to observe and record.

Jotting down a set of vital signs on the back of his glove, Kyle's lone coping mechanism was to murmur over and over, "He's just another trauma patient, just another trauma patient." Savagely shaking his head, he mentally screamed, "Stevens, concentrate man. Stay focused. Keep your mind on your job. You've got to keep these people alive!"

Security at the Canmore hospital had cordoned off part of the parking lot as a heli-pad. Immediately upon landing, Alex ran toward the emergency doors where a man stood waiting with a picnic cooler tucked under one arm. Squeezing on board, the surgeon went to work assessing both patients, then asked to speak to the pilot in charge. "I've got a patient back here who needs a central line started. If possible, I'd much rather do it while we're sitting on the ground."

"Weather's deteriorating real fast. Will five minutes be enough?"

"Five'll be enough," the doctor responded as he went straight to work threading a plastic catheter into Russ' neck. Besides blood, the IV would also give the medical crew a direct route for powerful life-supporting drugs if Russ' condition cratered during the trip.

Alex patched an urgent call through to Parkland Memorial Hospital. Handing the radio transmission over to the medics in the back, the pilot was eavesdropping to learn how Russ was doing when he felt a sharp rap on his shoulder. Dale was pointing a gloved finger at the front window. In their few minutes on the ground, a thick, sodden blanket of snow had totally obliterated the windscreen.

To try for Calgary now would be against everything either pilot had ever been taught. As if to emphasize the suicidal nature of the situation, a fierce gust of wind slammed into the BK, sending a spine-jarring shockwave reverberating through the fragile little craft.

Nearly flung from his seat, Kyle hurriedly wrapped up his call to Parkland. Alex flipped the radio back to the Flight Service frequency. "Calgary Flight Service Station, this is med-evac Charlie Gulf Papa Foxtrot Lima. How do you read? Over."

"Med-evac Charlie Gulf Papa Foxtrot Lima, this is Flight Service Station observer Calvin Hisand. Read you loud and clear. Over."

"Calvin, it's Alex Davis again. We're sitting on the pad at the Canmore hospital. It's snowing hard with winds gusting out of the west at sixty to seventy knots. Besides a wicked Chinook tail wind, what else can we expect en route to Calgary? Over."

"That's a negative Alex! Do not try for Calgary. The weather office has just downgraded their travel advisory to a blizzard warning. The RCMP have closed the Trans-Canada east and west and we are currently rerouting all incoming air traffic to Regina or Vancouver. Over."

Dale watched a large section of slush slide down his window. As captain of the aircraft, he carried sole responsibility for the safety of everyone on board. He activated his mike. "Uh doc, this is Captain Morgan. We have some mighty rough flying conditions between here and Calgary right now, and it's getting worse. If we remain here overnight, would the delay adversely affect either patient's chances for survival?"

"You want my honest opinion? We'll lose one, probably both. These patients need more than I can give them. They need an experienced trauma surgical team!"

The young physician looked up to find the two medics watching him anxiously. "Hey, I know what you people want me to say... 'Screw the weather. Let's try for Calgary anyway! This could be our guy's only hope!' Well that kind of macho hero crap is fine for the movies. If you want to risk it, go right ahead, only let me get out first."

A tomb-like silence settled over the helicopter.

"I know it was asking a lot," Darrel softly replied. "Thanks for putting in the central line for us. We'll be okay."

The doctor turned to stare at the storm raging against his window. The hospital was barely visible. "Look Morgan, you're the bloody captain. If, in your judgment, you feel it's unsafe to fly back to Calgary, then don't do it. Don't jeopardize four lives trying to save two! Be honest though, if it weren't one of your own lying back here, would you still want to risk it?"

Not waiting for a reply, the beleaguered doctor angrily motioned Darrel to surrender his helmet and exit the aircraft. Somehow, he already knew what the pilot's decision was going to be.

Struggling to keep control of his aircraft, Dale began tracking the east-bound section of the Trans-Canada. It was somewhere between the turnoff to Exshaw and a desolate stretch of scrub-brush prairie known as Deadman's Flats that the Aussie began doing something he was not supposed to do. He initiated instrument flight.

LIFE-STAR pilots were under strict orders to fly VFR or visual flight rules at all times. No exceptions. It was a rather ironic policy considering that a pilot had to have his or her instrument rating before being hired on by LIFE-STAR. They had to have it, but they were not allowed to use it.

Night flight minimums called for a cloud ceiling of at least 1000 feet above the highest obstacle on the flight plan. That ceiling had now dropped to less than 500 feet. While a fearsome tailwind had them zipping toward Calgary at nearly 200 knots, it was also pushing the small, egg-shaped craft off-course to the southeast.

With absolutely no visual ground markings to guide him, Dale's eyes never left the complex instrument panel. The altimeter and Horizontal Situation Indicator gauges had become his entire world. While the altimeter gave him a rough estimate of his altitude, it was the HSI, a high-tech compass showing his direction and heading, that would hopefully guide him home.

Because he had been forced to descend to less than 150 feet above ground in an attempt to minimize the effects of the treacherous crosswind, Morgan had entrusted his sharp-eyed co-pilot to keep him from splattering the million dollar aircraft into one of the sparsely lit highway overpasses that loomed up out of the darkness at irregularly spaced intervals. It was flights like this that made even veteran pilots cynically joke about what IFR really stood for: "I Follow Roads, Rivers and Railway tracks."

As Dale struggled to focus on his instruments, his thoughts kept going back to the report Kyle had given to Parkland regarding Russ' condition. "... fractured skull... blown pupil... decerebrate posturing... left leg nearly severed... pelvis smashed...." Even if by some miraculous act of God Russ somehow survived, what was his quality of life likely to be? An auxiliary hospital? A nursing home, maybe? So much for his sparkling personality and wit. So much for any kind of meaningful personality, period.

Fully aware that Calgary Dispatch would be pacing the floor, Dale waited ten long minutes into the flight before finally giving Alex the order to bring up the Provincial channel on the radio. Nearly half-way home now, the cunning Aussie knew the EMS dispatcher would be hard-pressed to order them back to Canmore.

Alex provided the dispatcher with a brief rundown of the situation, their present location and an ETA update, then asked to be patched through to Peter Lawson's home.

With the BK's nose crabbed 25 degrees to the left in order to maintain straight-ahead flight, as they waited for Peter to come on line, Alex heard his partner mutter, "I suppose I can always get a job flying for some drug cartel down in South America."

Amidst a burst of radio static, a gravely voice filled both men's headsets. "LIFE-STAR One, this is Peter Lawson. Come in. Over."

"Sir, this is Dale. We are currently inbound to Parkland Hospital with an ETA of fifteen minutes. We have two critical multi-traumas on board as well as a doctor we picked up in Canmore. Over."

As the wipers fought to keep the windshield clear of snow, tiny beads of sweat began to trickle down Dale's chest. Russ. The weather. The possibility of ice build-up. The God damn wind. The God damn visibility. Would Peter fire him? Would Peter kill him? Would he end up killing himself and everyone else on board. His mind a cluttered jumble of worries, the pilot was jolted back to reality by a roar of pre-transmission static.

"LIFE-STAR One, this is Peter Lawson. Dale, I copied your last transmission. What is the nature of your problem? Over."

"This is LIFE-STAR One. Sir... I uh... have some very bad news. Russ Andrews was hit by a car while on-scene. He is our second patient. The Canmore doc considers his injuries to be life-threatening. In view of that, I feel you should contact Angie and Russ' mom immediately and have them meet us at Parkland Memorial.

"We're following the Trans-Canada back and have just passed abeam the Ghost Lake Dam. We are presently experiencing strong crosswinds, poor visibility and icing conditions. It's taking everything we've got to stay on course, so this will likely be our last position report until touching down at Parkland. Over."

"I copy that, Dale. Please keep me advised if you have to divert from your intended flight path. I'll contact Angie and Mrs. Andrews and meet you at the hospital. I'll also notify city dispatch that we'll be temporarily out of service. Lawson out."

As the doctor continued to hyperventilate Russ, Kyle wedged his snowboot between the stretchers for balance as he reached forward to hang two more units of packed cells from the ceiling-mounted IV hooks. The doctor tersely reminded Kyle that he wanted a Mannitol drip set up as well. The powerful diuretic would hopefully decrease the mounting pressure inside Russ' skull. Before it could be infused, however, Kyle had to first attach a special filter into the IV line. On a calm flight, it was a piece of cake, but tonight, with his hands shaking and the chopper bouncing sideways across the sky, it was the equivalent to trying to thread a peti-point needle while white-water canoeing.

Collapsing back into his seat, Kyle wearily reached for his clipboard and set about catching up on his charting. Making note of the Mannitol infusion, the medic suddenly paused. His pen hovered unsteadily above the section asking for a brief inflight evaluation of his patient's condition. What was there to say?

Russ was not breathing on his own and had been showing decerebrate posturing ever since his head had cracked like a ripe cantaloupe against the car's windshield. With his arms and legs stiffly extended and his toes pointed downward, bleeding into the brain was causing his forearms to rotate inward to the point that the backs of his hands were pressed up tight against his hips. Even more unsettling was the involuntary shivering of his entire body, as if an invisible chill was constantly sweeping over him.

Kyle gently pried the grossly swollen eyelids apart. The left pupil showed a sluggish reaction, but the right was completely blown. Fixed and dilated to almost 6 mm, it was like staring down into a big black hole. The blown pupil indicated increasing intracranial pressure. Kyle knew it was an ominous combination of symptoms. The doctor knew it too. So did Darrel and Tracy back in Canmore. They all knew it, yet they also knew they had to try.

With the ghostly glow of Calgary's street lights growing brighter on the eastern horizon, the Canmore doc once again slid a suction catheter down Russ' endotracheal tube to clear it of blood and mucous. Russ showed absolutely no response at having the catheter shoved down his windpipe and into the extremely sensitive passages of the lungs. He didn't cough or gag—nothing.

The western edge of the city now in sight, Dale switched on the intercom. "ETA is two minutes. The wind is really kicking up, so make sure all your equipment is strapped down tight. I don't want anything getting sucked up into the rotor blades."

Kyle and the doc busied themselves connecting oxygen tubing to portable scout tanks, unhooking the pressure infusers from the ceiling and checking to make sure their patients' tangle of monitor cables were secured to the correct stretcher.

"We're sixty-five knots... five hundred feet... sink is five," Alex called out as Dale began his approach.

Parkland's pad had never rated among the LIFE-STAR pilots' favorite places to touch down. It was bordered by a steep drop-off to the south, a fully-occupied night staff parking lot to the east, and the hospital's power plant to the west. None of these hazards troubled Dale as much as the massive fortress which framed the pad to the northeast—the hospital's formidable west wing. He could almost feel the rudely-awakened patients glaring down at him from the upper floors.

While crashing into the building was a remote possibility, wind shear caused by the huge superstructure was creating absolute havoc with his usually flawless approach. One minute he was struggling to correct for a blustery northwest wind; a split second later, he and his helicopter were being savagely blasted sideways toward the four-story power plant as fierce crosswinds funneled around the main building from the east.

"Fifty knots... three hundred feet... sink is six. Forty knots... one hundred feet... sink is four."

They had reached the LDP or Landing Decision Point. With a mere hundred feet between his aircraft's skids and the ground, Dale had to decide whether to commit to the landing or abort.

"Going around!" the Aussie barked angrily as he was forced to swing the BK up and out over the river valley in search of less turbulent air. "Jesus Christ!" he cursed. "What's it going to take to get this damn machine on the ground?

"Alex, that visitor's parking lot around front is looking better and better. If I can't put her down there, we'll have to divert to the Mountainview." While it was not an accredited trauma facility, the Rockpile would have to do, as the Riverside Medical Center, with its equally-dangerous elevated landing pad, was out of the question.

The deserted parking lot, sheltered by the east wing, lay smothered beneath a sea of drifting snow. Dale set up for his approach one last time. "We're committed."

"Clear on my side," Alex said. "Power coming in... torque is fifty... torque is sixty... torque is steady at sixty-five."

At fifty feet above the ground, a white cloud boiled up around the aircraft. Flying blind, Dale did the only thing he could... continue with his descent. With his eyes glued to the artificial horizon as the helicopter sank slowly into the whirling maelstrom, he relaxed as he felt the right skid scrape hard against something. Gently easing the cyclic to the left to set the port skid down, the 'copter didn't level out. Instead, it began rolling onto its side.

As Dale shoved the cyclic hard to the right to prevent a catastrophe, an amber warning light on the instrument console started to flash. Seething with rage, he yanked up on the collective control. The helicopter rocketed straight up.

"Enough of this crap! I'm diverting to the Mountainview."

"No, wait! Look...." said Alex. The rotor-whipped snow cloud below had begun to dissipate and they could clearly see an off-white concrete parking divider sporting a foot-long scuff of black paint.

Thirty seconds later, with the cursed divider tucked squarely between the BK's skids, Alex peeled back the tight-fitting cuff of his Nomex glove. Squinting down at the gleaming Rolex beneath, he entered the time on his mission trip log sheet: 12:34 a.m.

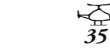

35
WORDS ARE NOT ENOUGH

Both patients were immediately transported inside to the Emergency Department's Code Room where two trauma teams were standing by. As doctors, nurses, respiratory specialists and X-ray and lab techs swarmed over each patient, Kyle Stevens had never felt more alone in his entire life. Always before he had felt palpable relief as his patient was transferred off the LIFE-STAR stretcher and onto that cold steel examining table. Not tonight.

Fighting to stay in emotional control, Kyle gamely stepped forward to give report. He got the first few sentences out, about the woman's car crash and her condition inflight. But as he began to describe his friend's accident and injuries, his husky voice took on an audible tremor. A basketball-sized lump squeezing off his windpipe, Kyle choked to a stop in mid-sentence.

"It's okay," the Canmore doc said softly as he placed a steadying hand on the paramedic's shoulder. "I'll finish report.

"Why don't you see if Russ' family have arrived yet," he added with just the right amount of firmness as he reached for the metal clipboard. "They're going to need someone to talk to... someone to sit with them. You've done all you can here... more than any close friend should ever have to do."

Kyle took a last look at his partner. Most of the trauma room staff had been so busy infusing blood, inserting drainage catheters, drawing lab work and setting up for X-rays that they'd failed to notice the ashen, quivering-lipped medic.

The nurse cutting off Russ' tattered flight suit sucked in a deep breath as she got a closeup look at the massive injuries underneath. Staring down at the uniform in her hands, she read the black leather name tag velcroed to the front pocket.

"Oh my God!" she gasped. "We know this guy! This is... is... Russ Andrews!"

Oblivious to time and place, his hands stained with his best friend's blood, Kyle aimlessly wandered the maze of corridors. Normally, he and Russ would be prowling the nurses' lounge in search of a doughnut and coffee right about now. Then Russ would toss a couple of bucks into the collection can and take two extra cups back for the pilots. But not tonight.

Kyle slumped hard against the wall. Tears cascaded down his whisker-stubbled cheeks. He'd begun to hear voices. Someone was calling his name over and over. Incredibly, it seemed to be coming from his own flight helmet which dangled like a severed head from his trembling hand.

Dropping the helmet to the floor with a hollow crash, the medic cupped his hands over his ears in a futile attempt to block out the voices that was growing steadily louder. "Kyle? It's Dale. Are you okay?"

With vacant eyes, Kyle slowly looked up at the chopper pilot standing over him.

Captain Dale Morgan knew only too well that thousand yard stare. While serving in 'Nam, he had witnessed the dreadful carnage of soldiers driven mad with battle-fatigue. The sound of their insane, psychotic laughter. Being forced to dive for cover as a mentally unhinged GI fired his rifle at anything that moved. No longer able to cope with the death and destruction that was just another typical day on patrol, few such men survived long enough to be airlifted out to a stateside mental facility.

It was during his second tour of duty, however, that Dale had picked up on something he'd never been able to fully explain. The men who broke down and cried after a hellish battle always seemed to fare the best, mentally that is.

The soldiers who hid their feelings away were a much different story. Those dead eyes. That far-away look reflecting a soul where life and death had lost all meaning and where overpowering human aggression was either positively channeled outward—as in slaughtering the enemy, or negatively inward—suicide.

While Dale passed himself off as a tough guy, he had cried his share of tears at the loss of a good friend. Nothing unmanly about showing a little emotion. Cleansed the soul. Forced you to deal with your feelings head-on. A lot better than harboring those tortured emotions inside you for the rest of your life.

Russ' accident had breathed new life into a hundred horrid memories from the veteran aviator's dark past. It was only by concentrating every conscious thought on flying that Dale had been able to keep his own feelings safely under wraps. But now, in the deserted hallway with the emotional wreckage that was Kyle Stevens, he could feel himself start to lose it.

One of the porters who had helped carry Russ' stretcher in from the parking lot had a story to tell the emerg nurses as they straggled into the lounge for their 3:30 a.m. coffee break.

"You know that LIFE-STAR medic who brought Andrews in... well, I saw him standing in the corridor down by Materiel Management just bawling his eyes out. One of the chopper pilots had his arms around him... trying to comfort him. But if you ask me, the pilot didn't look like he was holding it together much better. He was crying, too."

36
THE QUIET ROOM

Peter Lawson was directed to escort Angie and Mrs. Andrews to the E.R.'s "Quiet Room." This was a special waiting area for relatives of critically-ill emergency patients. It was a cramped, windowless room, but it contained all the essentials: a pull-out couch, soft chairs, TV, telephone, coffee machine, magazines, and boxes and boxes of tissues. Peter gave each teary woman a comforting hug before heading off in search of his insubordinate flight crew.

Checking in at the admitting desk, the worried LIFE-STAR manager was about to have his wayward crew paged when he spotted them coming down the hall with a doctor. Dale introduced the grim-faced neurologist to his boss. Learning that the Andrews family had arrived, the specialist immediately set off for the Quiet Room.

"Kyle," Peter suggested as he glanced at the medic's red-rimmed eyes, "would you go with him? Mrs. Andrews and Angie are pretty shook up."

As soon as Stevens was out of ear shot, Peter's icy stare settled on the two pilots.

"I'll have a written report on your desk within the hour, sir."

"That goes without saying, Captain Morgan," Peter shot back. "The last weather report I received said the blizzard warning for Calgary and area should be lifted around six a.m. As such, I've notified city dispatch that we will be back on line as of eight o'clock shift change...."

"I'm afraid that might not be possible," Dale interrupted. He moved his gaze from the floor to his employer's heavily-jowled face. "I accidentally set off the Mast Moment Indicator when we landed. That means the bolts connecting the rotor mast to the head will all have to be retorqued. I've already called Jim Forbes about it. He said it'd only take an hour or so to fix, but he won't be able to come in right away because he can't get his car to start."

Lawson silenced his chief pilot with a stiff, unfeeling shake of his head. "Oh, what the hell. Why don't you just fly over and pick him up?"

"Mrs. Andrews, this is Dr. Terry Hammon, Russ' neurologist," Kyle said. "And this is Russ' girlfriend, Angie Jackson."

Sitting himself down on the coffee table, the physician took the older woman's trembling hands in his. "Mrs. Andrews, your son was taken to the Operating Room about five minutes ago. His condition on admission was so unstable that we were unable to wait for you to arrive to give your consent for surgery. In such a situation, two doctors can legally sign the consent. In this case, it was myself and the trauma surgeon on-call.

As your son's neurologist, I've just been reviewing his CT scan and I'm afraid it doesn't look good. Russ has suffered severe bruising of his brain as well as a fractured neck. While the spinal cord appears intact, his brain is very swollen. Unfortunately, there is nothing surgically that can be done to alleviate this condition. As the physician in charge of your son's care, I must tell you this straight out. Russ' present neurological status is such that he may not survive the night."

The doctor paused, as if to give his first bombshell time to sink in. "In addition to the brain swelling, Russ has also suffered several other life-threatening injuries. He is bleeding internally, his pelvis is badly broken and his left leg was nearly severed at the knee. Blood loss has been enormous, but we've transfused him to the point that he now has enough blood pressure to withstand surgery."

The doctor turned to Angie. "Miss Jackson, it says on the chart that you're a flight nurse with LIFE-STAR and that you used to work in ICU. Is that correct?"

Silently, Angie nodded.

"Miss Jackson, sudden brainstem herniation within the next few hours is Russ' greatest threat. I'd place the odds at fifty percent. We're going to do everything in our power to prevent it, but if it does happen, total cessation of brain activity will occur. For right now, however, my greatest concern is that without immediate surgery, there is a one hundred percent chance Russ will bleed to death.

"Dr. David Blaines is the trauma surgeon on-call tonight. He and his team will attempt to pack off the open fractures of both the pelvis and leg. Once that's done, an exploratory lap will be performed to locate the source of the internal bleeding. As well, with the damage to Russ' left leg being so extensive, there is the very real possibility that they may be forced to amputate it. Dr. Blaines' primary objective is to control the bleeding, nothing more. I don't like having a patient with a severe head injury under anesthesia for an extended period of time. If further surgery is indicated, it can be done at a later date, when Russ is hopefully more stable."

As the doctor's words faded, Angie felt an awful numbness envelop her. It was only Kyle's crushing grip on her hand that kept her from losing all touch with reality.

The doctor picked up the yellow sheet of paper he had brought with him. "I know this may seem like a moot point with your son already in the O.R., but I'd like you to sign this. In the event Russ does need to be taken back for more surgery, we'll need your consent." Quickly scratching his name to the bottom, he handed it to Emily.

She stared blankly at the form. Eventually she signed her name on the line the doctor had marked with an X and handed it back.

37
IN SOMEONE ELSE'S MOCCASINS

Peter finally had to order Kyle to catch a taxi back to the hangar. More than anything else, Stevens wanted to remain at the hospital to learn how the surgery went, but with a mountain of blood-splattered paperwork awaiting him at the LIFE-STAR office, he also knew that Lawson was right. The heartless son-of-a-bitch was always right.

Thus it was while Kyle was back at the hangar, struggling to complete Russ' Patient Care Report, that his best friend was lifted off the O.R. table and taken directly to the Trauma ICU.

Outside the Trauma unit's automated double doors, was a tiny room tucked off by itself. It was the ICU's very own Quiet Room. At 2:45 a.m., it provided emotional shelter to three very tired and troubled women. Melissa, Russ' sister had just arrived. Two years younger than her brother, she'd been forced to roust her little girl from bed to drop her off at a friend's. Five months pregnant and with her husband out of town on business, Melissa sat slumped against Emily on the vinyl couch. Watching as mother and daughter consoled each other, Angie's worried thoughts drifted to another time and place.

She had always believed that twelve years of Intensive Care nursing had prepared her for almost anything the world could throw at her. She'd been wrong. Dead wrong.

Angie remembered back to all the times she had taken that long walk down to the Mountainview's Quiet Room so she could talk to a patient's family... either to tell them that everything was going to be fine or that things weren't looking too good and that the doctor would be in shortly to explain the situation in more detail.

That last line had always been difficult to say with a straight face. When an ICU nurse was forced to admit that "things weren't looking too good," it usually meant the rustle of angel wings had been detected in the patient's room and that the situation the doctor was about to explain involved letting the patient "go." That is, supportive care only. No heroic measures. No resuscitation. In other words... asking for the family's permission to allow the patient to die with some degree of dignity and respect.

If the patient met all the legal criteria, the most important being "no viable cerebral function," this was usually the point where the doctor would ask the patient's family about possible organ donation.

It was a difficult concept to talk about because most families didn't have a clue as to how the body functioned, let alone what brain death meant. They were usually in a state of shock, having gone for hours or days with little sleep or nourishment, and now here was the doctor whom they had entrusted to save their loved one's life... asking if he could have their okay to "pull the plug!"

Worse still, the doctor was actually seeking their permission to carve up their beloved parent, sibling, son or daughter so the organs could be transplanted into some total stranger.

Thanks to the inaccuracy of most TV medical dramas, a lot of families had some pretty weird ideas about what the doctor was really trying to say. Some even believed the doctor was throwing in the towel because they were poor, or without medical coverage.

In most cases, the physician didn't press the issue. What was the point? The family had every right to say no, but to the frustrated intensivist having to do the asking, it always seemed like such a waste. Thousands of perfectly good organs were being buried in the ground or sent to crematoriums on a daily basis while an equal number of desperate men, women and children clung to life... hooked up to dialysis machines or ventilators or aortic balloon pumps... waiting for that all important call that a perfect match had finally been located.

The doctor would do his best to explain all this to the potential donor's family. The patient's body would always be treated with respect. Yes, you could still have an open casket at the funeral if you wished.

Sometimes mentioning the fact that a part of their loved one would remain alive, helping someone else live a better life, was easier for the family to accept. Or maybe it was just the idea that some measure of good could come out of a senseless tragedy.

Angie was brooding over these morbid thoughts when a nurse knocked softly on the door. She stepped hesitantly into the room. "I'm looking for the Andrews' family."

"TELL ME HE'S STILL ALIVE!" Melissa cried out, clutching her mother for support. "I'M HIS SISTER... TELL ME RUSTY'S GOING TO MAKE IT... THAT'S HE'S GOING TO BE OKAY!"

"Russ is alive," the nurse reassured. "He was transferred down to us from the Operating Room about ten minutes ago. The surgeon Dr. Blaines is with him right now... helping us settle him into the unit. Before I go any further, I'd like to introduce myself. My name is Pam Lytle and I'm the nurse who'll be looking after Russ tonight."

"Hello Pam, I'm Mrs. Andrews," Emily replied as she got to her feet. "This is Melissa, my daughter and this is Russ' girlfriend, Angie Jackson. Please forgive us. We've all been though so much in the last few hours."

"Mrs. Andrews, there's no need to apologize. Before I take you in to see your son, however, I want to tell you a bit about what you're going to see. If you've never been in an ICU before, it can be pretty overwhelming. Russ' condition is extremely critical. The doctor had to make an opening in his throat, a tracheostomy, in order to help him breathe. Metal tongs also had to be implanted into his skull to stabilize his neck fracture. And I must inform you that unfortunately, the surgeon was unable to save Russ' left leg. He was forced to perform an above-knee amputation."

Walking her patient's family toward the double doors that guarded the entrance to the ICU, Pam Lytle reached out to slip her arm around Melissa. The show of compassion truly came from the heart. Knowing there was nothing more she could do for this family, Pam unselfishly gave them the only thing she could... her deepest sympathy.

Ushering the three women past bed after bed of patients who all appeared to be more dead than alive, Pam finally stopped at a jumble of bleeping, hissing equipment which surrounded bed number six. Russ' bed.

Sitting at the nursing station, a haggard surgeon in green O.R. scrubs looked up from his charting at the women huddled around his patient's bed. Staring down at the page of orders he'd just written, the doctor rubbed his bloodshot eyes. Rising from his chair, Dr. Blaines wearily flipped the chart shut and started toward bed six.

Mrs. Andrews bent over Russ. She reached down to touch his chest, formerly covered with dark hair, now shaved clean. His skin—more marble than skin—contrasted sharply with the colorful tangle of ECG wires, pressure lines and ventilator tubing strewn like party streamers across it.

"Honey, you're going to be just fine," she whispered, tenderly caressing her first-born. Melissa and Angie are here, too."

Her eyes filling with tears, Pam stepped forward to place a comforting hand on Emily's shoulder.

Angie meanwhile, stood all alone at the foot of the bed. Balancing on knees which were threatening to buckle, Angie clutched at the metal siderail for support as she inched her way toward the head of the bed. The color instantly drained from her face.

A thick dressing covered the right side of Rusty's head. Snaking out from under the multiple layers of white gauze, a gray intra-cranial probe cable stretched up to a pressure monitor above the bed. Two small holes had been drilled into his shaved skull, one just above each ear. A pair of thin steel rods, very much like old-fashioned ice tongs, had been tightly screwed into the holes. Attached by rope, via a pulley system, to a ten pound sandbag which dangled off the edge of the bed, the seemingly medieval contraption was needed to keep Russ' fractured neck in proper alignment.

A small plastic tube sprouted from just below his Adam's apple. Through a corrugated ventilator tube attached to it, Russ' chest rose and fell at precisely-timed intervals as the expensive life-support machine took over all the work of breathing for him.

Subconsciously, Angie evaluated Russ' status. The ashen, cadaverous skin. The bloated face. The fact that he was not assisting the ventilator. The extremely high cerebral pressure reading. The slow, plodding beat of his heart. The icy touch of his lifeless hand.

Who was this person with his thick, wavy hair gone and the gross purplish edema cruelly distorting his princely features? This couldn't be Russ Andrews. Not her Russ Andrews. Not her very best friend in the entire world. This could not be the same man who'd come within minutes of making mad, passionate love to her only a few short hours ago.

But as she cradled the stranger's hand in hers, Angie recognized the gold ring on his little finger. Though caked with dried blood, she could still make out its raised inscription: SAIT EMT-P.

Angie knew that Russ' pinky ring had become so tight he'd had great difficulty taking it off. She also knew that only one paramedic from his class had an emerald for a birthstone. As she lifted his limp hand to her face, the overhead light caught the gemstone at just the right angle, causing it to flash... a greenish flash.

A sudden rage swept over her. Determined to prove the doctors wrong, Angie pressed down hard against Russ' thumbnail. "Move! Just twitch! Come on, Rusty! Please!"

Russ' flaccid body lay perfectly motionless.

Angie glanced at the ventilator control panel. In order to hyperventilate and thus hopefully lessen Russ' brain swelling, the $30,000 machine had been set at 22 breaths a minute. She watched it cycle several times, hoping for some kind of miracle to take place, but the ventilator's assist light never came on once. Russ was not making any respiratory effort at all.

Kyle had earlier confided that Rusty had been real hard to bag inflight because he'd been biting down on his ET tube. Angie leaned over to check the airway gauge on the ventilator. It was registering a pressure of 20. A very nice, very respectable pressure for anyone on a vent. There shouldn't be any problem bagging him now. Russ wasn't seizing anymore. He wasn't making any chewing motions. He wasn't doing very much of anything anymore.

"Have you had to give him much sedation?" Angie asked.

Knowing exactly what her nursing counterpart wanted so desperately to hear, Pam sadly shook her head. "Since coming back from O.R., I haven't had to give him any sedation at all."

Without meaning to, Pam had pretty well summed up the story in Angie's mind. Deep down, however, Angie still had to know for herself. She had to be absolutely certain that what the life-support equipment and the pressure readings were trying to tell her... were in fact, the God-awful truth.

Leaning over the siderail, she gently pried her man's swollen eyelids apart. Both pupils were huge. Seven millimeters dilated and frozen at mid-line... like two bottomless black pits. They did not constrict down like normal pupils when exposed to light. The involuntary corneal blink reflex was also absent. Worst of all, they no longer had any sparkle... any vitality... any life.

Rusty had the eyes of a week-old corpse.

Pressing his hand against her cheek, Angie closed her eyes and cried. All she could think about was what his voice had sounded like... what his kisses had tasted like... what making love with him had felt like.

As she stood sobbing, a strange sensation crept over her. It was an unnerving awareness she'd experienced many times before while working in her old ICU. It was hard to explain, but Angie could no longer sense Russ' presence. His battered body might be lying on the bed in front of her... attached to a million tubes and wires, but his soul had taken flight. Clutching his hand to her tear-washed face, she could feel no warmth in it. No energy.

Rusty was no longer there.

Seeing his chance, the doctor stepped forward, motioning everyone to follow him away from the bedside. "Mrs. Andrews? I'm Dr. Blaines. I'm afraid I have very bad news. When the car struck your son, he suffered a critical closed head injury, resulting in a tremendous amount of brain swelling. The simple fact he was wearing a helmet is the only reason he survived as long as he did.

Angie felt her stomach contract. The doctor was talking in the past tense.

"During surgery," the physician continued, "the massive swelling caused Russ' brainstem to herniate down through the base of his skull. There was nothing any of us could have done to prevent it. The damage was just too extensive. The things that made Russ so unique... his personality, his smile, his laugh... have all been destroyed. If it's any comfort to you, according to the paramedic reports, your son was knocked unconscious on impact. He never suffered any pain."

"NO! IT ISN'T TRUE... YOU'RE LYING. RUSTY'S GOING TO MAKE IT!"

Angie was only dimly aware of Melissa's screams. The doctor's voice was echoing... as if down a long hallway. "No viable blood circulation to the brain... clinically dead... on life-support... no wallet found... did they know how Russ felt about organ donation?"

"Rusty never carried his wallet with him when he went on a flight," Angie heard herself answer. "But I know he has a signed donor card. I was his witness."

As the doctor hurried off in search of the necessary forms, Angie, Melissa and Emily went back to see Russ one last time.

Waiting until Russ' mom and sister had said their good-byes, Angie collapsed heavily against the bed's siderail. With her hot salty tears splashing one after the other upon his face, she gave Russ a final, lingering sweet kiss upon his swollen lips.

"Rusty... I love you so much. I wish I'd told you that more often," she whimpered. "Honey, I want you to know that you won't have to worry about me, okay? I'll be good. I promise. I won't have you to keep me out of trouble anymore, so I guess I'll have to be. I love you Rusty. I love you so much. I always will. Always."

Things moved along very rapidly after that. The consent forms were explained and signed. A lab tech was called stat so blood and tissue typing could begin. The results were then relayed by telephone to various provincial organ procurement programs across Canada. The search for that all elusive "perfect match" was on.

The Operating Room was notified of a multiple organ harvest, the ghoulish medical term used when several organs were to be removed for transplantation. Five good tissue matches had been confirmed. Hospital transplant teams were contacted and placed on emergency standby. Calls to the Calgary airport were made and private jets booked for immediate transportation of the organs to their various destinations.

LIFE-STAR 1 had occasionally been called upon to ferry the organ procurement teams to and from the hospital to save travel time... and this case would be no different.

The call came in at 09:45, just as Jim Forbes was retorquing the last bolt in the helicopter's mast assembly. The grieving pilots and medical crew on duty that fateful morning never once quizzed the surgeons with any of their usual questions: "What happened to the donor? Where are the organs being sent? How long had the recipient been on the waiting list?" They only stared bleakly at the three Styrofoam picnic coolers strapped to the stretcher. And they said nothing.

The temperature was minus 21 Celsius outside and it was not much warmer inside the helicopter, and yet for some strange reason, LIFE-STAR paramedic Michael Brown felt compelled to slide open his small side window on the pretext of letting in some fresh air.

While not one person would later admit to it, stale air was not the only problem plaguing the flight. A strange presence seemed to be among them... almost as if a fifth, unseen crew member was on board.

Was Michael hoping to let some fresh air in, or was he desperately trying to help something escape? Something that may have been left behind in the confusion of an earlier mission and now was not quite sure where to go?

A human soul... perhaps.

38
POMP AND CIRCUMSTANCE

Brilliant spotlights of sunshine streamed down from the pale blue heavens, glittering off the fluffy, new fall of snow with an intensity that was blinding. It was a Christmas card winter's day, perfect for a wedding celebration... not the sombre finality of a funeral procession.

It was a rather bizarre thing to be thinking about as she rode to the church with Kyle and Jennifer, but the department stores with their festive Christmas trappings reminded Angie of the present she had bought for Russ. A one-piece designer ski suit... bright red... for curving turns through the really deep stuff.

Like every good consumer, she had kept her receipt. That would not be a problem, but the clerk was bound to ask why she was returning it. What was she going to say... that it was the wrong size... the wrong color... her boyfriend had split for a warmer climate?

As Kyle drove off in search of a parking spot, Angie and Jennifer started toward the white brick church. A large number of people were already gathered out front. Though the service was not scheduled to begin for another half-hour, the small community chapel was rapidly filling to capacity.

Stepping inside, Angie was immediately enveloped by her family. Dutifully accepting their tearful hugs and words of condolence, she then walked over to express her sympathy to the Andrews family.

All the while, a steady flow of people were passing through the doors. Most were strangers, but as many were wearing their dress uniforms, it was not hard to figure out who they represented. Fellow medics Russ had worked with. Firefighters from the stations at which he'd been posted. Members of the local police force he gotten to know over the years. All had come to pay their final respects.

After hotly debating the issue with his second in command, Lawson had made the formal announcement that LIFE-STAR 1 would remain on emergency standby during the funeral service. It was then left to a furious Bateman to notify Calgary dispatch that the chopper's daycrew would be in attendance at the funeral. Should a scramble call come in, a police cruiser would be available to whisk them back, with lights and sirens, to the hangar.

As cold and insensitive as it sounded, Lord Peter was not alone in his opinion that the helicopter should stay in service despite the funeral. The rescue business was a dangerous job. Crawling around inside burning buildings, getting punched in the face by thankless drunks, fishing decomposing bodies out of the weir, worrying about powerlines and trees and other "rotor unfriendly" obstacles at two a.m. while setting down at the scene of a rain-swept multi-vehicle wreck.

To most police officers, medics or firefighters, the need for the occasional X-ray or suture was acceptable. But death was something rarely discussed. And if you asked any of them—even the bomb squad specialists—about the hazards of their work, most would stoically reply that more colleagues had been snuffed driving home than on duty.

At precisely two o'clock, an EMS ambulance rolled to a stop in front of the church. Kyle pulled on a pair of black leather gloves and went outside to join the rest of the pallbearers.

Along with Kyle, Dale, Alex, Howard and flight paramedic Michael Brown, there was Russ' former fire hall captain, Bill Scott—the man who'd signed them up for the training camp. Dale and Alex wore dark blue suits; the medics and firefighter the starched dress uniforms of their profession. As they took their positions to either side of the brown and silver casket, a brisk Chinook breeze brushed an airy hand through each man's neatly groomed hair.

Transporting Russ' body by ambulance instead of the traditional hearse caused raised eyebrows among the non-medical mourners. But to close friends of the cocky, egotistical paramedic, it was a symbol.

That shiny white ambulance had been Russ' home away from home. How many thousands of patients had felt the magical touch of Russ Andrews' caring hands... had their fears calmed by his confident smile... their pain eased through his expert medical skills... their tears acknowledged with compassion and reassurance? Using the ambulance as a hearse was an unspoken affirmation that Russ' career was his life, and that he'd made the ultimate sacrifice... unselfishly giving his own life to save another.

Because Russ had been a firefighter for eight years prior to becoming a paramedic, the Fire Chief had asked permission to provide an Honor Guard. Lining both sides of the walkway to the church, smartly decked out in their dark blue "Number Ones," forty firefighters stood at attention. An awe-inspiring sight, the Honor Guard also formed a barrier to hold back the crowd. Estimated at over seven hundred, friends, strangers, plus Emergency Rescue Personnel from all over the country spilled out onto the street.

As a lone bagpiper's rendition of Amazing Grace haunted the warm breeze, the pallbearers lifted the coffin and started toward the church. As the procession passed between their ranks, the Honor Guard suddenly saluted as one. Like the solitary piper, the salute was a time-honored firefighting tradition, a show of respect for a fallen comrade.

Inside, the straining pallbearers gently placed Russ' casket down at the front of the church. The six men momentarily paused. Then, taking one step back, they snapped off a crisp salute of their own. Final farewell acknowledgment of their friend.

The pastor made certain that all the prayers and hymns were done right. Then, to the surprise of nearly everyone, he handed the service over to one Peter Frederick Lawson.

Reading glasses perched on the end of his nose, his hands gripping the wooden pulpit like an old-time evangelist, Peter's eulogy took a look back at Russ' accomplishments and unfulfilled dreams. Slack-jawed LIFE-STAR employees could not believe what they were hearing. When the heck had Lawson had a heart transplant?

Nearing the end of his speech, Lord Peter paused.

Angie, seated in the front row and staring at a twisted facial tissue in her hands, immediately felt as if someone were watching her. Almost afraid to, she raised her head and found a misty-eyed Lawson staring back.

"Rusty's warmth and good humor touched many people's lives, but he saved the very best he had for the young woman in his life. She was his fire... his light... the reason for that special twinkle in his eyes."

Fishing madly through her purse for another Kleenex, Angie's fingers closed around a crumpled ball. Angie instantly realized what it was. Russ' paramedic class ring. His mother had given it to her. Unwrapping the thick gold band, she slipped it onto the third finger of her left hand.

Staring down at the specks of dried blood that still caked its deeply-molded crevices, the fact that Rusty was really gone and was not coming back hit Angie all at once. Her muffled sobs echoed through the chapel.

With a loud thump of his fist on the pulpit, and in a voice cracking with emotion, Peter drew his eulogy to a close. "See you later, Big Guy!"

The minister then stepped forward to perform the "ashes to ashes... dust to dust" ritual. The service was over.

Though surrounded by caring friends and family, Angie found herself struggling to keep her emotions under control as people lined up to offer their condolences. Forced to turn away for yet another fitful dab at her runny nose, Angie looked up to find a sorrowful Australian standing in front of her.

"Oh, Dale...." Bursting into tears, she felt two strong arms wrap themselves tightly around her.

Dale could feel her body shudder against him. It was a horrible sensation... almost as if he could feel her very heart breaking.

Using his hand to shield her tear-stained features as he cradled her in his arms, the gallant Aussie bent his head forward to rest his cheek tenderly against hers. "It's okay, luv. It's going to be okay."

39
EMILY MAKES A CALL

Dale and Alex were raked over the coals but good. First Peter, then the Transportation Safety Board had a go at them. Never mind attempting to fly home in a blizzard; among other things, they had flown IFR even though they knew their aircraft was not certified for it. In doing so, they had endangered not only the lives of their fellow crewmen, but also the flight program's continued existence.

As Chief Pilot, Dale had accepted full responsibility for his decision to fly back to Calgary, but it was not enough to spare Alex from the Board's wrath. In their eyes, Davis had been a willing participant. If nothing else, he should've at least attempted to stop his suicidal cohort.

The incident was duly noted on their flight records... along with a written warning from Lawson that any further blatant disregard for Standard Operating Procedure would be met with instant dismissal.

Angie spent a subdued Christmas at her parents' farm, then returned to Calgary. She was awakened Boxing Day with a phone call. It was

Mrs. Andrews. Could she drop by around ten for tea?

It was not an unusual request. The women had stayed in close contact following the funeral, reminiscing about all the wild stunts their Russ had pulled off in his brief life, and helping one another deal with the injustice of it all. What had hurt most was learning the truth about the mystery man found in the ditch.

Regaining consciousness in hospital, the man had initially pleaded amnesia. But it was later discovered that he had wandered away from a local house party and staggered out onto the highway... causing the woman in the car to swerve into the path of the oncoming pickup truck. It was surmised that, having seen what he'd done, he passed out from the shock. That was who Russ had been trying to help that night: a thankless drunk!

Her husband having passed away only a few years earlier, Mrs. Andrews understood the grieving process only too well. She knew Angie's pain. She also knew that, with time, the tears would eventually stop and the seemingly unbearable heartache eventually ease. Time truly was the great healer. Only trouble was, some people needed more of it than others. Sometimes, a lot more.

Emily came over that morning to ask a very special favor of Angie. It had to do with something that she and Russ had been so looking forward to. Something that her only son had diligently trained for by jogging twice-daily around Glenmore Reservoir; a large can of frozen orange juice hoisted proudly above his head. It was the Olympic torch relay.

Angie had all but forgotten about it. With Rusty no longer around for moral support, she had quickly reverted back to her old cynical self. As her own toughest critic, Angie had always demanded the very best from herself. Understandably, she had great trouble accepting anything less.

Being a top-notch Intensive Care nurse and earning the praise and respect of the nurses and physicians who worked alongside her meant very little. Since the vast majority of her patients left the unit with a toe tag, what real difference did her supposed talents make? While winning a Canadian luge championship had been a momentary high in her life, like always, that wondrous feat had been quickly blotted out by something else—her failure to make the Olympic team. Lumped together with Jeff dumping her and Russ dying on her, even her love life was on a depressing downward spiral.

Yep, she'd resolved as she cried herself to sleep one night, when it came to love, luge and life, Angie Jackson was a dismal failure.

What the heck did it matter, anyway? The only reason she'd been chosen to dance in the Games Opening Ceremonies was thanks to Russ' stellar footwork... not hers. And as far as the LIFE-STAR program was concerned, she could think of only one reason for her selection: a certain string-pulling, sweet-talking, fair-haired pilot named Dale.Floundering in the depths of a mind-numbing depression, Angie had even begun having morbid thoughts that maybe the only reason she'd had for living... had been reduced to a small metal container of ash sitting on a shelf in her living room.

When she failed a second time to show up for Two-Step practice, concerned committee organizers immediately phoned to find out why. There was no doubting hers was a heart-breaking story, but the Opening Ceremonies Committee was ultimately responsible for putting together a show-stopping spectacular that would have a viewing audience of two billion people worldwide.

To pull the thing off, they would need undying commitment from every person involved, something Angie no longer seemed to have. While a new partner could be found and the missed practices made up, Angie's total lack of enthusiasm was a different story. She just didn't seem to care anymore. About anything.

Everything had been going so great. She and Russ had finally found the love they'd been searching for all their lives. Not only that, they were each other's best friend, each other's soul-mate. They had jobs they loved. Russ was going to run in the Torch relay. They were going to be in the Opening Ceremonies of the Olympic Winter Games. They had even talked a little about getting married and having kids someday. Now all of that was gone. All her happiness. All her dreams. Why did it have to happen to her? Why couldn't it have happened to somebody else?

When Mrs. Andrews had notified the Torch Relay Committee of Russ' death, as expected, the official who took her call offered his most sincere condolences. Knowing she'd be catching him at a weak moment, Emily made a special request regarding her son's replacement in the run. The official hesitated, knowing there was a special waiting list for just this type of emergency, But, after listening to Mrs. Andrews, he eventually gave in.

Sipping a steaming cup of Red Rose in Angie's tiny flat, Emily smiled as her host. "I've given this a lot of thought, Angie. I'd like you to take Russ' place in the Olympic torch relay."

"You'd like me to what?"

"Honey," Emily looked Angie square in the eyes, "it was Rusty's dream to run the torch and you know better than anyone that if he were standing here today, he'd tell you there wasn't anyone he'd rather have take his place.

"I... " Angie's voice broke. "I don't think I could do that. I'd just fall apart. Russ showed me the route once. You should see it... it goes straight up the side of a mountain! Rusty was such a jock. I'd never make it. I'd only let you down. I'd let him down!"

Emily reached out to take Angie's hands in hers. "Angie, listen to me. Russ can't do it now. You're the only one who can, and when you stand on that mountain... with that torch in your hand, I just know that Rusty is going to be with you every step of the way. He'll be there cheering you on. He was always telling me what a tough little scrapper you were. That was one of the things he liked so much about you. But he also told me that sometimes you needed a push to get started. That's why I'm here, to give you that little push. I can't force you to do it. Nobody can. Just promise me one thing... you'll think it over. Okay? Promise me that."

Feeling the tears come as Emily slipped her arms around her, Angie wanted so desperately to scream, "NO PROBLEM! I'LL DO IT... GIVE ME THE BLOODY TORCH... I'LL RUN THE DAMN THING TO VANCOUVER IF YOU WANT ME TO."

Instead, the former Olympic hopeful buried her shameful face against Emily's shoulder.

40

WHEN PUSH COMES TO SHOVE

Citing "personal problems," Angie had taken an indefinite leave of absence from work. In a show of heart-felt compassion, Howard Bateman had been most understanding and agreeable, even though it meant utilizing all of his relief nursing staff to fill her shifts.

Each person was different and each person dealt with death in his or her own way. In Angie's case, however, she'd been off more than a month already. If she were to continue as a valued member of the flight program, she would have to get back in the saddle pretty damn soon. Or find herself another line of work.

Following a mandatory stress debriefing with Dale, Kyle had also been granted compassionate leave. But after a few days of moping around home, he realized that staying away from work was possibly the worst thing he could have done. With nothing to distract his thoughts, he started playing and replaying the fateful mission over and over in his head, torturing himself with unanswerable "what-ifs".

Jennifer was awakened from a sound sleep one night to find her anguished husband slumped at the kitchen table, crying. Truly frightened by what she saw, Jen picked up the phone and called the hangar. While talking with Dale had helped, what Kyle desperately needed was someone to confirm he'd done all the right things. That he hadn't let Russ down when he needed him most. And he needed to hear it from a fellow paramedic.

Michael Brown was about as compassionate as he could have been at 2:30 a.m. After listening to the medic's worries, he asked Kyle to drop by the hangar in the morning. They would go for breakfast and have a good talk then.

Six hours later, his omelet untouched, Kyle sat in silence as his co-worker read through the mission PCR.

"Kyle," Michael sighed as he tucked the paperwork back into its folder, "from what I see here, there isn't one thing I would've done differently. You did your best, man. How much more can you ask of yourself?"

Walking into Peter's office twenty minutes later with his head high and his broad shoulders barely clearing the door jams, Kyle Stevens informed his boss that he was ready to come back to work.

His first flight back was by far the hardest, but after that, it was business as usual. The workload had not changed. The endless paperwork had not changed. Nothing was changed except that Howard had hired on another full-time paramedic.

Checking in with Angie, three days later, Mrs. Andrews found her still undecided. Time was running out. The torch people would be forced to select someone else. Emily picked up the phone and began to dial.

Peter Lawson thanked Mrs. Andrews for her concern and wasted little time hauling Dale into his office for a little closed-door, off-the-record chat.

"Captain Morgan, I've been going over your Critical Stress Debriefing report regarding the Andrews fatality and frankly, I've got some questions that need clarification. First off, you've written here that you met on an individual basis with both Kyle and Alex, and that you also conducted two group sessions—one with the Canmore EMS providers and one with our flight crews. But I can't seem to find any mention of the person most directly affected by this tragedy—Angela Jackson. You did sit down and talk with her... didn't you?"

"Sir, I felt that uh... under the circumstances, it might be better if I uh... delegated Angie's debriefing to someone else. I spoke with Howard Bateman and he agreed to take on her case file."

"Dale, that doesn't make any sense. You've got your instructor's level in Stress Debriefing. You can teach the damn course. Howard's good, but he doesn't have nearly the experience you have. Good heavens, after all that poor girl's been through, I would've thought Angela deserved the very best emotional support we could give her. Why would you delegate that awesome responsibly to someone less qualified?"

Dale's embarrassed expression caught Peter by surprise. "Please tell me you've at least called her then. You know, a social call—to see how she's holding up... make sure she's still alive?"

Dale clenched his jaw.

"Good God, man, I can't believe this! I thought you and her were close! I can't understand how a friend could abandon....

The Aussie looked up from the floor to stare his boss in the eye. "You know why."

Peter's features softened marginally as he studied the troubled man seated before him.

"Look sir, I uh... Angie'll come through this okay. She just needs some time to pull herself together, that's all. She'll be alright!"

Peter ran a hand through his rapidly-thinning hair. "She's been off for over a month now. I've got nurses pulling two and three extra shifts a pay period to cover for her. This can't go on indefinitely. If Angie doesn't come back in the next week or two, I'll have to place her on long-term disability and that means filling her spot with somebody new."

"What about Kyle? Shouldn't he be the one in here? He's known her a whole lot longer than I have!"

Peter leaped up to glare his chief pilot full in the face. "Where the hell have you been? Kyle has tried! Jennifer's tried! Mrs. Andrews' tried! We've all tried, and so far nothing has worked. One of my program's valued employees is suffering through an emotional hell right now and I'd like to be able to say that I never gave up on her until I'd exhausted every possible option. You... Captain Morgan, are that last option.

"All I'm asking is that you go over to her place and talk to her. Look, more than anything else, she needs to hear the comforting words of a friend right now. Be that friend. We all know you like her. It's not a secret... trust me, everybody knows!"

The hard-nosed manager let Dale squirm a bit before continuing. "Dale, if you really do care about this girl, you'll go to her and try to help her through this."

Dale jumped to his feet. "Peter, have you thought about what you're asking me to do? If people find out I've been over to her place sniffing around, I'm going to come off looking like some kind of lusting vulture who just couldn't wait to start picking at the left-over pieces!"

"Who the hell cares what people are going to think? A friend's sanity is at stake here! She's shut herself away from the world. I got a call from Mrs. Andrews this morning. She seems to feel that something's gnawing at Angie... something that she won't tell anyone. That's why I need your help. I want you to find out what that something is.

"Just let her know you care. That we all care. You're a man of integrity. As both an officer and a gentleman, I know you'll treat this woman's fragile emotional state with the respect and dignity it deserves. I want you back in this office on Monday with a full update. Until then, good luck and good day, sir."

Taking his thermal mug along on the pretext of fetching fresh brew, Lawson closed his office door behind him.

Seated at Lawson's desk, Dale listened as Angie's phone seemed to ring forever, then Clint Eastwood came on the line: "PLEASE LEAVE A MESSAGE... OR ELSE!"

Following a hastily thrown-together plan, the crafty pilot blurted out a truly splendid yarn about spilling some nameless concoction all over his crisp white captain's shirt and how he was worried sick about removing the stain.

It was your typical "single male living on his own" tale of woe, but it worked like a dream. Within seconds, Angie called back. Over the course of the next few minutes, Dale was forced to call upon all his wily Australian charm to convince her that he must bring his shirt over that very night... before the stain set.

Rifling through his closet upon arriving home, Dale finally located what he was searching for... an old flight shirt from his Coast Guard days. Once his absolute favorite, he was now using it to wrap his collapsible fishing rod in.

As he paused to examine it more closely, the reason became quite obvious. An epaulette was torn away, three buttons were missing and a large purple wine stain covered the right sleeve.

Smiling to himself as he ran the sleeve under the tap to get it nice and wet, Dale momentarily debated whether to dignify the poor thing by placing it on a hanger. Mulling the idea over for a few seconds, he instead stuffed the dripping mess into a plastic bag and headed for his car.

41
CONFESSIONS

As Angie requested some time alone in her tiny kitchen to examine the "patient," Dale waited in the living room... performing an examination of his own.

From a distance, Angie looked the same as always—tight-fitting blue jeans, sweatshirt, hair pulled neatly back into a ponytail. But it was her face that gave her away—tired and drawn, with huge dark circles under her green eyes.

Wandering about the living room, Dale peeked at her crammed bookshelves. In addition to thick medical volumes were texts running the gamut from Understanding Egyptian Hieroglyphics, to Theories on Plate Tectonics to The Rise and Fall of the Russian Empire. Scattered among the books were awards: luge, basketball and slow pitch medallions, wall plaques for Physics 20, Chem 30 and track, and a 4-H horse club trophy for "High Point Rider of the Year."

Without a doubt, this A.Y. Jackson babe had all the makings of a twentieth-century Renaissance woman!

"I don't know quite how to break this to you," Angie said, carrying in the ratty shirt, "but I'm afraid your friend's condition is terminal."

If this decomposing rag was indeed Dale's best captain's shirt, then helicopter jockeys were not paid as much as she thought. Another mystery was how he'd even had the gall to show up for work wearing this thing! Bateman and his dress code had obviously taken the day off.

"I hate to say this," she continued, "but I think palliative care would be the most humane course of action."

"Palliative care? Isn't there something we can do?"

"Dale, if this shirt were truly a patient of mine, I would've unplugged its ventilator a long time ago."

At a complete loss as to what to say next, Dale found himself nervously shifting his weight from one foot to the other. Staring down at her hands, Angie began to pick at her one remaining unchewed fingernail.

"Darn... and that was my lucky fly fishing shirt, too."

"I don't doubt it attracted a lot of flies," Angie laughed. "By the way, did you know the fishing license you had stuffed in the front pocket expired last April?"

Relieved that the silly charade was over, Angie was genuinely happy that her favorite pilot had taken the time to stop by. In fact, she confided that she'd missed his warped sense of humor and colorful Aussie accent something awful. But her lighthearted mood quickly deteriorated.

"You know, in the last month, I've received a zillion sympathy cards, never mind all the food and flowers people have brought over. Thanks to everyone's kindness, I've packed on a whopping eight pounds. Even Howard drops by every week or so. It's as if he's on some sort of 'emotional pilgrimage' or something. Tries to feed me that old line about how the passage of time will eventually ease my inconsolable grief. I'm sure he means well, but I think what he really wants to know is when I'll be coming back to work.

"I should have said something the last time he was here, but I just didn't have the guts. I should've told him straight out that I've decided to hand in my flight suit. I've already called my old unit at the Mountainview about possibly getting back on there."

As if fully expecting it, Dale heaved a chauvinistic sigh. "It's probably for the best. With you being a female and all, the stress of coming back to work would've been too much for you to handle. Now say, heaven forbid, the tables had been reversed and sweet little you had bought the sheep station instead of Russ, why, that son-of-a-gun would've been back at work inside a week. He'd have hung his head for a few days in mourning, of course, but knowing that smooth-talking rascal as well as I did, he'd have been prowling the bars for a new squeeze in no time. Come to think of it, wasn't it Jodi who was always moaning about how he could practice mouth-to-mouth on her any time?"

Angie's screech could have been heard three blocks away. "How can you say such a horrible, disgusting thing? I'll have you know that Rusty vowed he'd enter a monastery if anything ever happened to me. But then how would you know? You never called once... or sent me flowers or a ham or brownies or anything. I could've starved to death waiting for a show of sympathy from you!

"And as far as going back to work is concerned, I would've coped just fine. It's just... uh... I don't want to, that's all. And that crap about Jodi... what an awful thing to say about her... you... you swine!"

"I said it because it's the truth!" Dale exploded. "Whenever the going gets a little tough, the first thing you do is run! Without Andrews around to stoke your ego, you all but curl up and die!"

"When the hell did God go on vacation and leave you in charge of my life, Morgan?" Angie screamed.

"Somebody had to, Ms. Jackson! Hidden away in your cave here, you sure haven't been doing such a shit-hot job of it so far!"

Angie responded with a string of filthy expletives.

"The truth hurts, doesn't it?" The Aussie went for the jugular. "You know something, Ange? I have never in my life met anyone with as much God-given talent as you. What a waste! You were one of the best flight nurses in the program, but we can forget all about that silly nonsense now, can't we? And the torch relay... and that Opening Ceremonies crap! You might as well chuck those two in your 'dead dream' file, as well. I've heard via the grapevine that you've already missed so many practices that the organizing committee won't lose any sleep when they finally give your wussie little ass the royal punt!

"Throw your life away if you want to, but before I leave here, I'm going to tell you something that should've been said a month and a half ago. The night of the Christmas party, before we flew over to pick you up, suddenly out of the clear blue, Russ started babbling about how he'd waited long enough... that he'd finally gotten the balls to ask his loving sweet girlfriend to marry him.

"That crazy, lovesick fool. He had it all planned out. Was going to take you out for dinner to some expensive restaurant downtown... wine you and dine you... before popping the question. Poor dumb bastard! He loved you so much and now here it is, what, only six short weeks after his untimely demise and the woman he wanted to share his life with is behaving as if she couldn't give a damn about any of his unfulfilled hopes and dreams. Yep, you must've loved Russ Andrews an awful lot!"

The room began to spin around her. Rusty had planned to ask her to marry him?

Dale was not through. "Stevens and Davis... they didn't want to say anything because they thought it would make you feel worse. At first, I felt the same way. But when I thought about it, I knew that if it had been me in Russ' shoes, I'd have wanted my girl to know how much I'd cared about her... even if someone else had to say it for me!"

Angie was crying now, partly over what she had been forced to hear, and partly because she knew Morgan was right. Everything he had said was true. About her having no drive, no motivation; about Russ at the Christmas party telling her of his plans for an intimate, candlelit dinner together that very next evening.

"You heartless bastard!" she retaliated. "I didn't need to know that! All this time I thought you were my friend. I thought you came over because you cared. You Aussies sure know how to cheer someone up. Why don't you just cut out my heart and be done with it?"

"If that's what it takes!" Dale yelled back. "Sometimes the only way to heal a festering wound is to lance it and let it drain. For God's sake, woman, I know you're hurting, but it's time to stop hiding away and start living again. Let your feelings out. Spill your guts if you have to. I'm here to help you through this."

"I don't want any help! Besides, why should I listen to someone who doesn't practice what he preaches? You say I've hidden away from the world, well what the hell's your excuse? I know divorce is rough, but how could you just take off and leave your family? Your own son? What wicked, evil sin are you trying to escape from, Captain Perfect? Poor old frozen Canada is about as far away from Cairns as you can get and still stay on the planet. What was the problem... no seats available on the frigging space shuttle?"

Angie had run out of words; it was time for action. Pursuing her startled quarry's rapidly retreating butt toward the kitchen, she grabbed the one thing she knew could inflict a lot of pain... her bug-splattered fly swatter.

Dale raced from room to room, trying to fend off his assailant's stinging attack. The seat cushions from the couch worked well for awhile. So did the pillow from her bed, the scatter rug from the hallway, the bath towel he found crumpled in the bathroom. Madly flinging things over his shoulder as he ran, most of his projectiles missed their target by a country mile. As her pain and rage dissipated into hysterical laughter, the mentally-unhinged woman stopped her mad swatting only long enough to fire every one of the projectiles straight back at his head.

"For Christ's sake... keep it down over there!" It was the Coopers from next door pounding on the wall.

Angie wondered briefly as to what they must've heard—a man wheezing, "Not so rough... I bruise easy!" and a woman gasping, "I always thought you macho Aussies liked it that way!"

With the fly-swatting crazy-woman hard on his heels, Dale abruptly changed course. Grunting like a old moose as his trailing leg sent the coffee table flying, he made a desperate spread-eagled leap over the couch. Using a combat roll to soften his landing, the winded pilot scrambled to his knees. Grabbing a nearby plant-misting water bottle, Dale bravely dug in.

Angie had not expected his sudden stop, and vaulted the sofa in hot pursuit. Smiling with sadistic delight, Dale watched as her momentum carried her past him, smack into a large potted plant.

"Oh no!" Angie gasped as she paused to examine her jaundiced-looking philodendron. Death had been instantaneous. Discovering its tinder-dry stalk snapped off at the roots, Angie cradled it in her hands like a dear and trusted friend.

Solemnly, Dale gave the plant a squirt with the misting bottle. "I'm afraid it's beyond even Holy water. If you ask me, it was a mercy killing." Reaching up to pluck a chunk of peat moss from Angie's hair, he added, "Maybe that's what you need... a good squirt of Holy water."

Choking back a giggle, Angie stared at the carpet.

"There... see? You can still laugh. It's time to come back to the land of the living, Ange. We all miss you so much... I miss you."

Angie's laughter faded as quickly as it had come. There was something else that had to be dealt with first. Something that'd been eating at her since the night Peter called with news of the accident. Something that, if she didn't confide to someone pretty damn soon... she was afraid would drive her insane.

"I've done a horrible thing, Dale... a horrible thing. I'm the reason Rusty's dead. I... I killed him!"

"How can you say that? You weren't even...."

With a wave of her hand, Angie silenced him. "I was off sick, remember? I was supposed to be on shift that night. And it won't help to give me that line about how it was a car that did poor Russ in, either. It wasn't any damn car... it was me! You've been on enough missions to know what Rusty would've had me doing at that call. We both know how much he loved extricating patients from wrecks. As the lowly flight nurse on board, he would've sent me off to help that female EMT with the drunk. I'm the one who would've gone back to pack up her equipment. I'm the one who would've been standing in that ditch when the car came over the hill. I'm the one who should've been staring into those headlights. It should've been me, Dale. It should've been me!"

Seventeen time zones and ten thousand miles from home, it was as if a ghost had just reached out and squeezed his heart. The past had finally caught up with Dale Morgan.

He tipped Angie's quivering chin so she was forced to look at him. "Luv, I'm going to tell you about something that happened to me a long time ago, when I was flying med-evacs in Vietnam. We were going in to pick up a patrol one night. It was darker than heck, no moon... no stars, and the LZ... the landing zone... was hot. Real hot.

"The Vietcong had the patrol pinned down in a crossfire. The last report we'd received was that, of sixteen men, only seven were still capable of returning fire. On the verge of being overrun, their lieutenant radioed for an immediate 'dust-off', that's the army's code word for med-evac. Anyway, he set up a strobe to help guide us in, but as soon as the VC saw that, they sent us a greeting of their own... in tracer bullets.

"Tracers always looked so damn pretty at night... so harmless. Just thin greenish-blue streaks of light zipping up toward us... with each one capable of blowing a fist-sized hole clean through the floorboards.

"I was flying co-pilot with a good friend that night. I'd known him since high school. His name was Brian James Cole, but he went by his initials, B.J. A great guy. Best damn pilot I've ever flown with. What made him good was not so much his skill, but that he knew his limitations—how far he could push himself and still get his ass and his aircraft back to base in one piece. B.J. flared his approach that night, planning to make a real quick touch-and-go. Nothing fancy. Just set the skids down, get the GIs and their wounded loaded on board, then get the hell out of there.

"Both B.J. and I had less than three months left in our tours. You'd have thought our luck would've run out long before then. Anyway, we were just about to land when my windshield exploded. I didn't feel the bullet hit, didn't feel any pain, everything just went black.

"The Huey's gear box must've taken a few rounds at the same time. We were only about thirty feet above the deck when we were hit. That's way too low to autorotate, so B.J. was forced to bellyflop the helicopter into the trees. The overhead rotors instantly disintegrated... sliced through the rear fuselage. Killed our port-side gunner. Fuel started spewing everywhere. Instead of trying to save himself, B.J. crawled out and ran around to my side. Our other gunner ran to help him and they were just dragging me clear when that Huey went up like a Roman candle.

"The gunner immediately wrote me off for dead. The entire right side of my helmet had been blown out. Ignoring the fact that I didn't appear to have a face anymore, B.J. claimed he could feel a pulse and started yelling for the platoon's corpsman. When he checked me out, the medic discovered that the bullet had caught me just above the ear and then followed the outline of my skull around before exiting out the back of the helmet. Nobody could believe it. My scalp was torn open from my ear all the way to my neck, but that was it. I'd simply been knocked cold. I wasn't dead.

"The lieutenant was forced to radio for a second chopper to do the dust-off. Ten minutes later, another good friend of mine, a guy named Ted Trevair, tried for the LZ. The VC did their best to light him up with tracer fire, as well. Killed his co-pilot just as he was flaring his approach...."

Dale stopped. Up to that point, it had been as if someone else were reciting the story, not him. Now his voice wavered with emotion. "B.J. helped load me into the cargo bay and was just climbing in himself when a sniper opened up. The round caught him under the left arm. Collapsed his lung. Severed his spine. He died on the flight to the aid station.

"Ange, the guilt I felt when I finally heard... it damn near destroyed me. B.J. was my very best friend. Anyone else would've left me to die after we crashed. My head looked like it had been blown off... yet he risked his life to drag me out of there. Then, when that second chopper touched down, he stayed behind to help load me on board. He didn't have to. Heck, he could've just climbed in and let one of the grunts do it. He saved my life twice that night. I couldn't cope with that. I kept asking myself, 'Why?'

"'Why was I still alive and he wasn't?' The awful guilt that I'd been the cause of his death never stopped haunting me. I wanted to die, too! I couldn't concentrate enough to brush my teeth, never mind fly. They had me scheduled to be shipped home as a mental case when a chaplain dropped by one afternoon to have a little chat. What he told me that day, nearly twenty years ago... I'm going to tell to you now.

"He said, 'Warrant Officer Morgan, your friend gave you the most precious gift of all. He gave you his life. Don't you dare waste it! You've got a lot of living left inside of you, and if you don't use it to the best of your ability, then you'll have not only throw your own life away... but B.J.'s, as well!

"Make the most of whatever time you have on this earth because someday you're going to meet up with B.J. Cole again... and he's going to want to know what you did with those years he so unselfishly gave you. When that moment comes, I pray to God that you'll be able to stand up straight and proud, look him square in the eye and tell him that you cherished every second of it!'

"Luv... someday you're going to have to give old Rusty a full account of what you did with all those extra years. He's probably in this room right now, listening to us. What are you going to tell him?"

Angie, whose tears had largely dried while listening to Dale's story, felt her eyes overflow again. "I don't know," she whimpered. "I don't have anyone to turn to anymore... to talk to. I'm all alone now!"

"Luv, you're not alone! You've got a bunch of good friends who want to help you through this. You're not alone!"

Dale scooped her up in his arms and she clung to him for dear life as her grief engulfed her. Waiting patiently for her to stop crying and blow her nose, the pilot pulled back to look her full in the face. "Well, woman... what's it going to be? Are you going to carry that damn torch or am I going to have to paddle your behind all the way to Creston with a fly swatter?"

Tears streaking her face, Angie stared up at her hero. "Would you come with me? I mean, that section of highway has an eight percent grade! What if I need a good swift kick to get me started? Please."

Dale's rugged features transformed into a shy smile as he tousled her ponytail. "Oh what the heck. I've always wanted to see where Kokanee beer was brewed!"

42
THE SALMO-CRESTON HIGHWAY

Dale had less than two weeks to whip Angie into a lean, mean jogging machine. She had always taken great pride in her physical conditioning, but after locking herself in her apartment for six weeks, she was now a chubby shadow of her former self. Ten pounds overweight and her endurance shot, just the effort of climbing the single flight of stairs to her flat left her winded.

With the advice of an aerobic instructor from a nearby fitness club, Dale devised an intensive training program that had Angie bending, stretching and pounding the pavement three hours every day.

Each morning she would diligently begin her day with pushups, sit-ups and several thigh-burning circuits of the ten-story stairwell. Thoroughly warmed up, she would then hobble outside to jog around the block. Carefully clocking each gasping lap with a stopwatch, she worked to lower her time by five seconds on every pass. Thirty minutes later, she would cool down with a brisk walk before returning to her apartment.

At two in the afternoon, and again at eight, she would wearily pull on her sweats and, with muscles aching and reeking of Absorbine Junior, repeat the agonizing process all over again.

Dale would drop by each evening after work. Parking his car across the street from her apartment, he would enjoy a coffee and doughnut as he kept track of her lap times. By the fifth evening, she was easily running a full ten blocks, barely breaking a sweat. By the tenth evening she was sprinting the entire distance.

The night before the torch run, Angie didn't sleep a wink. Toasting the dawn with a diet Coke and a bowlful of Cheerios, she stuffed an extra sport's bra, some Mole-skin bandages and a bottle of Aspirin into her gym bag before hurrying downstairs to meet Dale. She was coming prepared.

Seven hours, 300 miles and a gravel-cracked windshield later, Dale's salt-splattered Saab pulled into the tranquil retirement community of Creston, British Columbia. After checking in with the local relay organizers and snagging a quick bite to eat, Dale and his passenger wearily took to the highway again. Just past the town limits, a weathered sign announced, "SALMO-CRESTON SKYWAY... Next Right."

"Good Lord!" Angie exclaimed upon arriving at the summit. On a clear day, the view must have been spectacular. Today was not that day. As a dusting of ice particles sifted across the road in unrelenting waves, the endless stretch of frozen asphalt had a strange foreboding about it. Even the wind made an eerie moaning sound as it caressed the surrounding evergreen forest.

Angie stepped out of the car. Her warm breath instantly transformed into a frosty white cloud. With the thermometer hovering at minus 20 degrees Celsius, a stiff breeze out of the east made it feel twice as cold.

The car ride alone had been harrowing enough. But when Dale got out and promptly slipped on a patch of black ice, a very real fear swept over her. Was she ready for this? Was anybody?

After watching Dale nearly end up on his butt, Angie was extra cautious as she gingerly tiptoed around to the front of the car. Stepping onto what she thought was dry pavement, her feet suddenly shot out from beneath her.

"There's no way anyone could run up this section!" she sniffled as she crawled back into the car to press her fingers against the heater vents. "It's glare ice. All those toenails I lost training! All those blisters. It was all for nothing. The organizers are going to take one look at this section and cancel...."

"That's not going to happen!" Dale cut her off. "As far as we know, the relay is still a go, and until somebody tells me different, that's how we're going to approach this thing! We've got to keep positive here. Let me see your shoes."

Angie meekly surrendered a foot for inspection. "Good heavens, woman! How long have you been wearing these things? There's no tread left. We've got to get you some traction somehow." Dale pulled a U-turn and headed for town.

With an hour to spare before the caravan left with the torch runners, Dale dropped Angie off at the relay office, then sped away.

Incredibly, despite the weather, the run was still very much a go. As one of the chosen participants, Angie was presented with a spiffy red and white track suit and toque, then directed to a pre-run meeting which covered, among other things... how not to set yourself or your co-runners on fire, and what to do if the flame accidentally went out.

Dale meanwhile, cruising up and down Creston's main drag, finally located a hardware store and raced straight for the tool section. Three minutes later, a small package clutched in his hand, he was on his way back to relay headquarters. As he paced the lobby waiting for Angie, the Aussie soon found himself deep in conversation with one of the local caravan drivers.

"Yep," the driver drawled. "Reports have been coming in that the Skyway is getting a might slick. And that eight percent grade section leading up to the summit is by far the worst, but if she stays in the ditch and watches her step, your little lady shouldn't have any problems a-tall."

"Stays in the ditch?" Dale's voice climbed an octave. "Have you been up there lately? There isn't any ditch... there isn't any guard rail... the edge of the road just drops away... straight down... a thousand feet... to the flipping river!"

The grizzled old driver shrugged his shoulders. "Look sonny, from your accent, I'd say you're not accustomed to much snow. You're in Canada now. Up here, it's eight months of winter followed by four months of poor skiing. We Canadians are a resilient breed. Tough, feisty, and damn proud of it. The worse the weather, the more we want to go out and play in it.

"Don't get you knickers in a knot. That little missy of yours will do just fine. And don't you worry about me getting her up to the summit safe and sound, either. All the caravan's vehicles have tire chains on... just in case the going gets a bit slick."

As the official headed outside for a smoke, Dale muttered. "A bit slick? You'd probably like that, wouldn't you, Mate? Crazy Canucks!"

Returning from her briefing, Angie was a changed person, pumped and ready to run to the moon. She immediately dragged Dale outside to where the transport van was waiting to carry them up the mountain to their pre-assigned sections.

One after the other, each torch bearer was dropped at his or her position along the road. This was the moment they had all been waiting for... their chance to become part of Canadian Olympic history. Through their frozen hands would pass the spark that would one day ignite the fire in the Olympic Winter Games cauldron.

As the next-to-last runner was ushered out of the motorhome to await the torch's imminent arrival, Angie nervously looked over at her mentor. "Did you have any luck downtown?"

"I did indeed little missy," the Aussie grinned as he reached into his coat pocket and withdrew a staple gun. Holding her ankle between his knees as if he were shoeing a horse, he began pumping staples into the soles of her Reeboks.

Fifty-five staples were the magic that kept Angela Yvonne Jackson solidly on her feet as she was presented with the Olympic flame. Hoisting the Calgary Tower-shaped torch proudly in her right hand, Angie took up her position in the convoy. Led by an RCMP squad car, the torch runners' motorhome was next, followed by a car with two flickering miner's lamps mounted on the trunk just in case the blooming torch went out and had to be relit, then a media truck. Finally, there was Angie. Behind her was the command center motorhome, a van to pick up the previous runners, and then another police car.

Upon relating his heart-wrenching tale to one of the officials, Dale received the okay to ride in the media truck so he could video Angie's historic run as it unfolded.

As she timidly took that first step, Angie was riding a high no drug could ever produce. Gaining confidence when she realized Dale's staples were going to hold, she lifted the torch high above her head. With the icy wind stinging her eyes, she began to think about Russ and how he had wanted so much to carry this torch. If he could only see her now.

A mere thirty seconds of hoofing it up the increasingly-steep roadway, however, her enthusiasm began to wane. The frigid air scorched her lungs with each breath. The pavement stretched off into the clouds, and the blessed three-pound torch which had seemed so light, now weighed a flipping ton.

Her thigh muscles on fire, her cotton undershirt was already soaked with sweat. Angie was generating so much heat that Dale later swore he saw steam rising from the unzipped neck of her track suit.

Two minutes later, it was all Angie could do to keep the torch at waist level. The eight percent grade was taking its toll. Stumbling along, she struggled just to lift her feet high enough to keep from tripping.

As the intense cold threatened to freeze her watering eyes shut, Angie Jackson's grieving period was incredibly brief. Her only thoughts now were of a heartless jock named Russell Andrews. For crying out loud, how much further did she have to lug this damned thing, anyway?

Forced to jog head-long into the bone-chilling wind, Angie suddenly lost her emotional grip. "Andrews... you dumb creep! Why the hell did you have to pick such an awful place to run? What were you trying to prove anyway? How much of a macho jock-strap you were? This bloody road is heading straight up to frigging heaven. In a minute or so, you should be able to see me coming!"

Meanwhile toasty warm in the back of the media truck, Dale had been recounting Angie's tear-jerking tale to another amateur photographer. Touched by the story of devotion and undying love, the young fellow was just about to snap Angie's picture when the bedraggled woman abruptly cut loose. "Andrews... how could you do this to me? I don't deserve this shit! Damn it, are you listening to me?"

"I... uh... see what you mean," the photo hound sputtered as he stared at the fire-breathing female thundering up the highway toward them. With a fresh infusion of de-icing adrenaline coursing through her bloodstream, Angie's stapled runners bit viciously into the ice, sending up a shower of glittering ice fragments with every ground-pounding step.

As Dale would later confide to her over dinner, he simply could not believe this was the same pathetic flower who'd being crying her eyes out for weeks thinking she had been personally responsible for killing off her only reason for living.

As suddenly as it had come, Angie's anger faded. She'd been so caught up in cursing her former lover, she had almost forgotten where the heck she was. How could she have allowed her thoughts to sink to such a spiteful level? As remorse tore at her heart, sobs replaced her angry words. She had 500 yards left to go. Barely limping along now... head hanging, torch dangling sideways, Angie was on the verge of collapse when a curious feeling came over her.

Rusty.

She felt his presence! It was as if he were right there with her... his hand beside hers on the torch... helping her lift it up. Someone or something was telling her, "Hey, Ange, it's okay! We'll do it together."

Finishing with long, steady strides, torch and eyes blazing, Angie's historic run had taken less than ten minutes. She had started up that bleak mountain pass feeling very alone. By the time she handed the Olympic torch off to the relay official at the summit, she had come to realize the comforting truth that, while Russ may have crossed over to another dimension, she had not lost him.

For as long as she carried his memory in her soul, he would always be a part of her. He had been with her today. She had felt his presence. And yes, he had been very proud.

43
THE VOICE OF EXPERIENCE

The chain-smoking clerk behind the desk at the Sleep-Easy Motor Inn laughed out loud at Dale's request. "Separate rooms? Good luck! With the crappy weather and the torch passing through town, I've got one room left. It's a single, but I could drag a second cot in there if you want."

"Thanks, but I think we'll check somewhere...."

"We'll take it," Angie suddenly spoke up.

"It's okay... really!" she explained, walking back to the Saab with a mortified Dale to collect their luggage. "Look, nobody's going to know. We're both adults, aren't we? We should be able to share a room without feeling we're doing something immoral. If nothing else, think of the money we'll save!"

After a soak in the outdoor Jacuzzi, the two headed out for a late supper. Over a meal of succulent prime rib, Dale recounted his conversation with the photographer.

"Yeah, well I just pray you're be able to do some fancy editing with that tape when we get home," Angie giggled. "I really don't think Emily needs to see that part."

Arriving back at the motel, Dale was about to usher Angie inside when a blast of super-chilled air nearly knocked the bubbly couple off their feet. Incredibly, the gale seemed to be coming from inside their room. Searching the cramped unit for broken windows, Dale immediately discovered the real problem. The antiquated heating system had shut down and was now blowing ice-cold air.

Making a testy call to the front desk, Dale was curtly informed the cold temperatures had snapped a water line, and that the town wouldn't be able to get a repair crew out until the next morning.

"What the hell are we supposed to do in the meantime?" the Aussie shouted. "You either find us another room or I'm reporting you to the Better Business Bureau!"

"Look fella, I dare you to find another room in this whole damn town! This is ski season you know! If you want to check out, fine. But if you're planning to sleep somewhere other than your car, I'd advise you to stay put.

"I've told the other tenants to seal off the heating ducts with blankets or their suitcases... and by all means feel free to crank up the fireplace. There is one in your room, you know. Here's your big chance to get cuddly with that foxy dame who talked you into sharing a room. Who knows, maybe you'll get lucky and generate some heat of your own!"

"HOW WOULD YOU LIKE IT IF I CAME DOWN THERE AND GOT LUCKY WITH YOU TONIGHT?" Dale bellowed as he slammed the receiver down.

Upon debating the alternatives, the reluctant roomies decided it probably would be best to tough it out. Leaving Angie to deal with the air vents, Dale went out for firewood.

Returning with an armful, the former survival instructor immediately set about tossing several of the frozen logs onto the blackened grate. Using their motel agreement as kindling, a mere twist of the key in the gas outlet and a single match later, Dale Morgan had a snap crackling blaze any self respecting male would've been proud of.

Even with the fire going, however, they could still see their breath. Boldly unzipping his parka, Dale positioned himself so his back was flush against the side of the fireplace. Motioning Angie to lean back against his chest, the Aussie pulled his jacket around her. While it may have looked kinky to anyone scraping a peek through the frosted motel window, for the hypothermic individuals involved, it was pure heaven!

Sipping on coolers which the wine-loving Dale had brought along, their conversation soon turned to a subject that had long intrigued the Aussie. It concerned Angie's luge career and the terrible accident that had brought it to an end. "You made me tell one of my deepest, darkest secrets," Dale prodded. "Now it's your turn."

Picking at the label on her peach cooler, Angie began her story with the bare-bones—how she'd watched the Sarajevo Olympics on TV and been bitten by the wild and crazy luge bug. Knowing Calgary was to host the next Winter Games, and looking for a bit of adventure, she decided to give it a shot. It looked simple enough. All you had to do was lie on a little sled and slide feet-first down the hill. Right?

"I started sliding that fall. Luge was in its infancy back then. Most people had never heard of it. I told the nurses at work about what I was doing. One of them asked which event I liked best... two- man or four. She thought I'd taken up bobsleigh. The only person who seemed to have a grip on what luge was all about was my mother... and she was dead against it.

Anyway, to make a long story short, four months later I was the Canadian Senior Women's Natural Luge champion. Natural means we raced on snow. Nobody could believe it. I couldn't believe it. The media was all over me, writing stuff about how this luge thing was going to be my ticket to the Olympics. You should've seen the headlines: 'Local Girl Wins All. Sliding Phenomenon Takes Luge World by Storm!'"

Pausing to take sip of her cooler, Angie gazed into the flames. "Aren't you bored yet?"

"I want to hear it all... every sordid detail."

"You really are into S and M, aren't you, Morgan? Want me to spill my guts... make me bleed!" As if a huge emotional gate had finally been allowed to swing open, the story swept out of her.

"The Calgary track hadn't been completed yet, so they sent me to Lake Placid along with the rest of the provincial team to train on their Kunstbahn or Olympic-style luge course.

"We lugers used to laugh about it. If racing on snow is called natural luge, then Kunstbahn must be German for 'unnatural luge.' It's so much faster because it's on ice and has the high-banked curves. I was nearly blown away by the speed. Believe it or not, after only three weeks of training, I was sliding so well, my coach asked me to come back for more training in March and to compete in the Canadian Kunstbahn championships to be held then.

"Next thing I knew, four months had passed and I was back in Placid sitting in the start handles. My first three race runs were flawless. Nice clean lines. Quiet on the sled. My form needed major work, but my times were right up there with the national team girls'... an incredible feat considering I hadn't even learned to pull from the flipping start handles yet.

"I remember so clearly sitting on the start ramp, waiting for the track to be cleared for my fourth and final run. It had all been so easy. The sled seemed to drive itself. I was in fourth place. All the other racers had been sliding for years. The girl holding down second spot had represented Canada at the Sarajevo Olympics! I was racing against the very best Canada had to offer.

"Anyway, getting back to the race, curves five through eight were a breeze, but cruising through curve nine, I felt the sled climb higher on the wall than it had on any of my previous runs. I was just cooking! Curves ten, eleven and twelve whizzed past.

"Three curves left. My sled was just about to exit thirteen and I remember thinking about how great my time was going to be... and how my coach was going to be so impressed and how maybe... just maybe, I'd be asked to try out for the national team's summer program.

"That's how I entered curve fourteen—my helmet in the clouds and my bloated ego already at the awards ceremony. It damn near got me killed. Missed the entrance totally. My sled was still chattering merrily along in the gutter when it should've been seven feet up the wall. A split second later, when the looping law of physics finally kicked in, that Godless sled and I were sent rocketing straight up to the boards. It was like being strapped to the nose of an out-of-control rollercoaster.

"I lost all perspective of where I was in the curve. The walls... the deflector boards... the gutter... just one big blur. All of sudden, I ran out of wall to loop. I was six feet above the track when my sled just went sailing off into space. Next thing I know, my visor is exploding and I'm riding my face down the track.

"I don't remember a heck of a lot after that. The officials up in the timing tower said I really fought to hang onto my sled. Said it was a good thing, too, because if the dang thing had gotten away from me, my time wouldn't have counted. I don't remember doing it. What I do remember is tumbling backwards down the track. Melted a great big hole right through my racing suit... through my lycra underwear... left a lovely second-degree friction burn on my hip bone. I was only semi-conscious, but I sure the hell felt that! The heat was incredible. I had to get the sled back under me somehow. The timing officials said it appeared that's what I was trying to do when my leg flipped up over the edge of the track...."

Staring down at her left foot, Angie halted her narrative to take another sip of wine.

"I was probably still doing forty-five miles an hour when my ankle struck the edge of a vertical concrete support at the entrance to curve fifteen.All I felt was a tremendous jolt as the impact spun me around. When I regained my senses, I was lying on my side in the out-run. I had no feeling in my lower leg. Absolutely none. It was so weird. I actually had to turn my head and look back to make sure my foot was still attached.

"By this time, one of the officials was sprinting down the out-run to see if I was okay. Being a jock, I lied through my teeth. Told him I was just a little shook up... let him carry my sled to the finish dock while I gamely limped up the out-run behind him. For some neurological reason, my ankle had stiffened into a tip-toed position. I could put weight on it, but the entire foot felt like it was dead.

"Since my run had counted, I had to submit to all the usual weight and measurement checks. Once that was done, I snagged another slider to help me into the truck for the ride back to Ladies Start. I remember sitting in the back of that panel truck, asking myself... what the heck had gone wrong? What would my coach say? What would my mother say? What was I going to find when I pulled my racing bootie off?

"It's like the whole thing happened yesterday... hobbling into the start house... taking my usual seat by the window... reaching down to unzip my plastic racing bootie. That's when I noticed the blood seeping through the zipper. My ankle and foot were still totally numb. It was such an awful sensation, to know I'd hurt myself real badly and yet had no pain whatsoever.

"I tried to remove the bootie as gently as I could, but finally I just yanked the damn thing off. The girl sitting next to me ran outside to throw up. I nearly joined her. My Achilles tendon was staring up at me through a two-inch tear in the heel of my sock.

"I was right about one thing, though. I definitely would've set a personal best time if I'd been able to keep that stupid sled between my rear end and the ice. Even with the crash, I moved up to third position and won the bronze... wound up beating the girl who'd once proudly competed for Canada at the Sarajevo Games."

Angie paused to finish her cooler.

"And as my fellow teammates were on their way to the awards presentation, the great A.Y. Jackson was on her way to the Lake Placid hospital to have her mangled foot stitched back together.

"Thirty-six hours later, I was back home in Calgary with my swollen ankle in a hot saline foot bath, feeling real depressed, when I got a surprise phone call. It was the National coach. My race results had been good enough to get me invited to the National Team training camps that summer and fall! There was a God.

"The head coach set up a specialized weight-training program to strengthen my injured ankle. I worked so hard that summer. Seven months after almost slicing my achilles tendon in half, I was finally able to run again!

"While the training camps had gone well, when I met with the head coach for her evaluation, I was told I would be rejoining the provincial program. The reason? I needed more track time, in particular, I needed European track experience.

"As it turned out, not making the national squad was a blessing in disguise. I mean, dry land training was one thing. Racing was another. All summer long, the fact that I'd come so close to crippling myself secretly haunted me. The coach said to think of it as a freak, once-in-a-lifetime thing. But when I got back to Placid that fall, I found myself afraid of the track. Geez, just seeing the turn-off sign for Mt. Van Hoevenberg was enough to make my heart start pounding.

"I just couldn't get my head together—I was crashing or nearly crashing on almost every single run I made. Some of the sliders were even joking about placing bets on my chances of making it down the course without a Code eighty-one being called.

"The coach never gave up on me, though. Even sent me to Austria with the rest of the team to train on the track there. It didn't help. I was washed up as a competitive slider. My dream of representing Canada at the Calgary Olympic Winter Games had ended, not with a roar from the hometown crowd, but with a gutless whimper.

"Well, maybe not a whimper. I made what was to be my final training run on the same day the space shuttle was to launch. When I completed my run, an Austrian track worker came rushing over, waving his arms above his head. He only knew two words of English, but on this historic day, they were all he needed to get his message across.

"Challenger ka-boom... fraulein... Challenger ka-boom!"

Dale sat quietly for a long while. "When we all went sliding that night at Canada Olympic Park, you seemed so sure of yourself... so calm... so relaxed. Were you?"

His question brought a lopsided grin to Angie's face. "The only part of me that still likes to race is my heart. When I'm waiting up there in the handles, I swear to God sometimes it feels like the damn thing's beating so fast it's going to jump right out of my chest. In order to race, you have to be able to push yourself to the limit... right to the very edge. I know the price for straying over that fine line. Guess I'm just not willing to tempt fate anymore."

"Can I take a peek at the scar?"

"Just like a man!" The flustered flight nurse responded with an exasperated groan as she slowly reached down to peel her sock off.

In the shape of the letter "C" lying on its back, the scar extended four inches across her heel... completely encircling the base of the achilles tendon. "A quarter-inch higher and I would've had a permanent limp. Are you suitably impressed?" she needled, quickly pulling her sock back on.

"I don't blame you for not wanting something like that to happen again!"

"Enough about me Captain Morgan. Now it's your turn for show-and-tell. I want to see where that bullet altered your hairline."

Tugging her mitts off, Dale took hold of her hand and slowly guided it along the right side of his head.

"Oh my lord!" Her fingers were probing a ragged furrow that extended from just above his ear to the nape of his neck. Smoothing his thinning blond hair back into place, something she'd been wondering about suddenly came to mind.

"I don't mean to pry, but that friend you told me about, the one who was killed. His name was Brian James Cole. Isn't your son's name uh...."

The warmth of the wood fire seemed to move into the Aussie's eyes. Slowly, he nodded.

Dale began talking about the war, and how it had affected him psychologically. His wife had suffered through two excruciatingly lonely years without him. Upon his return, she immediately tried to change him back to the man with whom she'd exchanged wedding vows. She never could accept the fact that the unspoken atrocities of war had drastically and permanently altered his entire outlook on life.

Angie had by now finished her third cooler, and with alcohol clouding her judgment, uttered the heartfelt observation, "You know, in some ways we're very much alike... you and me—we're both unlucky in love."

Eventually shedding toques and gloves as they snuggled, one behind the other, their conversation turned to the delicate subject of relationships. As if he were a professor on the topic, Dale felt compelled to give the young woman nestled in his arms some expert advice. "This won't be for a long while yet, but someday, when you start having thoughts of maybe striking up a relationship with somebody new, make sure you're mentally ready for it. Dragging old baggage from one romance to another is something you should try very hard to avoid.

"My marriage was on shaky ground for a long time before we finally decided to call it quits. I still loved her with all my heart, but our lives kept drifting further apart. Whenever we'd try to talk about our problems, we'd end up in a screaming match. I didn't know what to do. I was so desperate for someone to talk to... someone to listen to me. One night, when I was out drowning my sorrows at the local pub, I ran into an old girlfriend.

"Suddenly here was someone who appreciated me for what I was. Someone I could tell all my innermost secrets to... someone I could trust... someone to hold me on lonely nights.

"One morning I woke up with Nancy asleep beside me. Looking down, seeing her there, I came to the shocking realization that I wasn't in love with her. That I never had been and probably never would be.

"Watching her make me breakfast that morning, I knew I couldn't let it go on without telling her how I felt. I wasn't ready to get emotionally involved with anyone. I liked Nancy an awful lot, but as much as I hated to admit it, I'd just used her. I couldn't live with myself. That's why I left. I had to get away. What with an ex-wife and an ex-girlfriend hounding me, I needed a fresh start. And that selfishness cost me my son."

Angie felt Dale tighten his arms around her waist as he nuzzled the back of her neck. Growing bolder, he allowed his lips to stray to even more sensuous territory... her velvety-soft ear lobe. "I bet that feels good, doesn't it?" he murmured. "Makes you feel safe... and secure... and warm."

Angie didn't know what to say. There was no doubt. Having a man wrap his big, strong arms around her was a nice sensation, alright. Feeling herself growing warmer by the second, her mouth suddenly went dry. What the heck did this crazed Australian have in mind, exactly? A fireside romp on the floor?

Dale continued as if Angie had said yes. "What's the matter, luv, cat got your tongue? I'll bet you really like having me hold you in my arms, don't you? And yet, at the same time, you're feeling guilty as sin because poor old Russ hasn't been dead three months, and you shouldn't be having these kind of feelings already. Am I right?"

Angie twisted to face him. "How the hell do you know what I'm feeling?"

"Because I've been there... that's why. Don't make the same stupid mistake. Until you're completely over this thing, don't let anybody crawl into the sack with you just because you're feeling cold and lonely. The sooner you get used to sleeping by yourself... the better off you'll be. Heck, when I first moved here, I nearly froze to death at night. But you know what? I went out and bought myself one of those electric blankets and now, whenever I get cold, I just crank up the dial and cuddle with it, instead."

"Come on!" Angie fired back. "What about all those hot-to-trot buckle-bunnies who were lusting after your body that night at Ringo's?You mean to tell me that not one of them got an invitation to follow you home?"

"Ms. Jackson, I'll have you know I'm a man of high moral fiber. That, plus the fact I was still suffering from that God-awful luge-induced leg cramp. I mean, a guy can't really give it his all when his leg's cramping up and... uh... getting back to the benefits of owning an electrical appliance, my blanket doesn't have cold feet, it doesn't snore, and I can respect myself in the morning."

Pausing as he gazed down at her innocent face, the pilot added thoughtfully, "You want to know something else, Ange? Someday you'll wake up one morning and find you won't have that guilty feeling anymore. When that happens, you'll know you're ready to get on with your life.

"You'll meet someone new. Or maybe it'll be somebody you've known a long time... only now you'll find yourself looking at him in a whole different light. The most important thing is not to rush into anything."

"What if I take too long, and by the time I'm ready, the guy's lost interest and is looking around for someone else to... uh... "

Dale laughed. "In that case, about all you can do is just be honest with the poor bloke and tell him that you need more time and if he still gives you some crappy line about how his juiced-up equipment will be irreparably damaged if he can't spend the night, well... he probably wasn't worth having around in the first place."

Having said his piece, Angie again felt the Aussie's arms tighten ever-so-slightly around her waist.

Glancing down at Dale's muscular hands, Angie couldn't help complimenting him on having such nice veins. "Good golly, nurses the world over would be drooling to get their fingers on these puppies!" she teased as she playfully palpated a particularly plump vein running down the side his forearm.

"That's how I met Russ. I was at a cabaret and he was the bartender. I must've gone up and ordered at least a dozen beers that night. He told me later that he thought I was an alcoholic. All I really wanted was to introduce myself, but I didn't know what to say, so I finally leaned across the bar and yelled, "Excuse me, sir, could I have another Big Rock, please, and by the way... do you know you've got the biggest veins I've ever seen?"

Having his veins stroked was something Dale had never experienced before in his life... and while he fought hard not to let on, there was definitely something very erotic about it. Especially when it was being performed by a certain fair-haired flight nurse.

Stifling a massive yawn, Angie checked her watch. "Two-thirty! Where the heck did the evening go?"

"Think we should call it a night?" Dale asked.

Angie nodded wearily. Helping each other to their feet, they shuffled off to their respective beds.

It was just after four a.m. when Dale suddenly awoke. Poking his nose out from under his wafer-thin, regulation motel blanket, the room was the temperature of a meat locker. Drawing his blanket around him, he headed for the fireplace to throw on more logs. Rounding the foot of Angie's bed in the semi-darkness, it was only then that Dale noticed it was empty. What the heck? Continuing toward the fireplace, he spotted her huddled in front of the smoldering embers, her threadbare blanket pulled over her head like a hood. She was shivering.

"Waiting for Santa?" he tried to joke as he knelt beside her.

"I used up the last of the logs," she answered through chattering teeth. "I also have a little confession to make—you're not the only one who sleeps with an electric blanket."

"Why on earth would you need an electric blanket when you had Russ to keep you warm?"

"He didn't live at my place, you know! There were some nights when I had to fend for myself!"

"I didn't mean for it to come out like that," Dale apologized, reaching out to pull the crestfallen woman to her feet. "I can be such a dope sometimes. Let me make it up to you, okay?" He turned to lead her toward his bed.

Angie, immediately getting the wrong idea as to how Dale intended to make up for his verbal blunder, pulled away.

"Trust me, it's not what you think," the Aussie reassured her. "Really. I can't sleep, either. Take a look at these rags they call blankets! You can practically see through the bloody things!

"Answer me this: Do you have cold feet?"

"Not when I'm wearing socks, I don't," Angie responded icily.

"Do you hog the covers? Do you snore?"

Angie raised an eyebrow. "I've never had anyone complain yet!"

"Okay," Dale continued, "if we're to survive this night, maybe we should try combining our blankets and our body heat."

"Excuse me, but isn't this what you just warned me not to do? I'm supposed to get used to sleeping alone... remember?"

"Yes... but no. This is different. Totally different. This is just two good friends who are trying to stave off the deadly effects of hypothermia. I'll be sharing your body heat, nothing more."

Her better judgment impaired by fatigue, Angie climbed into Dale's bed. Immediately assuming the fetal position as she slipped between the well-worn sheets, she felt Dale slide in right behind her. Wrapping his arms around her, he snuggled his sweatshirted chest against her back.

With both blankets pulled up to her eyebrows and the Aussie's bulging bicep resting comfortably across her waist, Angie lay in the dark with her eyes wide open. As she listened to the hushed sound of his breathing, however, she soon discovered that it had a very soothing sound; almost hypnotic.

Though the possibility of this middle-aged Romeo ravishing her body while she slept still occupied her thoughts, Angie could not deny the toasty warmth his lean frame radiated through to her shivering backside.

As she felt her aching muscles slowly begin to relax, Angie hated to admit it, but she did feel safe with these virile Australian arms wrapped around her. Within ten minutes, she was fast asleep.

Feeling her body sink against his in sleep, the Aussie smiled as he discreetly snuggled closer. If he died in his sleep tonight, he would die a happy man. And as he, too, began to drift off, a solitary thought flickered briefly through his brain. "This sure beat the heck out of an electric blanket."

44
NOW OR NEVER

One evening, a few days after returning from Creston, Angie found herself pulling into a parking spot in front of the LIFE-STAR hangar.

Hesitating outside the office door, she peeked through the window as Sue Dyer, the flight nurse on duty sauntered past on her way to the TV room. Angie's anxious features instantly transformed into a devilish grin as she watched the fiery redhead flop onto the couch with a glossy fashion rag and a bag of Doritos.

Catching Sue completely immersed in some mindless article about feminine hygiene, Angie silently crept up behind her. "Didn't your mother teach you all about that kind of stuff?"

Poor Sue nearly aspirated her corn chip. Spinning around to confront her attacker, the irate flight nurse couldn't believe her eyes. "Angie! Hey, I knew you couldn't stay away forever!" she exclaimed, greeting her friend with a big hug. "Gee, it's good to see you. How you doing, girl? You holding up okay?"

Snagging a chip, Angie nodded. "I'm doing okay. You know, taking each day as it comes. I was just driving by... saw the light on. Figured I'd probably find you guys kicking back... watching a movie or something."

"And just who is this young lady?" a voice thundered. Peter Lawson stood leaning against the kitchen counter, a pair of half-glasses dangling from his neck. "She looks an awful lot like that legendary nurse we once had working here. What was her name? Grandma Moses or Whistler's Mother or something? She was named after a painter, but I could never remember which one."

Lawson stepped forward so he, too, could deliver a welcoming bear hug. "We've missed you a lot, Ms. A.Y. Jackson RN," he added. "The place just hasn't been the same without you."

Peter filled his mug with fresh brew and gestured to her to follow him. Taking a seat in his office, Angie nervously picked at her fingernails. "Mr. Lawson, I missed you guys a lot, too. I was out driving tonight and I saw the light on in your office and I uh... thought I'd just drop in and say hi... you know... see how things were going."

"Really!" a wide-eyed Peter responded. "You were just in the neighborhood and decided to drop in and say hi? That was awfully sweet of you! Heck, you had me worried there for a minute. When I saw your car parked out front, I thought you were stopping by to ask about maybe coming back here to hang your stethoscope."

"Uh, well sir, now that you mention it, I was wondering if I could maybe talk to you about picking up a few shifts here and there. You know, maybe cover sick calls, short notice, that kind of stuff?"

Peter studied the earnest young woman seated before him. "Angela, absolutely nothing would please me more than to see your name back in the shift book. Only trouble is, the med-evac business doesn't play favorites. Those first few flights... they could be rough ones. Are you sure you're ready?"

"I think I am, sir. I've thought about it a lot over the last few weeks, and well, I think it's time I got off the dole and started earning my keep. In my entire nursing career, nothing made me feel more alive than pulling on my flight suit. I want that feeling back."

There was a knock at the door; Sue was all suited up. "Sorry to bother you, sir, but Kyle just phoned on the cellular from Parkland. We're being dispatched on another call... to Bassano for an MVA. As soon as they can get the Neonatal ICU team unloaded, they're coming right back to refuel. The pilots asked me to have all our downloaded equipment waiting at the hangar doors. Great to see you again, Ange. Wish us a good flight!"

Ten minutes later, the red helicopter purred into sight. No sooner had its skids touched down than the co-pilot cracked his door open to wave the fuel truck into position.

Kyle jogged over to help Sue guide the top-heavy stretcher across the dimly-lit tarmac. Within seconds, they had it hoisted aboard and locked into the floor's brown lining. With no time to fool around, the two medics immediately went about securing all the equipment that had been removed from the chopper to make room for the bulky NICU isolette.

Strapping himself in, Kyle reached back to plug in his helmet cord. Difficult to reach at the best of times, the radio jack was located on the bulkhead above and behind his head. After blindly probing the darkness, Kyle was about to triumphantly bury his plug to the hub when his female cohort let loose with a yowl. "Excuse me, but would you kindly get your plug the heck out of my hole?"

Co-pilot Jan Elliot flipped on the intercom to ask if his medical crew was ready for take-off. All he got was a giddy, high-pitched squeal. After several more seconds of what sounded like smooching, a breathless Kyle finally broke through. "That's a great big Roger Wilco, my good buckeroo! Permission granted to fly us to the moon!"

"What the heck is going on back there?" Jan demanded. "Stevens, are you and Sue sniffing the oxygen again?"

Going on the assumption that his demented medical crew was, indeed, ready, Captain Alex Davis pulled the aircraft into a low hover. Following a final check of his instruments, he gently eased his cyclic control forward, sending the BK careening across the short runway apron with nose down and tail high... rocketing up into the overcast night sky.

Jan came over the intercom again. "Stevens, have either you or Sue thought to contact dispatch with an update? You know, the usual BS... that we're en route, our ETA to the Bassano hospital, where to start looking if we don't show up?"

A female voice clicked on. "Swearing on the radio is a big no-no, Jan. You'd better hope that Lord Peter never finds out."

Leaving the mouthy co-pilot choking on his tongue, the female half of the medical crew switched from the intercom to the provincial frequency. "Calgary dispatch, this is LIFE-STAR one. How do you read? Over."

Unable to stand the suspense, Jan, twisting sideways in his seat, yanked aside the heavy curtains that separated the pilots from the medics. Whoever the woman was... and it sure the heck wasn't Sue, was now listening as dispatch acknowledged her transmission. Glancing in the perturbed flyboy's direction, she flashed him a big grin.

"Calgary dispatch, this is LIFE-STAR One. I copy that. We are currently outbound to Bassano. Our ETA will be approximately twenty-two-thirty hours. We will contact you on our return flight, over."

"Roger, LIFE-STAR One. Have a good flight. Dispatch, clear."

A.Y. Jackson had returned to face the music... and the world again.

45
A GHOST FROM THE PAST

One short week before the Olympics were to begin, a call came in from the emergency doctor at the Banff hospital. She wanted the chopper sent stat for a critically-unstable 45 year-old male anterior MI patient.

An uncomplicated MI, or heart attack, was bad enough, but an anterior MI was the worst type imaginable. Because it wreaked havoc with the heart's conduction system, and caused massive tissue damage to the left side of the heart, CCU nurses nicknamed it "The Widow-Maker."

If the patient was to survive the next few hours, his only chance depended upon immediate transport to a major cardiac care facility and placement on an intra-aortic balloon pump—a machine that would take over the workload of his badly-damaged left ventricle.

Handing the portable phone to Kyle, Alex hustled into the pilots' room where Dale already had the weather office on the other line. "We're a go," Dale yelled as he hung up the receiver, "but it's cold as heck up there today—minus thirty, so you and Angie had better have your winter woollies on!"

With Alex at the controls, the chopper touched down at Parkland just long enough to pick up flight physician Robert Markum. Having the doctor with them on this particular mission was imperative, for if their patient's heart suddenly decided to pack it in while they were two thousand feet up, it would take three sets of knowledgeable hands to conduct a Code—one to bag, one to do CPR, and one to give drugs and pray.

Soaking up the warmth as shafts of brilliant Alberta sunshine streamed through the windows, Angie and Kyle watched Dr. Bob eat his way through their entire bag of chocolate chip cookies. Her stomach growling in protest, Angie was about to ask the ravenous doc if he'd like a Gravol to top off his meal when Dale's Aussie drawl filled her headset.

"Folks, I'm afraid I've got some bad news for you. Banff hospital just radioed to cancel us. Apparently, their patient gave up the ghost five minutes ago. However, we've just intercepted an urgent radio patch from Yoho National Park. Seems three ice climbers got caught in an avalanche and the Parks Service is in the process of airlifting them off the mountain. As soon as I mentioned we had a doctor on board, the warden requested we nip on over there and fly at least one of them back with us."

"So we're headed for Supernatural British Columbia, eh?" Kyle said. "Have you radioed ahead and gotten us a 'P' number yet, Oh Great One?"

"Of course I've got a 'P' number," Dale replied. "Without a 'P' number, our program would be forced to financially eat this trip. Just to bring you up to speed, our ETA to scene shouldn't be more than twenty minutes. No, better make that twenty-five. I forgot Alex was on the stick today. Once he gets in the mountains, he can never tell which direction he's traveling... so we'll probably... have to drop down... and follow the... uh... highway like last time." Dale's last few words were disjointed, almost as if someone had been jabbing him hard in the ribs.

As bleak, glacial-scoured mountain tops swept past on either side, Angie, Kyle and Bob reviewed their plan of attack for when they arrived on-scene.

The Yoho wardens would be in charge of getting the victims off the mountain. They had a Jet Ranger helicopter for just such emergencies. Outfitted with backpacks stuffed with medical gear, specially-trained wardens could be suspended under the chopper by means of a sling and flown directly to the scene.

After triaging the victims and deciding who could wait and who couldn't, the warden would package and load the most critical patient into a Bauman transport bag. He and his patient would then be air-lifted down to the valley floor where the LIFE-STAR crew would be standing by.

Saving precious minutes by beginning treatment on the patient while the chopper was racing for Calgary, Angie and her co-workers envisioned a slick operation, a clear demonstration of how rescue programs could work together to save time... and possibly a life.

With any luck, they'd be back at the hangar in time for supper and the six o'clock news.

There was only an hour of daylight left as Alex swung the BK around to begin his approach to the landing area set up by the local RCMP. It was Standard Operating Procedure to circle the landing area at least once to check for hazards, and to leave the chopper's intercom open during landings and take-offs so the medical crew could keep a watchful eye, as well.

Glancing out her window as Alex set up to land, Angie was shocked to see another chopper rapidly approaching from above and behind them. Someone was swinging wildly back and forth beneath it like a spider on the end of a fragile thread. It was the Parks Service's Search and Rescue bird. But the chopper's flight path was completely erratic! Rolling and yawing violently from side to side, it appeared to be totally out of control… flinging the dangling warden every which way as he fought to hold onto a Bauman transport bag suspended horizontally across his hips.

"Alex," Angie screamed into her mouthpiece, "you've got a Parks Service helicopter descending above and behind you off your port side. It's coming down right on top of us!"

Immediately Alex put the chopper into a barrel roll to the right. With less than a hundred feet between his skids and the tree tops, Captain Davis had just enough room to bank sharply out of the way as the other chopper flashed past, and disappeared below them.

They had avoided a mid-air collision by less than fifty feet.

A split second later, a tremendous explosion rocked the LIFE-STAR helicopter. The shock wave nearly sent the BK autorotating into the thick blanket of spruce trees below.

When a pilot looks out his front window and sees nothing but an approaching blur of trees, the experience can be a deeply-religious one. Helicopters are delicate aircraft with super-sensitive controls; they don't like to be manhandled. A tribute to his skill, it was only Alex's calm, gentle touch on the controls that prevented LIFE-STAR 1 from becoming the subject of yet another chopper fatality inquiry.

As senior pilot on board, Dale ordered Alex to continue circling while those on the ground had a chance to deal with the situation. In an attempt to explain what had probably just occurred, Dale told his troubled crewmates of a similar occurrence in Vietnam.

"We were flying back to base with a fresh batch of GIs when the Huey in formation next to us took a mortar round through the cockpit. Even with its front-end blown off, that Huey continued to chug along for another four to five seconds before it suddenly pitched nose-down. That's when the smoke cleared enough for us to see one of the dead pilots slumped forward on his cyclic control.

"The body of a helicopter is suspended beneath the rotors, much like a giant pendulum," Dale went on. "Therefore, shoving the cyclic hard in any direction can have disastrous results. With the stick driven all the way forward, the Huey was forced into such an acute-angle dive that its tail boom section thrust upward into the overhead rotors.

"Its blades exploded into fragments as they sliced through the tailboom. There was nothing we could do except watch as that million dollar fireball plunged two thousand feet to the jungle floor. Took with it the lives of seven marines and two of my good friends."

By some awful twist of fate, it seemed as if a similar scenario had just claimed the Yoho Parks Service helicopter. As the lone pilot fought to regain control of his windmilling aircraft, hanging below, the warden and his patient were dragged along the snow-cushioned ground for a hundred feet before the cool-headed rescue specialist was finally able to cut his harness free.

Suddenly 380 pounds lighter, the chopper shot straight up into the air. Holding in a hover 150 feet above ground, the aircraft wobbled erratically for several heart-stopping seconds. Then, just like the ghastly spectacle Dale had witnessed twenty years before, the chopper went into a steep nose-dive, its tail boom disappeared into the main rotors, and, in an awesome display of just how volatile aircraft fuel can be, the chopper blew apart in mid-air.

With sheets of flame and blazing chunks of twisted metal raining down around them, the two wardens waiting on the ground risked their lives, running to help their fallen buddy drag his unconscious patient out of harm's way and over to the Parks Service's van.

Having seen enough, Dale contacted the scene commander on the ground.

"LIFE-STAR One, I read you loud and clear. This is Chief Warden Dennis Kallow. That was our Parks Service helicopter that just exploded. Both flight crew members are missing and presumed dead. The rescue specialist and patient they were slinging, however, both survived the crash, but they're pretty banged up. With forty-five minutes of usable daylight left, I'm forced to ask for assistance. Do you have anyone on board with rappelling or sling experience? Over."

"Warden Kallow, flight paramedic Kyle Stevens here. We have two people on board trained in rappel descents."

Angie immediately plucked at his sleeve. Who the heck was he kidding? Kyle might have had training in it, but she was the only LIFE-STAR medic to have actually done it with a real live patient. Unruffled, Kyle continued, "How many patients are involved, sir? Over."

"Three patients in all. One rescued, and two still marooned up on the mountainside." The head warden paused. "Uh, look LIFE-STAR, we have to get these climbers off the mountain in the next half-hour or we're not going to get them off at all. We have two options. Our first option has you flying up there to assess the situation. If you don't think you can get both victims off before we lose our light, you are to come straight back here.

"The temperature tonight is expected to go down to minus forty, so the second option isn't much of an alternative at all. It would involve lowering my already banged-up man and his survival gear down to the injured climbers to spend the night. I have him with me right now. He used to work in Calgary as a medic so he might even know some of you guys. He's still pretty sore, but, as he's not relishing the idea of freezing his nuts off tonight, he's offering his assistance with the rescue if you feel you're not up to it. Over."

One look at his partner's bugged-out eyes told Kyle all he needed to know. "You want to guess who that might be? Ange, do you really want that arrogant S.O.B. up here with us? For Christ's sake, girl, any idiot can do a simple rappel to the ground... even me!"

Angie was still thinking about the ramifications of ex-flame Jefferson Logan climbing on board, when Kyle blurted, "Jackson, don't sweat it, okay? I'll do the actual rappel, not you. All you'll have to do is sit on your pretty little ass and keep an eye on my rope. Think you can handle that?"

Her face a searing blend of outrage and defiance, Angie glared out her window as she keyed her mike. "Warden Kallow, this is LIFE-STAR One. We will not be requiring assistance from you at this time. We'll go up and take a look-see. If we find it's within our capabilities, we'll be toting you back a patient in very short order. Please give our kindest regards to Mr. Logan, though. LIFE-STAR One, out."

As Kyle clipped the tight-fitting rappel harness over his insulated flight suit, Angie tied a Purssik safety knot into his line. Within minutes, Alex had the chopper in a hover fifty feet above the injured men. Clinging to the forty-five degree slope, the motionless climbers lay side by side with a pale blue sleeping bag stretched over them.

Tiny by Yoho standards, a mere quarter-mile long and one hundred feet wide, the avalanche had still been powerful enough to strip away everything right down to bedrock. Trees, boulders, the seven foot-thick snow pack. From the air, the slide's classic fan-shaped path was unmistakable. So was something else. The slide's abrupt termination at the lip of a thousand foot cliff.

Why the experienced ice climbers had dared venture out onto such an unstable slope, and how they'd avoided being swept over the cliff to their deaths probably boiled down to two simple facts: they'd been incredibly foolish and they'd been incredibly lucky.

Kyle made it down to the climbers without incident, and immediately began assessing their injuries. The first man was shivering, but awake and alert with closed fractures of both femurs. "Everything's going to be fine," Kyle reassured him.

Then he peeked at the second victim under the sleeping bag. Barely conscious with an obviously depressed skull fracture, the climber's frost-bitten nose and ears were thickly crusted with pinkish-yellow cerebral spinal fluid.

"Oh wonderful," Kyle muttered. "If old Jeffy boy thought that either of these two was stable enough to be left behind, I don't want to know how badly off the other fellow must've been!"

A soft, swooshing sound made the medic swing around. Another small slide was careening down the slope fifty yards to his left. Scrambling to his feet, Kyle's crampon-studded boot caught on something. Hidden under the snow, two silver pitons with attached carabiners had been hammered into the bedrock. A gray climbing rope had been threaded through the carabiners and then tied off to each of the climbers.

That damn Logan had thought of everything!

Clipping himself into the safety line, Kyle took stock of the situation. There was absolutely no way he was going to get his head-injured patient onto the scoop stretcher and into the Bauman transport bag without some help from above.

The last thing he wanted to do was admit he'd bitten off more than he could chew. But, staring down at the patient, the medic knew he was only wasting precious time by delaying. Removing a glove with his chattering teeth, Kyle radioed the chopper. "Oh Ange, this is your good buddy Kyle here. Could I interest you in maybe popping down here for a bit? The patient I want to sling out first has a bad head injury, so I'll need someone to do C-spine. While you're at it, bring the Sager, the spare transport bag and a head roll, too."

Angie was already half-frozen from sitting on the floor of the hovering BK with one foot firmly planted to either side of the open door. She stared down at her radio in disbelief.

Before he had backed his self-assured ass out the door, Stevens had been most adamant that her only duty would be making sure his rappel rope did not slip through the ring bolted to the floor. She could have wrung her "good buddy's" neck.

"I'll be right down," the nurse answered, "just as soon as I find a silver bullet to load in my gun!"

"Ange, you don't have to do this, you know," Dale spoke up. "We can leave Stevens down there by himself for a few minutes while we fly back to get that other warden."

"If we do that, I'll have to put two bullets in my gun!" Angie retorted. "You guys just fly this cruddy bird, alright? It's up to us medics to handle all the real fun stuff. After all, eight months ago, I trained for a whole three hours for just such an occasion." As she spoke, Angie was madly yanking medical equipment from the nooks and crannies around her and stuffing them into her backpack.

Exiting the helicopter, Angie looked back at Dr. Bob. The usually bubbly emerg physician's face was a pale shade of green. "God, please don't let him woof on me on the way down!" Before stepping off into space, she mentally added, "And if the doc faints and lets go of my rope, I wanna land square on Kyle!"

Night was swiftly smothering the mountain peaks in pillowy shadows. If Kyle and Angie could not get the climbers packaged and ready for transport within the next 20 minutes, they would be forced to abandon the rescue attempt... and likely the lives of the two young men.

A mere six minutes after touching down, Angie and Kyle had the head-injured patient C-collared, restrained, bagged and ready to be air-lifted out.

As he carefully threaded a rope through the many loops on the Bauman bag, Kyle attempted to make amends. "Why don't you sling this one out, Ange? I'll stay behind and get this other guy packaged. I'll have him ready and waiting by the time you get back."

"Look Stevens, this patient is all yours! You found him. You keep him!" the testy nurse snapped. "If by some chance he becomes combative on the way down and feels the need to punch someone's lights out, I'd just as soon it was you tied to him, not me!"

Kyle began to protest, but Angie cut him off. "Get moving, will you? The sun's going down and I don't want to spend any more time in this frozen wasteland than I have to... so take off, eh?" Kyle radioed the boys above to lift off.

"Hurry back," Angie whispered as she watched Kyle, his patient and the chopper disappear below the cliff. All alone now, the flight nurse set about splinting her remaining patient's badly-fractured femurs. The cold had mercifully numbed the excruciating pain in his legs, but it had also dropped his body core temperature into the danger zone. That, coupled with the massive amount of blood he'd already lost into his thighs meant that, with each passing second, the poor guy was slipping closer and closer toward irreversible shock.

Using the sleeping bag, Angie gently eased the patient onto the backboard. Once she'd secured all the straps, it was then a relatively simple task to skid the backboard into the Bauman bag.

Calmly reassuring her patient that slinging people off a mountainside was all in a day's work, Angie gently tucked the sleeping bag around him before zipping the bag closed. She looked off to the northeast. What the heck was taking her "good buddy" so long?

Knowing that, during his descent, he would lose sight of Kyle and the patient swinging below as soon as the rotors started kicking up snow, Alex focused all his attention on a lone park warden standing in the middle of the highway. Signaling him in for a landing was Jefferson Logan.

Positioned with the blustery wind to his back, Jeff had warned everyone to stay well back until Kyle's feet made contact with the roadway. Swaying back and forth under a whirling helicopter was a great way to build up a static electrical charge, and until Kyle grounded himself by touching the road with his crampons, anyone foolish enough to reach up and touch him was in for one heck of a shock.

Fifty feet up the road, two wardens stood crouched, ready to cart the patient off to their van as soon as Jeff gave them the signal.

Its rotorwash blasting the highway free of snow, the helicopter hung in a hover above the LZ. Staring intently out his side window, Alex carefully lowered his collective control until he had Kyle and his patient safely on the ground.

Dr. Markum meanwhile, barely waiting until the aircraft itself had touched down, was out his door and running. Flinging a soggy cookie bag into the ditch, the ashen-faced physician rushed to help the wardens with their patient.

Kyle was so frosted up from his two-minute flight that his tearing eyes had frozen shut. It was as he was trying to gently pry his lashes apart, that Jefferson's bearded face suddenly swam into view. "Where's Angie?" he demanded, starting toward the helicopter. He poked his head inside, then spun around. "Dear Jesus, tell me you didn't leave her up there? Didn't you wonder why we didn't leave any of our guys up there? Didn't you see the two huge cornices still hanging above the chute?

With the snow pack so unstable, they could come crashing down any second. You've got to get right back up there and...."

The words caught in his throat as the frozen ground beneath his boots began to vibrate ever-so-slightly. The roar of the rotors was drowning out all sound, but as a million tons of snow suddenly lost its grip on a steep mountainside a half-mile away, its mammoth footsteps could be detected by anyone well-versed in the ways of the high country.

His unblinking eyes filled with terror, the warden watched as the spot where Angie and the climber had been, disappeared beneath a churning wall of snow.

There was nothing left on the slope after the avalanche passed. Only denuded limestone.

As the suffocating mass swept off the cliff and began its dizzying thousand-foot fall to the valley below, a shimmering cloud of ice particles spread out gracefully behind it like a billowing bridal train. Tumbling through the air in slow motion, the monstrous slide eventually impaled itself, roaring with fury, upon the evergreen forest below.

The sun meanwhile, had quietly slipped from sight behind the hulking silhouette of Mount Stephen. It was officially sundown, and the air temperature was minus 39 degrees.

Jeff grabbed Kyle by the throat and threw him against the helicopter. "You just killed her! Do you know that? By leaving her behind, you just signed her God damn death warrant!"

46
GONE, BUT NOT FORGOTTEN

There was no point sending the 'copter up for even a cursory look around. In scene commander Kallow's mind, with total darkness only minutes away, the only rational thing the grieving LIFE-STAR crew could do now was accept the truth, load the two surviving patients into the BK and hustle back to Calgary.

Eyes riveted to the pale green video screen, it was Dale who thought to use the FLIR Infrared Spotting Scope to scan the vast area below the cliff in the faint hope that Angie or her patient might have hung up on something. As the translucent veil of snow particles continued to trickle down from the barren slope above, however, only an endless expanse of cold, lifeless granite showed on the screen. There were no hot spots.

The Aussie switched the scope off and slowly turned toward the teary-eyed pilot sitting next to him. "Captain Davis, would you mind taking the stick on the return leg? I... uh, I'll owe you one."

Alone in the back of LIFE-STAR 1, Kyle, his face a mask of frozen tears, packed away his climbing equipment.

As he and Alex completed their pre-flight checks, Dale reached his hand down between the seats for the portable radio. Flipping it to channel seven, the frequency used for scene calls, the pilot squeezed the send button. "Angie... this is Dale. If you can hear me, luv, key your mike."

Except for the soft hiss of static, the radio remained silent. Repeating his plea twice more, the pilot was just about to quit the charade when his thickly-gloved fingers accidentally brushed against the radio's squelch knob. As the monotone hiss faded, a second sound, hidden beneath the first, made him instantly straighten up. It was faint. Probably his imagination. But as he and his flying partner sat in the cockpit... afraid even to think about the possibilities... over the radio came the unmistakable sound again. The sound of someone breathing.

Whoever was on that channel was holding their mike button down, preventing anyone from establishing contact. Dale almost dropped the radio as he switched to channel 1. "Warden Kallow, this is Captain Morgan! She's alive! Our flight nurse... she's alive!"

Busy organizing a search party to be sent out at dawn's first light, Warden Kallow had had enough death and destruction for one day. There was no point risking any more lives tonight, especially if the only thing his men would be looking for was bodies.

Forced to listen as the LIFE-STAR pilot, delirious with grief, ended his impossible spiel by brazenly asking permission to do a quick search of the cliff area, the warden's reply was explosive. "Are you out of your frigging mind? Permission denied! Your flight nurse is dead. She's buried under a hundred feet of snow. I don't know what you're picking up on channel seven, but trust me, it ain't her! Now, if you don't want to end up the same way, I'd advise you to have that machine of yours in the air and headed toward Calgary within the next five minutes! You got that?"

Having overheard Dale's transmission, Kyle used the cellular to dial Angie's voice pager. "Angie, release your mike button. If you can hear me, say something! Anything! I don't care how much it hurts. You've always been such a yappy little broad. Speak to me, damn it!"

Static spilled from the radio.

Kyle was raising his fist to slam it against the radio console when, above the static, a feeble voice crackled, "... hurting so bad. Please... don't leave me up here...."

Dale and Alex collided with each other as they leaped from their seats and raced around the front of the chopper to switch places. Only one man had the flying experience to go up and find Angie in the dark... and that man was just about to buckle himself into the Captain's seat.

Kyle jumped out the side door and raced into the night in search of Jefferson Logan. Jeff was stowing his rappelling gear into the back of Kallow's half-ton, and assumed Stevens had come to finish the fight. Balling up his fists, he was just about to land the first punch when Stevens grabbed him by the wrist. "For Christ's sake, Logan, would you grow the hell up and listen to me! I just talked to her on the radio... Angie's alive!"

47
WHEN YOU WISH UPON A STAR

It would have been such a beautiful evening to go flying. Gazing up through his overhead window, Alex could see the ghostly Aurora Borealis performing its spectral dance across the northern heavens... setting the velvety blackness of space ablaze with shimmering streamers of greens and purples.

The peaceful world beyond the helicopter's canopy was no match, however, for what was spewing forth from Alex's headset. Chief Warden Kallow had gone stark, raving berserk.

Piloting a helicopter was risky enough. Flying at night made the odds worse. Mountains didn't show up on radar, so attempting a helicopter rescue... at night... in the mountains... was suicide. Plain and simple. Besides taking the lives of three innocent crew members, if Dale succeeded in both killing himself and destroying his aircraft, who and what would be left to fly the two injured climbers back to Calgary?

"I don't know who the bloody hell you think you are, but if you don't turn that chopper of yours around immediately, I will see to it personally that you're grounded for the remainder of this life and quite possibly, for the duration of your future stay in Hell! Morgan... do you hear me, God damn it?"

Dale clicked his microphone button several times in rapid succession. "... hard to make out transmission... breaking up... radio malfunction... go to phonetic alphabet for further communication. Over."

Kallow was immediately back on the line and he did not use the phonetic alphabet to spell out what he thought of Dale and his bullshit radio malfunction, which was probably the oldest pilot trick in the book.

"Now, now," Dale chided. "No swearing on the radio. I'd love to stay and chat Dennis, but you see, I've grown rather fond of our flight nurse; promised I'd never return to base without her. Our ETA back to your location is unknown at this time. All I ask, is that you wish us luck. This is LIFE-STAR One, out."

Since Angie was still alive enough to talk... she obviously was not buried beneath the huge dump of snow at the base of the mountain. Therefore, the only other explanation was that she was hung up on the rockface somewhere below the cliff.

However, even after meticulously scanning the near-vertical granite wall for five minutes with the Spotting Scope, Kyle was no closer to pin-pointing Angie's whereabouts. "With that damn insulated flight suit on, she just isn't giving off any heat!" Kyle fumed. "Anybody got any better suggestions for locating her?"

It was Jefferson who spoke up. "Tell her to unzip her suit and face away from the wall if she can. If you still can't pick her up, tell her to take her helmet off."

"Are you crazy?" Kyle blasted. "She'll freeze to death."

Jeff slowly turned toward the lippy paramedic. "She's going to freeze to death anyway if we can't get her off this God damn mountain in the next fifteen minutes. I don't know how much fuel your pilots usually carry on board, but they must be getting awful close to the point of no return."

Dale was acutely aware of their fuel status. If they lit out for home right now, they might just make it. But that wasn't the only concern on his mind. It was so dark now, he had become wholly dependent upon the chopper's powerful Nite Sun spotlight.

Cautiously nosing his fragile aircraft closer and closer to the vertical rockface, the pilot's unblinking eyes were locked straight ahead. He had become one with the helicopter. He knew that the tiniest mistake could send them crashing into the wall, and from there, plummeting, rotorless, to the valley floor a thousand feet below.

Kyle contacted Angie and relayed Jeff's message about unzipping her flight suit and facing away from the wall. Very slow to radio back, her speech was noticeably slurred. But she still managed to tell the paramedic to kiss-off.

"Come on, Ange. Look, I hate having to ask you to do this, but I'm trying to pick you up with the Infrared Scanner and you're not radiating any heat. The sooner you unzip your flight suit, the sooner we can all go home."

Thirty minutes earlier, Angie had felt the bedrock shudder beneath her boots. Looking over her shoulder, she found herself staring into the face of death. A scant quarter-mile up the steep slope above her, a grayish-white cloud was boiling and seething, blocking out the last remnants of twilight as it began its descent toward her.

She had belayed her climbing rope through the twin carabiners and was in the process of lowering herself and her patient down the slope toward a small basin-like area fifty feet from the edge of the cliff. There, she reasoned, it would be easier for the helicopter to come in and drop her a line. Alex would have more room to maneuver and he wouldn't have to worry quite so much about clipping the unforgiving granite slope with the chopper's fragile rotors.

Now, however, she was hypnotized. As she gazed into the teeth of the murderous slide, Angie could already feel its corpse-like breath against her face. Knowing she had only seconds before the avalanche's preceding windstorm reached her, a deep-rooted survival instinct told her to run; to run as far away as humanly possible from this dreadful place. But where to? The slide thundering toward her was a half-mile wide. There was no place to go... not with a cliff behind her and a suffocating wall of snow bearing down on her from above.

Apparently, this time... there would be no Plan B.

Not knowing what else to do, she began madly dragging her packaged patient toward the sheer thousand-foot precipice. Disconnecting her Purssik safety line so she could run faster, her crazed mind did a strange thing. Suddenly it fragmented back... to training camp and the nurse who got herself hung upside-down under the eave during Dale's rappelling class.

With no time to put much thought into what she was about to try,

Angie heaved her neatly-coiled climbing rope out over the edge. Glancing back to make sure she was still tied into Jeff's piton anchors, she was about to lower her Bauman-bagged patient down the cliff face when her boots exploded out from under her.

Tumbling end-over-end as the avalanche's hurricane-force wind flung her through the air, the last thing Angie saw was the valley floor rushing toward her.

She'd been dangling 80 feet below the rim of the cliff for more than half-an-hour now, and with the minus forty degree temperature, Angie Jackson was not going to be staying with the program much longer. Bleeding profusely from the nose and mouth, Angie's probing tongue soon discovered the cause... two empty sockets where her right lower molars had been.

When the wind gust hurled her over the edge, her rappel rope had acted like a giant pendulum. The spine-jarring jolt of hitting the end of the rope had been nothing compared with slamming chest-first into the cliff wall on the inward swing. Her body had gone from 30 miles an hour to zero in less than one second.

Her numb, cold-stiffened fingers too clumsy to grasp the small metal zipper of her flight suit, Angie instead reached with an unsteady hand up toward the chin strap on her helmet. After failing several times to unsnap it, she cried out in frustration. What was the other thing Kyle had asked her to do? Huge blocks of snow suddenly began crashing down from above. Hugging her battered body tight against the rock face as the mini-avalanche roared past, Angie closed her swollen eyes and spoke to God.

"Please Lord, let me die."

Initially the crushing pain in her chest and the tremendous cold had been enough to keep her thoughts occupied. This was no longer true. Something sinister lurked in the surrounding darkness; something that would not be satisfied until it had sucked the life from her.

"Must be a Chinook blowing in," she muttered to herself. Incredibly, her teeth had stopped chattering. She no longer felt cold. How odd that her chest had quit hurting, as well. Come to think of it, none of her body parts seemed to have any feeling in them. Even the harsh, biting wind felt quite refreshing against her waxen, frostbitten-cheeks.

Reaching up with a rubbery right arm, Angie fumbled with the locking mechanism on the top of her helmet. It took her several tries, but she eventually managed to shove what was left of her visor back under its protective sheath. With nothing but black beneath her blood-spattered boots, Angie let her weary head fall back until she was staring blankly up into the black sky. "If you're going to take me, sir, then for God's sake take me now. Don't make me hang around here forever!"

She was drifting into a lovely, languid peace when a brilliant shooting star suddenly blazed across the heavens. Instead of fading away to nothingness, however, the solitary light grew steadily brighter and brighter until it seemed about to crash right into her.

Slowly turning her head toward it, the stuporous, barely-conscious nurse found herself squinting into the very face of God.

"How is it the Almighty can find me when no one from Search and Rescue could?" she pondered. "To be going to all this trouble to pick me up in person! He must really want my tortured soul in a bad way."

Suddenly, Angie's frozen brain began picking up disembodied voices from beyond. The voices sounded very excited as they all tried to talk to her at once. Someone was telling her not to move, while another voice, a voice that called itself Jeff, said, "Hang on, Babe, I'll be down to help you in just a few minutes!"

"Help me? What in heaven's name do I need help for?" she wondered. "I have God coming to take delivery of my mortal remains any moment now. I've had a rough life. I deserve to go to heaven, damn it! The last thing I need is some devil's disciple named Jeff to mess things up!"

Fighting to keep the wind-tossed BK under control, Dale and his formerly ecstatic crew gazed silently out their frosted windows at the motionless figure dangling a hundred feet away.

Like a Barbie doll cruelly strung on a wire, Angie's half-open eyes stared sightlessly. Her left hand, hopelessly tangled in the rappel rope, had been pulled up over her head at an awkward angle. All down the front of her red and white flight suit was a dark stain. A dark stain that had splattered down onto her white snow boots... turning them blood red.

Watching her limp body sway gently in the rotor's downwash, Kyle thought he saw something in the darkness twenty feet below her. It was the Bauman body bag. With half its support webbing torn away, the black bag hung vertically against the rock wall. Training the Spotting Scope upon it, Kyle reported somberly that while the main enclosure appeared to be intact, the poor guy inside had been hanging upside-down for nearly 45 minutes now. "Nobody could survive that."

Suddenly Angie and her patient disappeared behind a ghostly white veil, as yet another snowslide cascaded from above. Dale instinctively eased his aircraft away from the wall.

"Jeff, I'm looking at the fuel gauge right now and we don't have a whole lot of time to play with here. What do you want me to do? It's your call."

Warden Logan contemplated the situation. He was not about to rescue just any old climber. He was going after someone he'd once cared dearly about. Someone who, had the circumstances been just a little different, could very well have become his... well... who knows.

While flying up to the site, Jeff had quickly realized that he was in the company of three men whose emotional states went far beyond simply trying to save a valued crew member. These guys were putting their lives and their careers on the line for this woman. Against all odds, they had somehow found her in this nightmare of ice and snow, and now they were entrusting him, a much-despised former lover, with the job of bringing her safely off the mountain.

"Dale, I want you to line up straight across from her and then take us up. The only way I'll be able to stay in contact with the wall is if you hold in a real tight hover with the rotors overlapping the cliff edge. With so much snow still sifting off the slope, I'll have to follow the rope down to find her. I just hope it's still tied into the pitons and not just hung up on a rock ledge somewhere."

Jefferson Logan then did a very foolish thing—he asked Dale if he thought he could handle his assignment.

"I've been plucking people out of worse places than this since before you were born, Sonny!" the Aussie barked. "If we don't get her off tonight, it won't be because I was the one who screwed up! You got that?"

As Dale held his chopper in a hover above the black abyss that was the edge of the cliff, Jeff Logan began his descent to the barren slope below.

Thirty seconds later, his climbing boots made contact with the ground. He immediately went to check his piton and carabiner anchor. Dropping to his knees to brush away the snow, the warden let out a frosty sigh of relief. It had held. Angie's rappel rope was still looped through the double metal rings. He followed the taut nylon rope with his eyes as it disappeared over the cliff. It looked none-the-worse for wear; Jeff knew better. In stopping Angie's fall, tiny fibers inside the rope had stretched to the breaking point. Any added stress could cause the rope to snap.

Removing a jumar and a length of cord from his pack, Jeff quickly anchored the cord via a carabiner to a hastily-hammered piton before gently clipping the rectangle device onto Angie's fragile lifeline. Now, if the rope suddenly failed, the inverted jumar's pivoting cam would instantly grip the rope as it pulled through... holding it fast. At least he hoped so. Dear God, he'd never tried anything like this before.

Continuing his rappel down, 75 feet later, Jeff's boot brushed against something in the darkness. Thinking it was yet another rock outcropping, as he stepped on it to take a bit of a breather, he felt it move.

Fading in and out of consciousness, Angie had been just about to call it a life when Jeff's cramponed boot set down on her head. "Do you mind?" was all she muttered before lapsing back into her fantasy world again... to a dream that contained, of all things, a bottle of cheap wine, a roaring fire and a warm, cuddly Australian.

The moon picked just that moment to pop out from behind a snow-capped ridge. Two days short of full-term, it bathed the mountain valley in light. For the first time since he'd started down the jagged rock face, Jeff could see what he was doing.

Easing very cautiously down beside her, he immediately clipped Angie to his harness with carabiners. Screwing the threaded catch on the second carabiner down tight, the warden removed a plastic C-collar from his backpack to slip around her neck. That done, he cradled her floppy, bloodied body gently against his own. "I've got you, Babe. You're safe now. I won't let you go!"

Keying his mike, Jeff looked up at the chopper hovering overhead. "I've just tied into this feisty female of yours and as soon as I can cut her rope free, we'll be ready to go."

"Did you hear that?" Alex whooped. "He's tied into her!"

Staring intently out his side window, the taut as piano wire Aussie was fighting a losing battle to keep his aircraft from drifting off-line. His eyes were riveted to the cliff below as a massive slab of hard-packed snow tumbled over the lip.

Suddenly, he shifted his gaze to the darkened slope above. Something was wrong. Something was terribly wrong. As if waiting until it had the pilot's undivided attention, a tremendous downdraft slammed into the fragile aircraft... sending it cartwheeling onto its port side and over the cliff. The second cornice had broken away.

One hundred and ten feet below, Jeff got the picture right away. Watching the whirling rotor blades claw for air as the helicopter plunged tail-first past him toward the valley floor, the warden instantly reached for the survival knife on his belt. If he didn't cut himself free of the plummeting BK, he and the still-anchored Angie were going to be torn in half.

Suspended only by Angie's suspect life line now as he felt his own rappel rope suddenly go slack, Jeff's gloved fingers frantically yanked the knife from its scabbard. He yanked too hard. Listening in horror as the eight-inch steel knife clattered noisily against the rock face below, the warden heard something else whistling down from above. As he felt himself beginning to fall, he realized it was the jumar he had used to help anchor Angie's rope.

At 920 feet above the valley floor, Jeff knew he and Angie had about four more seconds of life before hitting the frozen ground. He had once flippantly promised that his last wish was to die in her arms. For once, Jefferson Logan was about to keep his word.

Thrown forward in his seat by the crushing G-forces, it was all Dale could do to keep his boot in contact with the left floor peddle. As the plummeting 'copter continued its lethal tail-first dive into oblivion, the vertical rotors were unable to provide any lift. Bent nearly double, the Aussie clamped the cyclic between his knees as he grabbed for the base of his seat with both hands. Reefing back with everything he had, he forcibly jammed the left peddle into the floor.

The aerodynamic effects were instantaneous. Feeling the BK immediately start to pivot to the left, Dale maintained full peddle while shoving the cyclic all the way forward. It was a do or die gamble. It pitched the helicopter abruptly nose-down.

The shimmering moonlit outline of the Kicking Horse River was clearly visible through the front window, snaking its silvery way along the valley floor. A small herd of elk near the water's edge stood with necks craned, their red, glowing eyes staring spellbound at the commotion overhead.

Dale shouted, "Can you see them at all? Stevens, is there any tension on Logan's rope?"

Lying flat on his belly with both hands clutching the floor-mounted anchor ring in a death grip, the medic scanned the surrounding darkness for all of a nanosecond. "I CAN'T SEE A GOD DAMN THING! WHO THE HELL CARES ANYWAY. WE'LL ALL BE DEAD IN A FEW SECONDS!"

Blocking out Stevens' crazed observations, Dale slowly pulled back on the cyclic control. As the front of the helicopter grudgingly began to lift, a mechanical tremor reverberated throughout the delicate aircraft. With the overhead blades whirling at nearly 300 RPMs, hauling back on the cyclic had placed an incredible force upon the rotor mast.

Even with his vision totally distorted by the skull-rattling vibration, Alex knew exactly what was happening as an amber warning light on the instrument panel began to flash. "We've got a 'Low Rotor Speed' alarm! You're pulling too much pitch! Back it off! The blades are going to stall! Back off!"

Dale braced his feet evenly against the floor pedals as he continued to haul back on the cyclic with everything he had. As if already in its death thralls, the shuddering chopper felt like it would break apart any second.

It was especially difficult to judge distances with any accuracy at night, but the pilot guessed the terrified elk scattering below to be less than 300 feet away now. Adding to that the 75 foot-high canopy of spruce trees, and the 110 feet of rappel rope he was trailing behind—if by some divine grace of God, Angie and Jeff were still tied into it—that meant he had only a hundred feet to somehow coax this doomed bird out of its suicidal plunge and into forward flight. As the ground rushed to greet them, the BK's nose sluggishly inched upward.

Alex leaned forward to assume the crash position. Staring down through the window beneath his feet, the co-pilot gasped. There, spinning like a child's top in the moonlight, was the Bauman bag, and twenty feet above it, a couple cradling one another in a loving last embrace.

It was Chief Warden Dennis Kallow who guided the BK in. Even through the dense cloud of rotor-whipped snow, both pilots could see the inferno blazing in his eyes.

Two wardens scurried toward the Bauman bag as Dennis directed Dale to back his ship off to the left so that Jeff and Angie didn't end up crash-landing on top of his men.

As soon as he felt Angie's snowboots contact the highway, Jeff waved for help. Within seconds, Angie and the climber were being hustled off to the Parks Service van. An ambulance from the town of Field, with the other two critically-injured patients on board, sat idling beside it.

Crawling between the stretchers, Dr. Markum immediately went to work assessing his two new patients. While the ice climber was alive, though just barely, and Angie's chest injury was considered life-threatening, after only a few seconds of deliberation, it was the emerg doc's decision that the two patients waiting in the Field ambulance were to be flown out first.

"I want that first pair loaded on board the chopper right away. Once that's done, these two are to be transferred into the ambulance and transported with lights and sirens to the Canmore hospital. We'll try for as quick a turnaround as possible in Calgary, refuel and fly right back and meet you there. Let's move, people!"

As the paramedics began to scatter, the doctor grabbed Jeff by the arm. "I want you to accompany Angie and this patient back to Canmore. Looking after them both is going to be too much for one medic. The climber's in big-time shock. No BP. Faint carotid. I'd estimate he's already lost half his circulating blood volume into his pelvis and thighs. The only reason he hasn't totally bled out is because of his severe hypothermia. Feel free to pile on the blankets, but I don't want you to warm him up too much. Understand? Intubate him as soon as you can. Then put a nasogastric tube down to decompress his stomach. The last thing you need is for him to vomit into his lungs. Once you get that done, try for a jugular line. If you can't get it, go for a femoral. The Field medics brought four units of O negative blood with them. Lay them on the heater vents to warm them up first, then pump them in as fast as you can. They won't fix what's wrong with him, but they might buy us a blood pressure.

"Our girl Angie here, has broken four, possibly five ribs on the left side. She doesn't have a flail, but she's got one hell of a pulmonary contusion for sure... probably a cardiac contusion as well. She's also got a ton of blood draining down the back of her throat from her sinuses. Elevate the head of the stretcher as much as you can without losing her pressure... and be damn sure to have the suction ready in case she aspirates. Slap a non-rebreather mask on her and watch the air entry to that left lung. If you're lucky, all she'll develop is a tension pneumo... for which you have my permission to treat with a simple needle decompression. If she really starts bleeding into her pleural space, however, there's not a heck of a lot you'll be able to do about it. Watch her ECG for ectopics. You can bolus her with Lidocaine, but only if she starts having runs. Get two large-bore IVs into her and hang some Ringers at one hundred c.c.s an hour. I don't want you to give her too much fluid 'cause it'll only make the pulmonary edema worse. One more thing, she's also suffering from extreme hypothermia so don't be afraid to strip down and use your own body heat if blankets alone aren't enough to raise her core temp. Do the best you can and I'll see you in Canmore in ninety minutes. Any questions?"

Four minutes later, LIFE-STAR 1 was skids up and on its way back to Calgary.

48
BACK WHERE IT ALL BEGAN

Angie awoke to find herself laid out on a very hard, very uncomfortable bed. It could mean only one of two things: She was either still alive, or she had not ended up in heaven, after all.

Her wandering fingers brushed against a metal side-rail. She was in a hospital bed, alright, but in which hospital? As her thawing brain slowly began functioning again, she became aware of something pressing against her face. Her immediate reaction was to push the offending object away.

"No you don't!" a voice called out sharply as the oxygen mask was repositioned on her face. "Come on, Ange... open those eyes for me. You're back home and you know how we run things here. It's an unwritten rule that none of our ICU patients are allowed to sleep more than twenty minutes without being woken up for some damn thing!"

Gritting her teeth with the effort, Angie finally pried one of her swollen eyelids partway open. As her Morphine-constricted pupil accommodated to the dim light, a sympathetic face slowly drifted into focus. It was Becky Dexter... one of her former Mountainview buddies.

Angie's eyeball wavered unsteadily as she took in the scene around her. From what she could make out, her outlook did not look very promising. She had been placed in a private room. That was a very bad sign. Only people who were dying got private rooms. Even worse, there were four IV poles standing at attention around her bed.

In ICU, it was an undocumented fact that the more IV lines a patient had, the worse their final outcome was likely to be. Anyone with more than five IVs was almost always labeled a future bag-and-tag candidate.

Above her head, a cardiac monitor showed an irregular sinus tach of 127 beats per minute. "Poor devil," Angie mumbled as she analyzed the tracing. "Must be an MI patient. Look at all those PVCs!"

Her good eye followed the ECG cable down from the monitor and up again until it disappeared into the sleeve of her hospital gown. Dear God! This was not looking good... not at all.

The room started spinning. As she shakily held her right hand up in front of her face, Angie found a clothes pin-shaped device clipped onto her index finger. Recognizing it as an oxygen saturation probe, the RN twisted her head in a determined effort to see the bedside monitor it was attached to. In the process, her mask fell off again.

"Angie! Would you just lie still and leave the nursing to me, okay?" Becky scolded as she gently replaced the mask and brushed a strand of damp blond hair from her patient's frightened eyes.

Angie reciprocated by making a desperate lunge for the stethoscope slung around Becky's neck... an action that nearly decapitated the ICU nurse. "Becky... is id really you? I'm so glad you're here. I didn'd wand to die alone!"

"Hon, you're not going to die," Becky wheezed, disentangling herself from her paranoid patient. "You're doing just fine."

Angie's glazed eyes did another wavering check of the room before staring back up at Becky's sweet face. "I wasn'd bord yesderday you know!" Her protest was barely audible as she braced her aching chest. "They've pud me in a private room. There's four IV poles around my bed. My hard's skipping along ad a hundred and fifty miles an hour and the lefd side of my chesd feels like someone adtacked me wid a sledgehammer. Becky, I'm nod an idiot... I'm a critical care nurse and I should know if I'm dying or nod!"

"Angie, you're back home at the Mountainview Hospital. Parkland didn't have any beds, so they flew you over here to visit us. You used to work here. Don't you remember? All our ICU rooms are privates, hon. Feel your neck. No central line. No Swan. Take a look at your arm. You've only got two IVs. One's just a saline drip and the other's plain old D-five-W with a little Lido to add some pizzazz. Trust me. You don't have four IVs. Your blurry little eyeballs must be seeing double."

For some strange reason, Becky's reassuring spiel had quite the opposite affect on her patient. Angie's eyes were like a trapped animal's as she clutched at her nurse's hand. "Two IVs! Good God... only two IVs? The docdors have given up on me already! They knew there was no hope so they didn'd even bodder ledding the residents pracdice pudding a centdral line in me!"

Clawing her way up the front of Becky's scrub suit, Angie hauled herself into a sitting position. Even though she was almost passing out from the horrendous pain in her chest, she had to know. "They haven'd made me a 'No Code' yed... have they Becky?"

There's an old saying that nurses make the worst patients in the world, second only to doctors, and it took two doses of IV Valium and an awful lot of sweet-talking before Becky was finally able to convince her patient that: #1... she was not dying, #2... the doctors had not given up hope on her and #3... she was still very much a full "I WANT EVERYTHING DONE" Code!

Seven hours later, as day-shift nurses meandered out of morning report with Styrofoam coffee cups in hand, Becky wearily signed off her charting. Angie's parents and siblings had taken turns holding a tearful vigil at her bedside most of the night and Becky had got to know them quite well. Stopping by the quiet room on her way home that morning, the nurse was gratified to deliver the reassuring news that Angie's heart rhythm and vital signs had stabilized over the last few hours and she had drifted off to sleep.

Angie's family had not been the only ones to spend the night worrying if she was going to pull through. Dale had phoned in so often and with such genuine concern, that one of the night staff—a nurse of Kiwi extraction and the only RN on shift that night who could understand his distraught Australian accent—eventually clued in and wrote his name down on Angie's kardex under the heading, "Significant other."

49
VISITING HOURS

For the first two days, Angie was so drugged and out of it that only her immediate family was allowed to visit. Hourly injections of Fentanyl had taken the edge off her pain, but because the potent narcotic tended to depress her already shallow respirations, the chest physiotherapist decided to try some TENS on her.

A small orange box the size of a deck of cards, the TENS unit's spidery-thin monitor wires were taped directly over her broken ribs. The TENS reduced a patient's pain because the body's sensory nerve pathways can carry only one message or sensation up to the brain at a time... either hot, cold, pain, touch or pressure.

What the TENS unit did was inundate the underlying nerve fibers with electrically produced "tingling-touch" sensations. With all the "phone lines" to the brain tied up in this manner, the "pain messages" from the broken ribs could not get through.

As an added benefit, the TENS unit also stimulated the body's own production of endorphins, the naturally produced "Morphine-like" pain killers. Within minutes, Angie's discomfort markedly decreased.

Those first 48 hours had been the most critical. As her oxygen saturation percentages gradually crept closer to the normal range, and her daily chest X-rays showed steady signs of improvement, by the morning of her third day on the unit, Angie was actually looking forward to her breakfast tray. Considering it was hospital fare, and she couldn't smell or taste anything anyway, her doctor viewed this development as a very good sign, indeed.

As fate would have it, the nurse who came in to pick up her breakfast tray that morning wasn't just any old nurse. It was her former Nursing Unit Supervisor, Jean Wallace.

The NUS fought to maintain a stern face as she slid open the heavy glass door. "Angela, when I said 'drop by and visit sometime,' I never meant like this!"

Having received another blissful shot of Fentanyl a scant five minutes earlier, Angie was struggling to focus her fogging eyes on the disembodied face floating at the foot of the bed.

"I'm nod supposed to tell anyone this, but I'm actually working undercover for the hospital. I'm here to ged the inside poop on how well you're running this insane asylum."

"Well, in that case, I'll make sure your primary nurse snows you with plenty of Valium. You won't remember a blessed thing."

"Fine, but see if I leave you guys any goodies when they kick my keester oud of here!" Angie giggled. "Valium induced amnesia is the main reason ICU nurses never ged any chocolades. We bust our budds keeping patients alive and when they finally regain their faculties out on the regular ward, guess who ends up with all those boxes of Turdles? The ward nurses, thad's who! How's thad old saying go: "Time flies when you're sedated!"

Pulling a chair up to the bedside, Jean let out an exasperated sigh, "Angela, first there was the sky diving lessons and then the luging and now this air rescue thing. Where is it all going to end? In a body bag?"

"I uh... I can'd... da... quid now," Angie replied, her tongue thickening by the second. "It would uh... be such a waste. I'm uh... jusd gedding the hang of id."

Jean shook her head. "Ange, I don't know if you're aware or not, but Connie got her wish. As of March fourteenth, she'll be taking over as the hospital's new Assistant Director of Nursing. That leaves me with a vacant Assistant NUS posting to fill. You know, for an experienced nurse, someone with a solid knowledge base, confident in decision-making, it could be a sound career move."

Angie's scrambled thoughts momentarily cleared. "I know whad you're asking and I've very honored—fladdered really!—bud you know charge nursing has never turned my wheel. Believe id or nod, I'm really happy doing whad I do. I love the challenge, the adventure, maybe even the element of danger. To tell the truth, I'd much rather cash-in on a mountainside somewhere, trying to sling a climber to safety, than rock myself to death in a nursing home."

As they weren't immediate family, they had to call and get permission first, but later that afternoon, some very close friends dropped by to check on the progress of their accident-prone colleague. Had Jennifer and Kyle arrived 45 minutes earlier, they would have met up with the person directly responsible for Angie's admission to an ICU and not a funeral home. A devilish rake of a fellow, toting an armful of long-stemmed red roses, Jefferson Logan.

Even as he bent down to give her a tender peck on the cheek, Kyle's probing eyes were assessing his partner's injuries. The multitude of crusted-over scrapes and abrasions. The bruises. Her grossly misshapen nose. The pallor of her skin. The bluish tinge to her lips and fingernails despite the high-flow oxygen mask.

Clearing his throat in preparation for baring his tortured soul, Kyle found himself beaten to the punch. "You know something Kyle? This place has gone to heck in a hand basket since I left. They did a whole series of scans on me yesterday and the only thing the tech could tell me afterwards was thad I wasn't pregnant!

"Id's not as bad as id looks. Really," Angie added. "All I did was crack a few ribs and bang up my poor old shnozz again. Geez, I felt worse than this last year when you tried to kill Russ and me by almost smacking thad freight train."

The medic winced as he reached for his partner's hand. "You're one damn smart cookie, you know that, girl? Rappelling down the cliff to duck under the slide. I'd never have thought of that."

"Don't sell yourself short, Stevens," Angie's eyes boldly locked onto his. "All I was trying to do was ged away, thad's all. When you look up and see a mountain of snow aboud to crash down on you, everything kind of stops, switches to slow motion. I jusd knew I had to try something. Anything!"

Kyle shifted in his chair. "You know, after all you've been through in the last couple of months, I mean, if you did decide to pack it in... no one would blame you. We'd all understand."

Jennifer Stevens, having taken a chair in the corner, had not said two words since her arrival. Angie glanced over to get her reaction to the statement. Jen immediately turned away, but her eyes said it all. They were red and puffy; like she'd been crying for a long time.

"Pack id in? Who said anything aboud packing id in? Whad happened to me wasn't your fault, Kyle. It was an act of God. Thad's how you have to look at id. It wasn't your fault.

"To be honest, I don't remember much aboud whad went on up there. Jeff filled me in on a few details, but I want to know everything. First off, have you heard how the injured ice climbers are doing?"

"I knew you'd ask, so I called Parkland this morning," Kyle's face lit up. "They're all alive, even the guy who was hanging out with you. The one with the skull fracture's still in a coma, but the other two are awake and expected to do well.

"Which uh... speaking of doing well, is more than I can say for Captain Morgan. You know, we were all prepared to accept the consequences for disobeying Warden Kallow's order to return to base, but it seems Dale is the only one who's going to end up paying the price for it.

"His commercial license has been yanked for three months by Transport Canada, for, among other things, violating a bunch of safety regulations, gross misconduct, endangering his crew, endangering his aircraft, endangering Park wildlife—you name it!

"Just finding you was miracle enough. Then, when that second cornice broke free and flung us tail-first over the cliff, it was, without a doubt, the finest piece of flying Jeff or I had ever seen."

Kyle paused as his eyes settled on the oxygen sensor on Angie's finger. "You know, the damn fool Aussie put all our lives on the line to save you. I guess, in a way, the suspension was justified. But it's going to be a black mark on his flight record that'll follow him for the rest of his career."

Angie slumped visibly back against her pillow.

Seeing her reaction, Kyle abruptly changed subjects. "Just to let you know, I haven't forgotten about our dance practice tomorrow. I'm so honored that you asked me to take Russ' place. I've been working real hard, getting my timing down. Jen's been helping me."

As he and Jen got to their feet, Jennifer finally found her tongue. "Ange, if you think his dancing's bad, you should see him try to skate!"

Peter and Dale were the next to visit. With his chief pilot, soon to be ex-chief pilot, waiting in the wings, Peter greeted her with a smile, then asked the usual visitor questions: How was she feeling? Did she need anything? When did she expect to be released?

"I'm ready to ged oud of here right now!" Angie retorted, her eyes twinkling above the oxygen mask. "I don't have time for this. I've god things to do, places to go. Jusd give me a second and I'll pack up my stuff."

"Whoa girl, you've got plenty of time. The Olympics are still a whole week away and they're going to be the only show in town until the end of February, so you just concentrate on getting better, okay?"

Peter bent to kiss her softly on the forehead. "There's another fellow here who wants to say hi so I think I'll just nip down to the cafeteria for a coffee."

50
PRAYERS AND PROMISES

Dale was about to sit down in the chair left vacant by Kyle when Angie patted the bed. "You can sit here... if you like."

As she had frequently been lifting her mask to converse with her earlier visitors, the amount of oxygen filtering into Angie's blood stream had dipped to an all-time low. As a result, just as Dale was settling himself onto the bed, the oxygen saturation monitor's low alarm started bonging.

A respiratory tech rushed into the room. After silencing the alarm and checking to make sure her oxygen tubing was still connected to the wall outlet, the RT turned toward his non-compliant patient. "Look Ms. Jackson," he said grimly, "you're down to eighty-seven percent again! If you keep pulling this stunt, you're going to end up arresting and if that happens, we'll have to call a Code and start doing chest compressions on that tender little chest of yours! So you just keep that rib-cracking vision in mind the next time you think about taking your mask off. Understood?"

As he left, the RT flashed a wink at the shaken fellow perched on the edge of the bed. "Don't worry, she's not in any danger. These pain in the rear-end type of patients always pull through! Well, nearly always."

As soon as the RT left the room, Angie reached for Dale's hand.

Removing the saturation probe from her index finger, she stealthily clipped it onto his. Then she looked up at her gallant, grounded hero. "I know all aboud your suspension," she said. "I just can'd understand. Any sane, rational person would've called id a day and gone home. What made you keep looking for me?"

Dale gazed deep into her questioning eyes. "I just asked myself one simple thing. What would old B.J. have done in this situation?"

A timid smile crept across his face. "Besides, I couldn't have just left you dangling around up there. Heck, the paperwork alone would've taken Alex and me a week to fill out."

Angie shyly returned his smile, but she did not laugh. "Id's just nod fair. Why did they single you out? What aboud Alex or Jeff? How come nothing's going to happen to them?"

"Because Chief Warden Kallow filed a complaint with Transport Canada, that's why. The Inspector they sent out was real nice, though. Pretty lenient considering the circumstances. He could've yanked my license indefinitely. As it was, I only got handed a three-month suspension."

"Three months! What are you going to do in the meantime?" Angie wailed. "If you can'd fly, how are you going to support yourself? How are you going to pay your rent? How are you going to eat?"

Dale rolled his eyes. "You really are something, you know that? Here you are, lying in a hospital bed looking like you just went ten rounds with George Foreman... and all you're worried about is how I'm going to pay my rent? You nut bar. I haven't slept a wink in the last three nights, but it sure the heck wasn't about being evicted!"

Dale rested his hand on hers. "Don't you worry about me. I'm a big boy, I can take care of myself. I'll just have to be extra careful the next time I visit Yoho National Park, that's all. You should have been at that Transportation Safety hearing yesterday. Herr Kallow was demanding that I be taken out and shot. Even told the inquiry board that he had a gun in his truck and that he'd be more than happy to oblige as soon as they gave him the okay.

"Following that little performance, I got booted out of the room so the big boys and your old flame, Mr. Logan, could discuss my aviation future. Lawson must've gone to bat for me because my 'immediate' suspension doesn't go into effect until after the Games are over. I don't know what he said to the board, but it must've been one heck of a sell job."

Angie shook her head. "Peter may have gone to bat for you, but id was Jeff who appealed for your suspension to be delayed."

Dale stared at her.

"Id's true. Jeff dropped by this morning to see how I was doing. Even brought me some flowers," Angie added as she pointed a shaky finger toward the window ledge and a vase filled to overflowing with gorgeous roses.

Catching sight of the lovely bouquet, the empty-handed Aussie suddenly looked sick. Logan obviously wasn't wasting any time. Why hadn't he thought of something caring and thoughtful like that?

"Dale," Angie continued, "apparently after you left the room, Jeff reminded the board thad four people were alive today because of your flying ability. He also told them thad the cold must've affected the chopper's radio because id kept cutting out and id was impossible to say whether you actually heard Kallow give the order to return to base. Can you believe thad?"

As Dale sat with his mouth hanging open, Angie gently caressed his arm. "You know whad else Jeff said before he headed back to Yoho and his pregnant girlfriend? He said you gave him the distinct impression thad if he'd screwed up and came back without me, you would've flown extra low on the way back... as in, to maybe snag him on a tree. You wouldn't have done thad... would you?"

Dale exhaled loudly. Logan had a girlfriend... and a pregnant one to boot. There was a God! His visit to Angie's bedside had been for old time's sake and nothing more. With this happy thought messing up his head, the pilot struggled to answer Angie's question. "Well, it was dark and the tree tops can come up at you pretty fast... and it's really hard to judge distances at night and... well, HELL YES! If Jeffy boy had failed to rescue you, I most definitely would've given him the ride of his life!"

Struggling not to laugh, Angie's line of questioning switched to a more serious note. "Did they ever find out whad caused thad Parks helicopter to crash?"

Dale's flushed face turned sombre. "Rumor has it the pilot probably suffered a heart attack. One of the wardens testified he'd seen the pilot popping a whole handful of antacid tablets just before taking off. The ironic part is that the guy passed his medical with flying colors just last week."

Angie pondered Dale's answer. "Now thad you mention id, in all the years I've worked Intensive Care, I can'd remember ever admitting a pilot. Not one!"

"And you probably never will," Dale replied sadly. "That pilot would never have passed his MOT physical if he'd confessed to having chest pains. You can lose your commercial ticket for simply having high blood pressure, never mind heart disease. I know it sounds terrible, but some pilots would rather die at the controls than risk losing their license."

"Is thad how you're planning to check out?"

"Heavens no!" Dale laughed, an embarrassed smile creasing his rugged features. "I plan to succumb in the arms of a blissfully satisfied woman!"

"Well, if id's euthanasia you need, just give me a call. You're not allergic to Morphine... are you?"

As the shy couple broke into laughter, Angie nearly passed out from the pain. Splinting her chest with both hands, at times, it was hard to tell whether she was laughing or crying.

"Good God, woman, I leave you on a hillside for five minutes and look what happens! Got to keep my eye on you every second," Dale teased as he built up his nerve. "You know, when I was out in the waiting room, I got to reading a pamphlet about heart attacks. With you being a cardiac nurse, maybe you can answer a question for me. If you did an ECG on a normal healthy guy, would you be able to tell if he was in love with you?"

"Well uh, I... I'm good Dale, bud I'm nod thad good," Angie sputtered. "I'd probably... have to see if he had any other uh... telltale symptoms. To be perfectly honest though, if this guy could hide his feelings so well I had to do a flipping ECG on him to find out if he loved me or not, well... I don't think I'd waste my time on him."

Taking her hand, Dale interlaced his fingers with hers. Giving her hand a tender squeeze to remove all doubt from her mind, slowly, gently, he felt Angie's fingers tightened around his.

"You know, that poor old ticker of yours has really taken a beating lately. Do you think maybe a little TLC might help it heal? I mean, when I watched the avalanche crash down, I thought you were gone forever. I honestly thought I'd missed my chance to let you know how much...."

A faint rap on the window interrupted him. It was Peter signaling it was time for them to go.

Besides her broken ribs and badly-bruised heart and lung, Angie's nose was strictly for appearance's sake now. "I'll probably have to give up kissing as a contact sport because of the risk of suffocation," she jokingly lamented.

The soft-spoken Aussie couldn't help but grin as he got to his feet. "Trust me, luv, there are plenty of places a guy can kiss a girl other than on the lips. I'd be happy to give you a little demonstration, if you'd like."

Angie laughed and immediately grabbed for her chest. "God, the person who coined the phrase, 'to die laughing,' obviously had broken a rib!"

Dale leaned forward and delivered a lingering kiss to the only uninjured patch of skin he could find... a lip-sized spot just below her right earlobe.

Slipping the oxygen sensor back onto her finger, Angie did not seem surprised when the monitor let out an ear-piercing squeal. The respiratory tech came flying back into the room.

"Eighty-five percent!" the tech yelped as he silenced the monitor alarm. Immediately placing his stethoscope on her chest, the RT was just about to holler for help when he saw Angie flash her visitor a wink. Instantly putting two and two together, the tormented tech had finally had enough. "Sir, I'm afraid I'll have to ask you to leave! And I would advise you to say your final good-byes right away because Ms. Jackson obviously doesn't have much time left.

"We'd better get some gases on her right away!" the RT hollered to another tech who'd rushed in carrying a bagging unit and a plastic package that Angie knew contained a very long, very sharp needle.

Her eyes the size of tennis balls as she clamped her oxygen mask tightly to her face, the flight nurse started doing some yelling of her own. "Get away from me with thad thing! I feel fine. I was just horsing around, thad's all! I promise I'll be good from now on... okay... okay guys?"

51
STAGE FRIGHT

Three days later, Angie was released from the unit and allowed to go home. She wasn't exactly released... she signed herself out against medical advice.

"Look Dr. Stewart," she explained, stuffing her meager belongings into a plastic hospital bag, "I'll be just fine. Really."

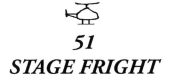

The doctor's trained eyes observed Angie wince as she slipped her jacket on. A trivial activity, it left his patient gasping for breath.

"Sir, I'm... fully aware... of the extent... of my injuries," Angie fought to get her breathing back under control. "I know what to watch out for... and I know I've got to take it easy for awhile. I know my limitations. I won't push myself. Thanks for everything you've done, I really appreciated it, but I've got a zillion things I've gotta... I'll be okay."

The jaded physician stared back at her. He had seen many bruised lungs suddenly develop pulmonary edema... even days after the initial insult. When that happened, the patient got into big trouble, real fast.

"This is totally insane, but I can't do a thing to stop you short of declaring you mentally incompetent... a thought which has crossed my mind, young lady!"

Pausing to look straight into her defiant eyes, the doctor's tone softened. "Look Angie, you're just barely getting by on one lung right now. I'll let you sign yourself out, but only under these conditions: there'll be no flying, no driving, no long walks, no prone sex, no nothing. Understand? Take your incentive spirometer home with you and make sure to use it every single hour to do your deep breathing exercises. I want you to go straight home and stay there and if you feel the need to leave your apartment during the next week, it had better be because the building's on fire. If you think your breathing is becoming the least bit compromised, I want you to dial nine-one-one and get yourself hauled to the nearest emergency ward. Do I make myself clear?"

Angie leaned heavily against her bedside table. "Doctor Stewart, I promise I'll be good and I promise I'll be careful and I promise I'll see you in your office on Friday. I give you my word."

If you included the twenty minutes it took Jennifer to drive her to her apartment, Angie followed her doctor's instructions to the letter for almost half an hour. Once inside her apartment, however, she was on the phone to the hangar and asking for the head push.

After informing Lawson of her earlier that expected release from captivity, Angie casually mentioned that she probably wouldn't be available for shifts until the middle of next week.

"The middle of next week?" Peter responded. "Funny, I just got off the phone with a Doctor Stewart. He claims we should nail the door of your apartment shut and mark you off sick until the middle of May!"

Clutching her aching chest with one hand while trying to pop the tab on a diet Coke with the other, Angie replied that he just might be surprised by her recuperative powers.

"There's absolutely no point in rushing things, Angela! You're lucky to be alive. Enjoy your time off. Take it easy! You'll be back on line soon enough." Peter ended his fatherly spiel by stating that everyone at the hangar was thinking about her and that they were all wishing her a speedy recovery... but not too speedy.

"Tell them I really appreciate it, sir. It's nice to know I haven't been forgotten. Oh, by the way, Kyle left a message on my machine. If it's not too much bother, could you put him on?"

Not fifteen minutes later, Angie was pulling her Chevette into the LIFE-STAR parking lot. Audibly distraught, Kyle had pleaded with her to come to the hangar. With the big event less than four days away, Mr. Confidence had apparently developed a terminal case of stage fright and couldn't remember how to do a simple little dance that had only two steps in it!

Out of the corner of his eye, Peter caught a glimpse of someone trying to sneak past his door. "Jackson! Didn't I just tell you to stay home and count your blessings?"

"I am! I mean, I will. I just dropped by to see Kyle. The Opening Ceremonies are on Saturday and he's having trouble getting his timing down. Besides, if I do suffer a relapse, I can't think of a better place to do it!"

Peter tried to look disgusted as he walked over to give her a hug.

"You call that feeble thing a hug?"

"I was afraid I might hurt you!" Peter replied. "It's like cradling a cracked egg—I'm scared to death all your insides will come oozing out!

Hearing the phone ring in his office, Lawson reluctantly shooed Angie on her way. "You'll find Stevens out at the helicopter."

Watching as she stole a sideways peek into the pilots' room as she headed down the hall, Peter added softly, "By the way, you just missed Captain Morgan. He's working nights all this week."

Angie could feel her face flush a hot crimson. "Oh... really!" was the snappiest comeback she was able to concoct as she backed toward the hangar door. Her heart suddenly started to race.

Had the mere hint that something might be going on between herself and Dale brought it on? Nah! She'd just over-exerted herself, that was all. It couldn't be something as silly as... as... was it possible that something really was going on between herself and Dale?

Angie located her Two-Step partner sitting on a 'copter skid, waiting for an Ian Tyson tape to rewind in his portable boom box. As she watched him stumble through the tune, "Four Strong Winds" with Jodi Munro, the flight nurse with the misfortune to be on shift with him, Angie wondered how this man had ever managed to get his wife pregnant.

As Jodi did her best to keep up with his seizure-like movements, he elbowed her in the forehead, not once, but twice. It was too brutal to watch. Feebly waving her arm, Angie motioned for Kyle to shut off the tape player. Simultaneously, a voice message erupted from both Kyle's and Jodi's beepers. They had a mission to Drumheller for a NICU baby transport. Rubbing her aching head, Jodi immediately laid sole claim to the flight.

"Don't waste your time on this clown, Ange!" the flight nurse muttered callously as she ran to fetch her helmet and jacket. "When I get back I'll give you my brother's phone number. He teaches Two-Step lessons at Ringo's and he'd kill to dance in the Opening Ceremonies!"

With the chopper pulled outside, Angie was left to search for a new roost. Watching as Kyle headed off to snag her a chair, she could tell by his hurt look that his morale had hit rock bottom.

He returned with a chair and a spare scout cylinder of oxygen. "No offense intended, but you look like you could use a few whiffs of this stuff," the medic quietly remarked as he attached a mask to the tank and handed it to her. Nearly ten minutes passed before her overwhelming feeling of fatigue and breathlessness finally began to ease.

Slipping an arm around her partner's neck, a revitalized Angie fervently assured him that, come hell or high water, it would be their footwork, his and hers, that would dazzle the world in four days time.

"You know what your biggest problem is? You're trying too hard. Pretend you're at home. Amanda's finally asleep. You've got Jennifer in your arms. Willy Nelson on the stereo. The lights down low."

As if someone had flipped a magical switch, Kyle's stilted movements softened. With his anxious thoughts distracted by the wondrous imagery of old Willy crooning a love ballad as he and Jen swayed to the music, the medic's frenzied footwork relaxed. Instead of floundering a half-step behind, he was unconsciously matching Angie step-for-step as she gasped her way through the complicated routine.

Breaking into jubilant applause as they finished their dance, the smile on Kyle's face quickly faded as he assisted his wheezing, blue-lipped partner back to her chair. He had seen week-old cadavers with better color.

Her battered rib cage heaving with each breath as she hungrily sucked back another ten minutes of oxygen, Angie eventually found the strength to flash Kyle the "thumbs-up" sign.

A faint shade of pink coloring her cheeks, she smiled at her worried partner. "This time, I want you to do the driving."

Moving in sync as they pranced around the oily entrails of a dismembered Pratt and Whitney engine, Angie found herself remembering another place... another dance partner.

And as Kyle twirled her about, for a moment, it was Rusty's arms that were around her... holding her... guiding her every step.

52
LET THE GAMES BEGIN!

February 13 was the mythical date for which Calgarians had waited seven long years. Seven years. It had always seemed far off in the future. A day to fantasize about... but never to realize. As the rising sun chased the wispy remnants of night over the mountains to the west, the last of the torch runners were being dropped off north of the city. With each hand-off, the flame moved one kilometer closer to McMahon Stadium... the waiting Olympic cauldron... and history.

Kyle and Jennifer had been most fortunate to snag tickets to the Opening Ceremonies, so when Kyle ended up having to dance in the televised extravaganza, it seemed only natural to offer his seat to Dale.

Arriving at their seats, Dale and Jennifer were surprised to find tightly wrapped bundles waiting for them. Quickly pulling on the bright red ponchos, they discovered that their section was a mere red splotch in an ocean of white. Only later did they discover that their section had formed the center of a huge Canadian maple leaf.

Pulling their toques down over their ears, Jen and Dale sat back to enjoy the pomp and pageantry of an Olympic Winter Games Opening Ceremony.

One by one, the fifty-seven countries participating in the Games proudly paraded past. Blowing on his frozen fingers as he zoomed in on the athletes with his telephoto lens, Dale abruptly sat up. The powerful

Italian team had marched into view... and there, smiling and waving from the front row were lugers Klaus Stockner and Manfred Burghart.

In keeping with Olympic tradition, the host country of Canada brought up the tail-end of the procession. As the crowd responded with deafening applause, a boisterous group of performers, introduced as "The Calico Dancers," ran hooping and hollering into the stadium.

Due to the fact Kyle had told his wife exactly where to look for them in the large formation of dancers, it did not take Dale long to get his camera trained on Angie's radiant smile. For the next ten minutes, as they snapped off an entire roll of film, Dale and Jennifer nearly burst with pride as they watched their mates dance several variations of the Two-Step in a performance broadcast live to the world. Against her partner's steel-blue slicker, Angie's hot pink jacket and skirt were a striking contrast. Trimmed with fake white fur, her fuchsia mittens and bonnet, together with Kyle's black-and-white neckerchief, black gloves and black cowboy hat, perfectly accented the romanticized rendering of a western couple.

Her puffy honker notwithstanding, in Dale's love-blinded eyes, Angie was, without a doubt, the cutest cowgirl on the field.

Their first dance was to a piano instrumental and as they stepped and whirled in unison, Angie and Kyle were having the time of their lives. "I can't believe we're doing this in front of sixty thousand people!" Kyle whispered nervously as he swung his partner in a graceful arc.

Out of breath, but deliriously happy, Angie just smiled. Good Lord! How would he react if she reminded him of the billions watching on TV?

As the first dance ended, Ian Tyson and Gordon Lightfoot stepped up to the microphone with their guitars and started singing "Four Strong Winds," followed immediately by "Alberta Bound." The hypothermic crowd came alive, clapping their mittens and tapping their mukluks in time with the music.

The culmination of two years of weekly practice sessions, the dancers finished their program and galloped off the field. The time had come to get down to business. Following a slew of well rehearsed and politically correct speeches, the 15th Olympic Winter Games was officially proclaimed open. Accompanied by a mighty cheer from the crowd, the Olympic flag was unfurled as several thousand homing pigeons were released into the air.

The poor man's 'Doves of Peace' had purposefully been starved overnight so they couldn't do what pigeons were famous for doing, especially with over 60,000 possible targets sitting directly below.

Following the pigeons, there was more singing and dancing and a mini-Stampede featuring lantern-jawed Mounties, stern-faced native Indians in ceremonial garb and even some wildly-careening chuckwagons. As the horse poop was hurriedly scooped up, a thousand screaming children raced onto the field, their assignment—to act out all ten of the Olympic events by using their bodies to form huge picturegrams of each individual sport.

With the entertainment portion of the Ceremonies completed, a hush fell over the crowd. All eyes were suddenly trained on the south end of the stadium. As the last of the torch runners jogged into view, the crowd went nuts. Taking the final handoff, a small girl representing all future Games competitors ran with it up the steps to the base of the cauldron where she paused to salute the athletes before lighting the spectacular flame.

In a thrilling finale, the Canadian Forces "Snowbirds" aerobatical team thundered overhead. As an increasingly stiff west breeze dissipated their rainbow-colored contrails, Calgary's two weeks in the world's sport spotlight was officially underway.

Dale and Jennifer had already bolted their seats. At a prearranged spot in front of the Volunteer Centre, they knew Kyle and Angie would be waiting for them.

After snapping off several close-ups of the handsome couple, Dale called out to a passerby. "If it's no trouble, could I get you to take a picture for me?"

Their emotions reflected in their beaming faces, Kyle and Angie slipped their arms around Jennifer and Dale respectively. It was a photo that all of them would treasure for the rest of their lives.

53
EVERYBODY LOVES A LUGER

As luge was one of the first events on the Olympic program, and Angie ground-bound with nothing but time on her hands, it was a heads-up play on Dale's part to ask if she would like to go to the men's singles competition with him. How could she refuse?

She seemed to be personal friends with just about everyone involved with the race, from the lowly athlete escorts to the lofty race chairman himself, and after awhile, Dale lost count of the number of well-built European and Canadian males who came over to plant a kiss on her.

Chatting it up with Dale's former doubles partner Manfred Burghart, they received the awful news that Klaus Stockner had injured his shoulder during one of the mandatory pre-race training runs. As an ex-racer, Angie's heart immediately went out to Klaus. Luge was a sport of upper body strength and at this level of competition, all things being equal, a strong pull from the start handles meant the difference between first place and fifteenth.

Rather than meekly withdrawing from the race, however, Klaus Stockner showed the true champion he was. Denied the glory of the medal podium, he would race simply for pride. Not his own, but that of his beloved country... Italia.

Because the Calgary Games were to be Klaus' third and final Olympics, it was with a great deal of sadness that Angie listened to his name being called to the Men's Start position for the very last time.

The friendly Italian had always been a huge crowd pleaser, and as he coasted to a stop amidst an impressive spray of ice chips, he leaped to his feet and began blowing kisses to the mob of adoring female fans.

"Angela!" Klaus cried out as he spotted her in the crowd. "Mein sweet kitten, come now as I slide not again."

"I think you're being paged," Dale laughed as he gave her a playful nudge toward the waiting Romeo.

"I don't want to make a scene," Angie whispered.

"You don't want to make a WHAT!" Dale nearly choked. "Get that shapely butt of yours over there! You're holding up the race!"

Feeling like the eyes of the entire planet were upon her, Angie timidly pushed her way through the dense crowd as Klaus motioned her on. With the refrigerated track elevated three feet above her head, a delighted cheer rose from the throng of flag-waving onlookers as Klaus leaned over the safety railing to take her hand.

And so it was, while balancing in an almost upside-down position, that the studly Italian landed a big, exuberant kiss on Canada's unofficial first lady of luge.

54
H.O.P.E.

Three weeks after her near-encounter with God, and just days before the Games were to close, Angie arrived at the LIFE-STAR hangar, suited up and ready to work. While Peter had reluctantly given her his blessing to return to duty, he hoped her first shift back would be a nice, quiet one.

It was not to be. A mere 45 minutes later, LIFE-STAR 1 was skids up and en route to the Olympic venue of Nakiska. The on-scene medic's report didn't sound good. During a timing check prior to the start of the women's downhill skiing event, one of the race forerunners had skidded off the course and collided with a tree.

"Unconscious. Fractured skull with brain tissue exposed. This patient's definitely of the 'load and go' and 'fly real fast' variety!" Kyle announced over the helicopter's intercom as Dale and Alex prepared for lift-off from the ski hill.

Nine minutes into the return flight, as her partner was radioing Parkland to have their neuro/trauma team standing by, Angie had a second large-bore IV line up and running. Pausing to make sure her patient still had a pulse, she began pressure-infusing a 500cc bag of Mannitol in the hope it would reduce the brain-crushing pressures building inside the young girl's skull.

"Russ must've looked a lot like this when you flew him back," she stated quietly.

Kyle stared at their teenaged patient. Angie was right. It was Russ all over again. The blood-soaked dressings. The pinkish cerebrospinal fluid oozing from the nose and mouth. The rapidly-dilating pupils.

Angie glanced out her window at the Trans-Canada Highway fifteen hundred feet below. "You know, it was so beautiful up there today with the warm weather and sunshine and all! Rusty was such a ski nut. He would've given anything to be there with us."

As Kyle numbly contemplated his partner's words, a brilliant idea occurred to him. It was definitely off the wall, and if Lord Peter ever found out, well... Captain Morgan would be having company down at the unemployment office.

Both pilots meanwhile, had been covertly listening in on Kyle and Angie's private conversation. After discussing the pros and cons of Kyle's idea at great length, Dale switched the intercom on. "You can count us in, too, Stevens... or are you planning on flying this glorified eggbeater yourself?"

"I know you guys mean well, but if Peter ever caught us... it's just that I don't want you to get into any more trouble than you're already in," Angie said.

"Ange, how on earth can I get into any more trouble? I'm already suspended, they can't suspend me again!" Dale laughed. "Don't you worry about us, okay? Just fill out a Patient Care Report like you do on every mission. Use lots of fancy medical terminology and make it look real authentic. Maybe write down that the patient had HIV or hepatitis or something and then prick your finger and smear a few drops of blood on the sheet. Knowing how squeamish Bateman is regarding that kind of thing, he won't want to touch it... never mind spend a lot of time entering it into that old computer of his."

The next morning, with sunrise still a good half-hour away, LIFE-STAR 1 was pulled from its cozy hangar and readied for flight. Upon receiving clearance from the tower, the helicopter gracefully lifted into the air and after skimming over the airport's outer boundary, quickly gained altitude as it headed due west across the slumbering city.

Following standard protocol, Kyle notified Calgary dispatch of LIFE-STAR 1's destination and about the fact that, should another call come in over the Trauma Hot Line, they were to be contacted stat with the particulars. "Dispatch, we can abort our present mission at any time, so don't hesitate to give us a buzz if we're needed someplace else."

Signing off, Kyle surveyed the sleepy, smiling faces around him.

Helmets and seat belts securely fastened, Russ' sister Melissa was seated across from him while Mrs. Andrews was in the jump seat next to Angie. With 50 mgs of Gravol pumped into each of their behinds, both women were actually holding up quite well, considering the mission they were about to undertake.

Twenty-five minutes later, Dale eased the helicopter into a lazy circuit above Nakiska. Reluctantly surrendering to the dawn, the wispy scarves of mist still clinging to the rock outcroppings of stately Mount Allan were beginning to vaporize in the morning sun.

"Anytime you're ready, Ange," Alex's voice crackled over the intercom.

Prior to lift-off from Calgary, Russ' ashes had been carefully poured into a tube-shaped container which Alex then duct taped to the right rear landing strut. Attaching a short length of nylon cord to the tube's spring-loaded lid, the co-pilot fed the other end up through the sliding window on Angie's side of the aircraft. Pulling on the rope would open the top of the container slightly and allow the ashes to fall out. Releasing the rope would close the lid again.

Everyone was now waiting for her to give that first pull. Angie's hands trembled as she held out the coil of rope that had been resting on her lap. One by one, Kyle, Melissa and Emily placed their own unsteady hands on top of hers. It was time.

As the chopper passed over each Olympic site, the four people in the back took turns pulling on the rope. It took almost an hour, but when they were finally through, a little bit of Russell Patrick Andrews had been scattered over every single sporting venue. His dream of attending the Winter Games had become a reality.

As they flew from venue to venue, the emotion of the people on board mirrored the true spirit of what they were trying to do. Instead of surrendering to overwhelming sadness, everyone was soon laughing and reminiscing about the man who had touched all their lives so profoundly in the brief time he'd been among them.

"I'm sure Rusty is with us right now, and he's enjoying the show immensely," Angie said softly. "This kind of thing would've been right up his alley!"

"I have a little secret to share with you all," Mrs. Andrews suddenly spoke up. "An official with the HOPE program called me the other day. She read to me several Thank-you letters she had gotten from the people who had received Russ' organs. I thought you might like to know that it was two elderly ladies from Calgary who received Rusty's corneas. Apparently, they'd both been legally blind for years and were so completely overwhelmed that they just had to write to express their gratitude to the program.

"The HOPE program also got letters from a farmer near Saskatoon and a teenager in Lethbridge who received Russ' kidneys," Emily continued.

"And... oh gosh, brace yourself, but it was a young man from Edmonton who received Rusty's heart. Apparently this poor fellow had gone to all the Eskimo and Oiler games before he developed some kind of degenerative heart disease. He'd been waiting for a new heart for months, and his time had just about run out when he finally got the call. I'm still having trouble believing it. To think my son's heart is now beating in the chest of an Edmonton sports fan!"

Their mission complete, Dale was making a bee-line back to the hangar when a local radio station's helicopter traffic reporter spotted the chopper passing below them. "If you're traveling on the Deerfoot right now, I hope you're being courteous to your fellow motorists. I just saw the LIFE-STAR air rescue helicopter headed north toward the airport, and I hope none of you will ever have to ride in that big red machine. With that in mind, let's all drive extra-carefully today, shall we?"

Peter Lawson was one of those listeners motoring up the Deerfoot. So his crew was returning from another successful mission, eh? He was delighted with the news. The more flights LIFE-STAR 1 made, the more evidence he had to prove the effectiveness of his program. "Did LIFE-STAR really save lives?" In Peter's mind, there was no question. And he had the stats to prove it!

Upon reaching the hangar, Peter found to his utter astonishment that his hard-working night crew had already finished the usual half-hour of paperwork that accompanied every mission and, according to a suddenly preoccupied day shift, had promptly vacated the premises for home... and/or places unknown.

While finding that rather odd, Peter was nevertheless in a very chipper mood as he cracked open the mission book to check the number of calls they had had for the first three weeks of February. They were already ahead of January's total for the entire month!

Yes, today had all the makings of a great day, and as he waited for the coffee machine to produce some fresh brew, Peter did something he usually left for his assistant. Pulling the most recent PCR off the top of the February mission pile, he cheerfully began to enter the statistical information into Bateman's database.

55

SOME ENCHANTING DEPOSITION

On the eve of the official Closing Ceremonies, a "Thank You" party was held at Canada Olympic Park for all the medical services personnel.

Except for Bateman, off sick with the flu, the rest of Peter's Posse dressed up in their colorful Olympic apparel for the last time as they prepared to party the night away in an emotional farewell to the 15th Olympic Winter Games.

Sipping on her third pre-dinner cocktail, Angie's empty stomach wasted little time absorbing the white wine and sending it off in search of a liver to detoxify it. Because it didn't know exactly where the liver was located, however, the alcohol had to first take a complete tour of all the body's organs, with the brain number one on the travel agenda.

As a result, Ms. Jackson was soon philosophizing her viewpoints on such thought-provoking topics as "Why was Australia called 'The Land Down Under?'

"Down Under what?" Angie babbled to no one in particular. "Any astronomer worth his telescope will tell you that there's no up or down in space. So like, who decided to make the North Pole the top of the world anyway? The way I figure it, the person who started that little rumor was just trying to get a patent to simplify his map-making business, that's all. For all we know... or don't know about the universe, I think the South Pole should demand equal billing."

Dale was naturally the most fascinated by the paradox. The question had never crossed his mind. After all, every atlas that had ever been printed had placed Australia down there at the very bottom. The more he thought about it, the more he wondered if Angie just might be onto something.

Angie, meanwhile, had moved on to another pet peeve of hers. "And that crazy von Trapp family—from *The Sound of Music*. Captain von Trapp was an officer in the Austrian navy, right? Well, the thing I could never understand was, Austria is a land-locked country. It doesn't border on any ocean or sea... so just where the heck was its navy based? On the Danube River or what?"

Jodi took a cautious sniff of her colleague's half-empty wine glass. "How much of this stuff have you had?" the rangy nurse demanded.

The waitresses had just begun serving the usual banquet fare of roast beef, mashed potatoes and veggies when Peter fished into his jacket pocket. With a dramatic gesture, he set a crumpled sheet of paper on the table.

It was a Patient Care Record.

"Angela, speaking of stuff that doesn't make sense, I was wondering if maybe you and Kyle would be kind enough to fill me in on what exactly transpired on that early-morning mission you two went on yesterday?" Peter inquired as he scraped hesitantly at one of the PCR's many red splotches with his dinner knife.

"I've read over... God I hope this is just tomato juice spilled on here... this PCR of yours at least a dozen times and to be quite honest, it wins the prize as the most poorly-written and confusing Patient Care documentation I have ever had the displeasure to read. Since this is your dyslexic signatures scrawled at the bottom, would either of you care to explain this slip-shoddy effort?"

Angie and Kyle blinked at each other with virginal innocence. Even with Dale's assurance that Peter never read PCR forms, they had wisely thought to cover their rear-ends by concocting a clever cover story... just in case.

"Let me try and clear things up for you, sir," Angie began in a strong, confident voice.

With their food growing cold in front of them, everyone at the LIFE-STAR table sat transfixed as Angie detailed a gripping yarn of how she and Kyle had received an urgent call from the Nakiska ski patrol to pick up an unidentified, badly dehydrated, 35 year-old male... who had a prior history of serum hepatitis, was HIV positive, and was also suffering from genu varum, traumatic epicondyle periostitis and the always life-threatening hallux valgus.

Angie spread it on with a trowel as she gave her boss the low-down on a whole slew of imaginary particulars pertaining to the hellish flight in question. When she was finally through, she submissively bowed her head and apologized for the poor documentation, assuring Lawson that both she and Kyle would be much more attentive to their charting in the future.

Peter leaned across the table and, doing his best Mr. Spock impression... cocked a lone eyebrow in outright fascination. "That was a positively enchanting deposition, Angela. But I've still got a few nagging concerns about this call that will need clarification before Howard can send the paperwork to the government for reimbursement. Since we've got a few minutes before the speeches begin, maybe you and your associate could clear up a few details for me right now?

"First off, Ms. Jackson, what exactly is a genu varum, a traumatic epicondyle periostitis and a hallux valgus?"

Angie looked around the table at the sea of expectant faces and with no assistance forthcoming, ended up staring intently at her plate... as if the answer had been secretly tattooed onto the roast beef somewhere.

"Uh, sir, if it's okay with you, I'd rather tell you after dinner. It's pretty gruesome material and these people are trying to eat."

Peter rolled his bloodshot eyes. "Come on, Angela, we're all adults here. I think we can handle the gory details. So please, do tell us what a genu varum really is, and for those at the table who are medically uninformed, I'd like you to use English subtitles."

Angie would have gladly swallowed a cyanide capsule instead.

"Uh... it means... that uh... the patient... uh... had bowed legs."

"And traumatic epicondyle periostitis?"

"Uh... well, I guess uh... he also had... uh... uh suffered from tennis elbow?" was Angie's barely audible mumble.

"And hallux valgus? Ms. Jackson, please tell everyone gathered here tonight exactly what a hallux valgus is?"

Angie was praying for a bolt of lightning or, barring that, a meteorite of any size to crash through the ceiling and strike her dead.

"We're waiting!" Peter said.

"Uh... well sir... I think it means that... uh the poor guy had uh... uh a... had a...."

"Can you repeat that last word, Angela? I didn't quite catch it."

"... bunion."

Not missing a beat, even with all the stifled laughter around him, Peter pressed on with his brutal cross-examination. "Bowed legs, a tennis elbow and a bunion. Good Lord! I can see why the medics at Nakiska wanted this guy airlifted out right away. Considering how critically ill he was, I noticed that under the 'vital signs' section you wrote down that you were unable to obtain any. Why was that?"

Her vocabulary liberally sprinkled with hems and haws, Angie valiantly attempted to explain that the patient not only did not have a palpable pulse or blood pressure, but that he also lacked any visible respiratory effort.

"So the patient was a full arrest when you arrived? Is that what you're saying?"

Angie glanced over at Kyle in the hope that he would jump into the conversation and save her. Instead, he just nodded his head slightly... as if encouraging her to continue.

"You did Code this patient... didn't you, Ms. Jackson?" Peter grilled, his gruff voice taking on the ruthless, cold-blooded reptilian characteristics of a courtroom prosecutor.

"We thought about calling a Code, sir, but the patient was circling the drain when we landed. I mean, with both hepatitis and HIV, his condition was considered terminal. We had to give him credit, though. Apparently, his last wish had been to ski all the 'Black Diamond' runs at

Nakiska before he died. To Code him would've been inhuman. He was already 'on his way out' when we showed up... if you know what I mean."

"No BP, no pulse, no CPR done because the patient was terminal. Do you mean to tell me that we're spending our limited financial resources picking up supportive care patients with bunions and a 'Black Diamond' death wish now?

"I take it you did try to tube the patient, didn't you Kyle?"

"Well no, I wasn't able to intubate him, but I did give the guy lots of air... uh... oxygen. Did I mention the fact that he also suffered from emphysema. Must've been a bad Carbon Dioxide retainer too 'cause as soon as I started the oxygen, his condition immediately cratered! Just sort of faded right out of the picture."

"So you gave your emphysemic patient lots of air, did you Kyle? That was nice of you. Since he wasn't tubed and you make no mention of having thought to use any type of oxygen mask, how exactly did you accomplish that wondrous feat... open a window?"

As Kyle sank into his chair, Peter turned his gunsight back on his female accomplice. "Angela, you've written here that your patient appeared severely dehydrated. If that was the case, why didn't you start an IV on him? Didn't you think he might've benefited from a few litres of something wet... even if he was 'on his way out?'"

"I was unable to find a vein, sir."

Peter could not help laughing out loud. "You... the great A.Y. Jackson, couldn't find a vein! I find that extremely difficult to believe. I've always been told that you're so good at sniffing out veins, Venus de Milo's nurse would've asked for you personally!"

Kyle came to Angie's rescue. "Uh, sir, your little comment regarding Ms. de Milo wasn't that far off the mark really. The reason Angie couldn't find a vein was because our patient didn't have any uh... arms."

"What the heck do you mean? He was one of those amputee skiers?"

"Well... sort of, only he... uh, didn't exactly start out that way. You see, we... uh, inadvertently left out another important piece of information... that the patient had fainted while riding the chair lift, pancaked the ski run below and was then accidentally run over by a snow blower."

A snow blower, for God's sake! Angie winced. They were doomed. Unable to just sit and listen, she leaped back into the conversation to explain that yes, their patient had lost both his arms after colliding with a run-away snow-making machine.

Behind heavily-hooded eyes, Peter was starting to enjoy himself. "A snow-making machine ran over him, eh? I always thought those things were pretty stationary, what with the water hoses and all. I didn't know they could be moved once they were hooked up?"

"It was a prototype, sir," Kyle shakily added his two cents worth, "brought in just for the Olympics. You see, after he was run over, the patient was uh... accidentally kind of sucked into one of the air inlets. It wasn't a pretty thing to have to see."

Angie gave her partner in crime a look that screamed for him to keep his big trap shut.

"Now let me get this straight. Your terminally-ill patient fell off the chairlift, pancaked the ski hill, was run over and then accidentally kind of sucked into a moving snow blower. Is that right? I want to make sure I've got all the facts straight."

With God as their witness, both Kyle and Angie raised their right arms into the air as they solemnly stated that yes, that was exactly how it had happened.

"Did you two trauma specialists ever think to try the MAST pants to get some kind of blood pressure on your patient, or no... don't tell me, he didn't have any legs either, did he?"

"You should know us better than that!" Angie responded as if her professional integrity had been questioned. "You're correct about the fact that the guy didn't have any legs, but believe me, sir, if he had had anything remaining down there, you know I would've wrapped something around it!"

Everyone at the LIFE-STAR table cracked up at Angie's poorly-worded retort. Struggling to keep a straight-face, Lord Lawson cleared his throat as he redirected his attention toward the two pilots who had flown the mission.

"Captain Morgan, you have on your report here that you flew directly from Nakiska to Parkland Memorial... via the Riverside Medical Centre. If that is indeed the case, could you please explain how LIFE-STAR One could've been observed flying up and down the Banff-Calgary corridor that morning... from Nakiska to Canmore to Canada Olympic Park to the Saddledome, for heaven's sake? Don't try and weasel your way around it either, because the RCMP have video of you passing over every single sporting venue. They paid me a little visit after you dumped the 'copter back at the hangar and scattered like rats. They grilled me for an hour... wanted to know if I thought you could belong to some terrorist organization! Tell me the truth, do you normally circle the Saddledome and then make a few passes over the Olympic Speed Skating Oval before you set up to land at the Parkland pad?"

Dale was quick to remind his boss that it was Standard LIFE-STAR Operating Procedure that the pilot must always circle the landing area at least once while he and his crew checked for hazards below.

"With the Olympics in town, you can never be too careful. I wanted to be sure that I wasn't about to land right in the middle of a hostage-taking incident or something."

"You honestly want me to believe that story, Dale... that by flying over the Saddledome, you could detect a terrorist plot being hatched in the back parking lot of a hospital four miles away? I don't have time to hear your excuses right now, as I have another little problem with your report. I've noticed that you failed to record the time you touched down at Parkland. How come?"

"Well, sir... the patient... uh... didn't quite 'make it' to the hospital... and Alex and I... we couldn't see the point of landing if we didn't have a patient to unload so we just decided to uh... you know... call it a day and head back to the hangar, instead."

Peter cradled his head in his hands. After what seemed like a very long time, he raised his head to take a cold, hard look at the people across from him.

He had been onto their little game from the very beginning, ever since he had read, with latex-gloved hands, Angie and Kyle's ketchup-spattered report. But after listening to their unbelievably far-fetched cover story, the idea of soaking the entire crew with jet fuel and then flame broiling them was appealing.

What they had done was bad enough... using the company helicopter to spread a person's ashes, but what if they'd had another call? A real call. What would they have done then?

"Sir, we'd thought about that, too, and Angie and Kyle had it all worked out," Alex reassured him. "If another call had come in, we would simply have taken Emily and Melissa along for the ride."

"You had Mrs. Andrews and her daughter up there with you? Dear Lord, tell me you had them sign a release form? Please tell me you did that much?"

Upon learning that they had, the worried expression on Peter's haggard face relaxed, but only for a moment. He had a real dilemma on his hands. Yes, they had broken all the rules, but as he looked down at the

PCR form that had been Russ Andrews' last official flight aboard LIFE-STAR 1, he just couldn't bring himself to berate his gutsy employees.

With their paramedical careers on the line, they had taken it upon themselves to pay their final respects to a dear colleague in the way they knew Russ would have wanted. Surrounded by his closest friends, they had taken him on one last ride and in doing so, had set his spirited soul free.

While the interrogation had been going on, the Olympic Organizing Committee had been busy presenting several key figures within the medical services area with special commemorative plaques... thanking them for their hard work and dedication toward making the Olympics a success.

Peter was in the midst of lecturing his employees about coming to him the next time they had the urge to use his multi-million dollar helicopter as a fertilizer spreader, when he suddenly heard his name being announced over the PA system.

"... and thus it is with great pride that we present Mr. Peter Lawson with this plaque as a tribute to his commitment toward the Games, toward improved pre-hospital health care and toward his invaluable Shock Trauma Air Rescue program... LIFE-STAR."

Peter bashfully headed for the podium as the announcer continued with the accolades. "Peter has the cream of the province's paramedics, nurses and helicopter pilots working for him, so let's give all those good folks sitting over at the LIFE-STAR table a big hand of appreciation. I'm sure that I speak for Peter when I say how very proud he is of this dedicated group of highly-trained professionals."

Peter got a standing ovation from everyone in the room, but the people who jumped to their feet first and applauded the loudest were the very ones he had the hardest time keeping under control—his very own hand-picked group of "HAVE HELICOPTER-MOUNTED FUNERAL URN... WILL MAKE YOUR LAST DAY ON EARTH AN EXTRA SPECIAL ONE" ash distributors!

56
BOYS WILL BE BOYS

The awards ceremony concluded the dinner portion of the evening, and when Peter returned to his table after picking up his plaque, he found his entire squad in a feeding frenzy. With busboys waiting to clear their table so dessert could be served, the famished medics did manage to stop chewing long enough to warmly congratulate their wonderful and, hopefully very-forgiving, leader.

One by one, as his loyal employees abandoned the table to stretch their legs, a much humbled Angie and Kyle were the last to get to their feet.

All the while staring at the floor, Kyle finally summoned the courage to speak. "Sir, I take full responsibly for what happened. Angie's not to blame. Dale and Alex had nothing to do with it, either. They just wanted to help out. It was all my idea. If anyone is to be punished, let it be me."

"There's an old saying," Peter said quietly as he studied the crestfallen pair, "'It's always easier to beg forgiveness than ask for permission.' You know, Howard Bateman's been on my case since day one to be tougher on you people. He's always telling me that I give you guys too much rope and that one day, you're going to end up hanging me with it.

"Mr. Stevens, I understand that you acted with only the best of intentions, but I still can't publicly admit that I condone it. Ours is a dangerous business and while I hope that we're never again faced with a similar situation, Russ unfortunately wasn't the first, nor will he be the last, to die in the line of duty. Off the record, I wish I could've been up there with you. As Base Manager of this organization, however, I can't just let you off Scott-free. Thus as of tomorrow morning, you're on two weeks unpaid vacation."

The relieved offender looked like he was going to drop to his knees and kiss His Lordship's ring for being so merciful. As Peter swatted off the medic's subservient gratitude, he left Kyle with one final piece of advice. "Oh, and Stevens, one more thing—Angela almost had me believing that half-assed story of hers until you threw in that part about the motorized snow blower! Couldn't you come up with anything more inventive than a flipping snow blower?"

For sixteen all too brief days and nights, the sprawling cowtown of Calgary, Alberta had reigned as the undisputed "Winter Sport and Social Capital" of the civilized world. Within hours, that wondrous fairytale would be drawing to a close. Though safe in the knowledge that Calgary had indeed pulled off the most successful Winter Games in history, everyone at the party was also acutely aware that their city probably would not host another Olympics until well into the next century. As a result, most people were overjoyed and depressed at the same time, and at one point, the farewell soiree was in danger of becoming "The Manic/ Depressive Capital of Canada." That all changed, of course, once the bar reopened.

Sporting a wine cooler for his wife, it was as Kyle was on his way back from the bar that he spotted Angie at the banquet table, happily heaping her plate with a tasty assortment of finger sandwiches, cheeses, crackers and dip.

"Are you going to smuggle that home in a king-sized doggie bag?" the medic inquired.

"It's not for me, it's for Dale. I don't think he's wintered very well. Haven't you noticed how thin he's gotten lately? I'm kind of worried about him. He needs to put on a few extra pounds of insulation or he's never going to make it till spring."

"You don't have to worry about that 'cause he's not going to be here come spring."

Angie looked dazed. "What? He's not thinking about going back home... is he?"

"He's way past thinking about it," Kyle replied. "Alex told me they had a pilots' meeting last week and Dale got up and announced that he was leaving to go back to Cairns on March first. It didn't appear like he was planning on coming back in the near future... if at all. Some kind of family problem, apparently."

Suddenly aware that the hand with which she'd been holding the snacks was quivering, Angie set the plate down. Her "good buddy" might not have been aware of most of what happened around him, but he spotted that tiny detail right away.

"Geez, I thought he would've told you. He's been hanging around you like a virus for the past month. Didn't he mention anything about it?"

As Angie stood at the buffet table, in a room milling with people, she suddenly felt totally alone, as if she were the only person left alive in the entire world. It was Russ' funeral all over again. The sound of people laughing and talking all seemed to blend together until it was just one big, confusing rush of noise.

Kyle had been right. She and Dale had spent a lot of time together during the past month. There'd been that hand-holding thing at the hospital. The Opening Ceremonies. The luge event. Pin trading on the 8th avenue mall. They had had great fun together, but there had also been something else.

While attending the medal presentations one evening, Dale had accidentally brushed up against her. Maybe it was only static electricity, but the feel of his lean body against hers had almost sent her heart into atrial flutter.

On top of all that, she'd caught him sneaking peeks at her when he thought she wouldn't notice, and the gentle expression on his face and in his eyes seemed to reflect her innermost feelings exactly.

How'd that old saying go? "Loving eyes can never see." With Kyle's stunning revelation smacking her square in the face, it was obvious she needed to have her eyeballs examined immediately.

"Gosh, has it ever gotten hot in here. I think I'll just step outside for a few minutes to cool off."

"I don't like the sound of that one bit," Kyle said.

"I'm okay... really. It's just that there's so many people crammed in here, that's all. I think I'll uh... I need some fresh air."

Angie hurried off in the direction of the coat check. As she fled the room, she plucked an unopened bottle of wine and a plastic champagne glass off a table. If ever she needed a drink to numb the ache in her heart, she needed one now.

Waiting in line with Alex at the bar, Dale did a double-take as he saw Angie scurry for the exit with her parka under her arm. Not liking what he saw, the pilot made straight for Kyle who was still standing at the snack table.

"Where the heck is Angie going?" he asked Kyle.

"She said she was going for a little walk and that she was coming right back, but I rather doubt she will. I think she was kind of upset about something. Before she left, she told me to give this stuff to you. She didn't think the harsh Canadian winters were agreeing with you."

Dale stared at the plate of tempting morsels, but he made no move to take the plate from Kyle's monstrous mitt. "It's freezing outside. What would make her so upset that she'd want to risk frostbite by stumbling around out there in the dark?"

"I think I may have said something that I shouldn't have."

"What the hell did you say? I hope you didn't tell her I was leaving? Please tell me you didn't say that?"

Kyle slowly set the plate down. He had been waiting a long time for this confrontation. "Well someone had to, for Christ's sake! You know, she didn't have the faintest idea that you've been planning on splitting all along. When the heck were you going to tell her anyway? From a pay phone at the Cairns International airport?"

"I had my reasons for not telling her, alright! I've been trying to organize an urgent trip back home for the past couple of weeks and a whole lot depended on if I could swing some things here first. As usual, you don't have a frigging clue about what's really going down."

The lanky chopper pilot had always been impressed by Kyle's sheer size, but now, with his chest all puffed out and his high-heeled cowboy boots on, the paramedic seemed to tower over him... and the look in his eyes was not sweet.

"Don't go playing innocent with me, Morgan. Once Russ was out of the picture, you couldn't wait to fill his jock strap. How could you take advantage of a woman like that... and now that she's finally getting her act half-way back together, you're going to take a hike. Isn't that just peachy? I'd always heard that pilots were the 'love them and leave them' type! What the hell was your prime mission objective this time around Captain Morgan... to boldly go where no Australian male has gone before?

"And while we're on that subject, what made you come to Canada in the first place? I heard a rumor that you were running away from a girl or a marriage or something. It figures. Obviously you have quite a track record back home, as well. It's a damn shame philandering isn't an Olympic event... you'd have taken the gold medal!"

"You don't know what the hell you're talking about!" Dale shouted. "I've never cared more about a girl in my life. I was the one who dragged her kicking and screaming back to reality. If you were so bloody concerned about her emotional welfare, where were you when she needed someone to talk to... to show her that life was worth living? You don't know the torment that girl's been through. I do. And because of that, we've both had to come to terms with a whole lot of things... things that neither of us wanted to face... things I doubt you could possibly understand."

Out of the corner of his eye, Dale could see Kyle flexing his massive fists. "So that's the problem, is it? You think I'm trying to replace Russ in Angie's life? Well if it is, then wake the hell up. Nobody's trying to replace anyone. I don't want to play second fiddle to any man... living or dead, and the last thing I want is to get some girl on the rebound. I want Angie to want me for myself, not as a last minute substitute for somebody else."

Dale was almost afraid to look away from Kyle's menacing glare for fear of not seeing that huge right hand when it started to come for his face. Kyle meanwhile, calmly held his tongue as he listened to Dale's lecture on morality. He had it all planned. He was just letting this foreigner say his piece and then he was going to punch his Australian lights out. Simple as that.

"Kyle, I miss him too, we all miss him. Russ was your best friend and believe me, I know what you're going through. A long time ago, I lost a close friend, too. He was in the process of saving my life when he took a bullet in the back for his efforts. The guilt nearly destroyed me. I didn't think I'd ever get over it. As hard as it may be for you to accept, Russ' death was an accident... an act of God. It wasn't anybody's fault. One morning you'll wake up and realize that... that you've simply been asking too much of yourself... too much of anyone!"

Returning from the bar with a beer in both hands, Alex found his flying partner pulling on his coat and gloves. "First Angie... now you. Where the heck is everybody going? Is there a fight outside or what the... sweet Jesus man, what happened to your eye?"

"That dumb-ass Stevens stuck his fist in it!" Dale snapped. "He opened his big yap and told Angie I was leaving. She apparently didn't take the news very well and now I've got to try and find her so I can explain. I don't even know where the heck to start looking. Christ, she could've jumped in her car and be half-way home, for all I know."

"You've got no one to blame but yourself," Alex replied with an air of authority. "If you'd just leveled with that poor girl in the first place and told her what you had planned, she wouldn't be out there right now... probably sitting in a snow drift somewhere, crying her eyes out."

"Thanks for the moral support, Captain Davis. I've always known I could count on you in time of need. Now if you'll excuse me, I've got the whole damn city to search."

"You know Dale, for someone as smart as you are, you hide it very well. Look around you, man! We're at Canada Olympic Park! If you were a washed-up former luger and you thought you'd just been 'dumped on' yet again, where would you go?"

57
DESTINY

Finding Angie's Chevette still in the parking lot, Dale hopped in his car and pointed it in the direction of the luge track. All the while cursing his own stupidity, the Aussie rolled down his frosted window and stuck his head out for a better view.

The snow-making equipment on the adjacent ski hill was roaring at full capacity, and a delicate breeze floated the dense cloud of man-made snow pellets across the park. Drifting past the track's towering light standards, the sparkling ice crystals took on a rich golden hue, bathing the entire hill in an incandescent fairytale glow.

As his good eye frantically scanned the luge track's twisting contours for any signs of life, the constant drizzle of falling snow only added to Dale's misery.

Continuing up the road, the heavy-hearted Aussie was just about to turn around and circle back when a flash of movement caught his attention. Bringing his Saab to a stop, he patiently waited until whatever it was moved again. Fifty yards to the south, someone emerged from beneath the out-run's shadowy overhead walkway. Whoever it was seemed preoccupied with viciously flinging something high into the night sky. After pausing to scoop up material for a second snowball, the person resumed his or her aimless wandering down the track toward the loading dock.

Dousing his car lights, Dale pocketed the keys and started toward the desolate, windswept platform.

Balancing on the track's three-foot concrete sidewall, Angie Jackson solemnly hoisted her plastic glass aloft, in tribute to the spotlighted Canadian flag rippling at the top of the hill. "A toast to the end of the Games," she whimpered. "To the end of Russ' dream. And to the end of a romance that never was... and never will be."

Dale watched her refill her glass with wine. With his quarry momentarily distracted, he silently climbed the wooden steps leading to the dock. She was facing away from him, but from the sounds of her muffled sobs, she was hurting, big time.

"What are you doing, luv... drinking a toast to the luge gods?"

Angie whirled around and lost her balance. Waving her arms about as she teetered on the narrow ledge, she sent her glass sailing into the darkness. Nearly following it into the black abyss that bordered the elevated track, it took several seconds of frenzied arm flapping before the unbalanced RN finally reestablished equilibrium.

Reaching up to brush away her tears, Angie was suddenly stuck by the futility of it all. What was the point? This damn Australian already knew she was a hopeless basket case, anyway.

"A toast to the luge gods? Heck no. I was just... uh... you know, the Olympics wrap up tomorrow and I guess I'm just kind of sad about everything coming to an end. It was fun while it lasted."

Watching as the pilot slowly advanced toward her, she jumped down from the sidewall, pulling up the collar of her parka to shield her face. The last thing she needed was for him to find out she'd been crying.

"It was fun while it lasted, eh?" Dale echoed as his eyes moved over her tear-streaked face. "Something tells me you're not just talking about the Olympics when you say that. What are you doing out here, woman? I was just about to relate your incredible snow blower story to the bartender when I turned around and saw you racing for the exit with a bottle of bubbly crammed under your jacket!"

As he spoke, the pilot gazed solemnly into the surrounding darkness. Cleverly utilizing the age-old ruse, his shuffling feet soon had him standing directly behind her. Knowing she couldn't help but feel his chest against her back, the fact that she made no effort to move gave hope to the shy Aussie.

"It was so hot in there," Angie fidgeted. "I just stepped out for some fresh air."

"Considering your usual frigidity, I find that hard to believe."

Spending the next five seconds mindlessly picking at the wine bottle label, the broken-hearted nurse finally could stand the agonizing suspense no longer. "Kyle told me that you're going back home... and that you're leaving next week... and that you're... you're probably not coming back."

"I was going to tell you. I was just waiting for the right...."

Having heard enough, she spun around to face him. "It's okay. I knew you couldn't stay forever. You want to be with your son. Nobody can blame... Oh my God! What happened to your eye?"

"I'm having an allergic reaction!" Dale replied testily as he gently fingered his swollen cheekbone.

"To what? Something you ate? I didn't know you were allergic?"

"I'm allergic all right... to your good buddy's right fist. Forget about my eye. I have to tell you something. Over the past few months, I've watched as an emotionally-bankrupt girl slowly transformed herself into a strong, self-confident woman. I never told you, but I marveled at your spirit. Rusty's death... not to mention having to face your own mortality... a lot of people would've given up. Not you. You had the courage to look into the future and knew that in order to get there, you'd have to conquer your fears first. I so admired that. It was what gave me the strength to deal with my own problems."

"Well that's just frigging wonderful!" Angie yelped. Pausing to gaze up into the overcast night sky, she decided it was time for a little chat. "You know something, God? I was actually beginning to think that maybe, just maybe, my life was finally changing for the better. Seems I was dead wrong again. Apparently just because I nearly froze to death trying to haul my butt up an ice-encrusted mountainside, and then had the unmitigated gall to dance the Two-Step in front of two billion couch potatoes, I've somehow given this mild-mannered guy here the strength to hop on a plane and leave. Thank you very much, God! That was a really great reward!"

Morgan's laughter probably could've been heard all the way back to the Volunteer Centre. After a bit, Angie found herself joining him.

"Dale," she eventually asked, "do you think you'll ever come back to Canada?"

"To be truthful," the Aussie's voice wavered with emotion, "there's nothing to hold me here. No family. No ties. Never mind the fact that my work visa expires in a few weeks. Don't get me wrong, though, I've really enjoyed flying for Peter and I've got a bunch of real good friends here, but it's not enough. If I were ever to come back to stay, it would have to be for a very special reason."

Dale could not have been more subtle if he'd whacked her over the head with a jar of Vegemite. With her heart hammering against her still-tender ribs, Angie knew the time had come for her, too, to lay her cards on the table.

"Would a certain girl with Canadian citizenship papers be a good enough reason to stay?"

"It might. You wouldn't happen to know anyone willing to take a chance on an over-the-hill, unemployed chopper pilot... would you?"

Knowing that within her hands rested the power to control not only her own, but Dale's destiny, as well, a little voice deep down told Angie to trust her feelings and follow her heart.

Melting into Dale's waiting arms, it was as close to heaven as Angie Yvonne Jackson was likely ever to get.

Dale meanwhile, closed his good eye as he, too, savored the delicious moment. Angie's attractively-packaged body fit so nicely against his that it was almost as if she'd been born with just that purpose in mind.

Tenderly kissing the tip of her nose, the Aussie suddenly pulled back. "Are you able to breathe through that thing yet?"

Angie couldn't believe her ears. "You want to know if I can breathe through my nose?" she asked, taking a superficial sniff of the crisp night air. "It's not terrific, but I can breathe through it a little bit."

"Well, in that case, I want you to take a couple of nice deep breaths. What do you medics call it? Hyper... hypervent...."

"You want me to hyperventilate?" Angie blurted. "What are you planning to do to me, Morgan? I think you should let me know right now if you're into any of that kinky exotic stuff."

"Kinky exotic stuff!" Dale laughed. "Ange, it's just that I've been waiting for this moment for such a long time that I didn't want you to suffocate, that's all. I mean, once I get started, I may not want to stop."

Pulling her to him, the love starved pilot wasted little time getting down to business. His body surging with a passion he had not felt in a long, long time, Dale's hot, burning kisses carried with them the promise of more, much more.

Angie's response was less than subtle. As her buttery-soft lips pressed hungrily against his own, the Aussie was nearly consumed by the raging fire he'd ignited in this feisty Canadian girl.

Forgetting about the bottle of locally-produced vino in her hand, Angie reached up to caress the back of her favorite pilot's neck. The bottle slipped unnoticed from her grasp and dropped into the snow. But the cheap, sugary booze had worked its magic.

"Wow!" Dale exclaimed as he came up for air. "Your kisses do, honest-to-God, taste sweeter than wine!

"By the way, luv," he smiled as he pulled something from his coat pocket. It was two airline tickets. "I had no intention of leaving without you."

The End

GLOSSARY

ACLS: Advanced Cardiac Life Support. An advanced skill level which allows paramedics to intubate, defibrillate and administer cardiac stimulating drugs to patients who are breathless and/or pulseless.

Algorithm: A step-by-step problem-solving procedure. Algorithms are frequently used by medical staff to help remember the correct sequence of treatment and drugs to be given during stressful emergency situations.

AMC: Air Medical Crew.

Black trauma Patient: Same as Code 32, patient found dead at scene.

BLS: Basic Life Support. Allows a certified rescuer to perform basic CPR skills on a patient who is breathless and/or pulseless. Does not cover advanced life support treatments or medications.

BTLS: Basic Trauma Life Support. An advanced skill level covering emergency procedures related to traumatic injuries. Areas covered include advanced airway skills such as needle decompression of the chest and cricothyrotomy (the cutting of an emergency opening in a patient's throat).

BVM: Bag Valve Mask. A collapsible bag used to assist a patient's breathing. Mask portion can be removed, allowing bagging unit to be attached directly to an endotracheal tube.

Code 32: Patient pronounced dead at the scene of an accident.

Code 81: A crash on the luge track in which the slider is uninjured.

Code 82: A crash on the luge track in which the slider is injured and requires medical assistance.

Code 99/Code: Medical lingo for a patient found without spontaneous respirations or a heartbeat. A cardio-pulmonary arrest, it is also frequently referred to as a "Code."

Collective Control: The method of control by which the pitch of the main rotor blades is varied equally and simultaneously. Held in pilot's left hand, pulling up on the collective causes aircraft to raise into the air. Lowering causes aircraft to descend.

CT Scan: Computerized Tomography. A computerized X-ray scanner used for diagnosing injuries undetectable with regular X-rays.

Cyclic Control: Changes the pitch of the main rotor blades individually during a cycle of revolution to control the tilt of the rotor disc, and therefore, the direction and velocity of horizontal flight. Held in pilot's right hand, the cyclic is used to maintain directional control of aircraft, ie... moving control to the left causes aircraft to move to left, etc.

ECG: Electrocardiogram. A routine heart tracing.

EMS: Emergency Medical Services. Denotes pre-hospital care and transport by either ground or air ambulance.

EMT: Emergency Medical Technician. Does not have as much medical training as a paramedic. Most ground ambulance units consist of one EMT and one EMT-P (paramedic).

EMT-P: Emergency Medical Technician Paramedic.

ETA: Estimated Time of Arrival.

ET or ETT: Endotracheal Tube. A plastic tube inserted into a patient's windpipe to help them breathe. This procedure is called intubation.

Extrication: Term used when a patient trapped in a vehicle is removed through the use of hydraulic tools and other specialized equipment (such as "The Jaws of Life")

FLIR: Forward Looking Infra-Red. A heat sensitive spotting system which detects the amount of heat given off by an object. The more heat an object gives off, the clearer it shows up on the monitor.

Foot Pedal Controls: Controls inherent torque created by rotation of main rotor blades. Pressing on the left pedal increases torque on the tail rotor blades causing tail to swing to right and nose of aircraft to the left.

G Forces: Gravitational Forces. Centrifugal force allows a luge sled to glide suspended through a vertical walled curve without falling off.

Glasgow Coma Scale: A medical scoring system which indicates a patient's level of consciousness. For example, an alert, orientated patient would score 15, while a patient who is unconscious and unresponsive to any form of stimulation would only score a 3.

Green Trauma Patient: A stable patient with minor non-life threatening injuries. Classified as walking wounded, patient can walk and thus doesn't require a stretcher. Could safely be transported by car.

HOPE Program: Human Organ Procurement and Exchange program.

ICU: Intensive Care Unit. A specialized hospital unit in which majority of patients are critically ill or injured.

IFR: Instrument Flight Rules. Conditions under which a certified pilot is allowed to fly an aircraft solely by reference to flight instruments and radio navigational equipment (usually during times of reduced ceiling [cloud height] and visibility).

Large Bore IV: An IV in which a large sized catheter is inserted into the vein. The larger the gauge (bore or diameter) the faster IV fluid can be infused into the patient. Critically injured patients usually have two large bore IVs started.

Lidocaine: Drug used to decrease the excitability of damaged heart tissue. Lessens the risk of a patient developing a life threatening arrhythmia such as VT or VF.

MAST Pants: Military Anti Shock Trousers. Inflatable splint used to stabilize fractures of the pelvis and legs. Their use in the treatment of shock, is presently under review.

MI: Myocardial Infarction. A heart attack.

MOT: Ministry of Transport.

Mottled: A purplish or grayish discoloration of the skin. Usually indicates poor blood circulation to the area. Common in patients suffering from shock.

Mounties: Royal Canadian Mounted Police. Canada's national police force. Also known as the RCMP.

MVA: Motor Vehicle Accident.

NRB Mask: Non-Rebreather mask. A type of oxygen mask (with an attached oxygen reservoir bag) which delivers a higher concentration of oxygen than does a regular face mask.

NUS: Nursing Unit Supervisor. Formerly referred to as the head nurse.

PALS: Advanced Pediatric Life Support. An advanced skill level which allows paramedics to intubate, defibrillate and administer cardiac stimulating drugs to infants and children who are breathless and/or pulseless.

PCR: Patient Care Record or report. The form medics fill out on each patient they transport or care for.

Port: Left side of aircraft.

PVC: Premature Ventricular Contraction. Also known as an ectopic. An abnormal heart beat frequently seen following a heart attack. Three or more PVCs in a row is called VT and can be life threatening.

Rapid Sequence Intubation: Used when a patient has to be intubated in a hurry. Specific rapid acting drugs are administered to sedate and chemically paralyze the patient. Most commonly used when the patient is in respiratory distress yet is still conscious enough to fight the procedure by clamping jaws together, coughing or gagging.

Red Trauma Patient: Patient either has sustained or has the possibility of having sustained life threatening injuries. Mechanism of injury plays a big part in Trauma color classification. If the patient was ejected from the vehicle; the accident was a rollover with unbelted passengers; one or more patents were found dead at scene; any deformity of the steering wheel; major damage sustained to interior of vehicle etc., there is a high probability that the patient may have suffered severe and possibly life threatening injury. For example, at the scene of a high speed MVA, even if the patient's injuries initially appear minor, great care would be taken to assess, package and transport the patient to hospital as quickly as possible. As a lengthy transport time often can mean the difference between an alert, talking red patient and a fatality, the majority of red patients are transported to hospital with lights and sirens or are air-lifted.

Roger Wilco: Will Comply.

RRT or RT: Registered Respiratory Therapist. Manages the respiratory and oxygen needs of a hospital patient.

Scoop Stretcher: An aluminum stretcher which can be disassembled lengthwise into a left and right portion. The two halves are then slid under the patient from either side and snapped together. Scooping a patient eliminates the need to lift or roll the patient. Frequently used if spinal or pelvic injuries are suspected.

Starboard: Right side of aircraft

Stat: Immediately.

TENS: Transcutaneous Electronic Nerve Stimulator. A external device used to decrease a patient's pain by blocking pain transmission to the brain.

TSB: Transportation Safety Board.

Ventilator/Vent: Machine which takes over the work of breathing for a patient. A patient attached to a ventilator is said to be on life support.

VF: Ventricular Fibrillation. A potentially fatal heart arrhythmia. If not treated immediately, patient will die.

VFR: Visual Flight Rules. Allows a pilot to fly an aircraft by maintaining adequate visual reference to the ground.

VT: Ventricular Tachycardia. A potentially life threatening heart arrhythmia. If not treated, can deteriorate into an even more deadly arrhythmia... Ventricular Fibrillation or VF.

Yellow Trauma Patient: A patient who cannot be classified via the trauma color scale as green, red or black. Injuries are such that patient requires a stretcher. ie... broken leg, etc. Though injuries are considered non-life threatening, a yellow patient would be monitored frequently for any deterioration of condition and transported to hospital as soon as possible. It is not uncommon once the initial shock of the accident wears off, for the patient to begin complaining of other injuries. ie... headache, back pain, increasing shortness of breath. EMS medics are always watchful of the fact that a yellow patient has the potential to deteriorate into a red patient.

A crisp, autumn afternoon. A speeding sports car. A teenaged driver. A moment of distraction. Seconds later, the car is upside down in the ditch. One boy lies dead at the scene. Another, still trapped in the wreckage, is critically injured.

Speed kills!

In the traumatic world of emergency medicine, however, speed can sometimes save a life. Written by veteran helicopter flight nurse Pat Jensen, SHOCK TRAUMA is the first novel ever to focus on the life and death world of air ambulance transports. Semi-autobiographical, Pat draws on her own personal experiences to craft this incredible story.

Set against the spectacular twin backdrops of Canada's Rocky Mountains and Calgary's Olympic Winter Games, SHOCK TRAUMA revolves around Angie Jackson, a burnt-out Intensive Care nurse who risks her ground-bound existence for a chance to fly the skies with LIFESTAR, a fledgling air rescue program.

Teamed with dashing paramedic Russ Andrews and macho Aussie chopper pilot Dale Morgan, Angie soon finds herself caught up in a series of sometimes hilarious/sometimes tragic misadventures that will keep you turning pages to the very end.

SHOCK TRAUMA allows the reader to explore a world few 'outsiders' ever see. A world where a good day is when your patient doesn't die on you and where a bad day can haunt you for the rest of your life.

The Cell phone is ringing. Quick, grab your helmet, pull on a flight suit and buckle yourself in. The medical crew aboard LIFESTAR-1 are waiting to take you on the adventure ride of your life!

About the Author...

Pat was born in High River, Alberta, and grew up on a farm west of Okotoks. A graduate of the nursing program at Calgary's Holy Cross Hospital in 1978, she has worked as a helicopter flight nurse with Calgary's STARS Air Ambulance since 1989. She also enjoys the challenges of nursing in the high arctic, having worked at the Nursing Stations in Aklavik, NWT, Fox Lake, Alberta, and Deline, NWT. In addition to STARS, Pat works as a flight nurse in Cambridge Bay, Nunavut.

Sportwise, Pat won both a gold and a bronze medal at the 1985 Canadian Luge Championships. She served as the Luge competition's 'Chief of Finish' at the 1988 Calgary Olympic Winter Games and has twice been decorated by the International Luge Federation for her outstanding contribution to the sport. In 1989, Pat received the Canadian Bobsleigh and Luge 'Volunteer of the Year' award.

Her other literary credits include scripting several screenplays. One of which 'Arctic Circle,' was selected as one of four finalists for the 2004 Writers Guild of Canada's 'Jim Burt' script writing prize.

When she is not flying, writing or working in the Arctic, Pat is married to EMS helicopter pilot Gordon Jeffery, and lives in Calgary, Alberta.

ISBN 978-0-9681956-0-4

9 780968 195604

Canada	$18.95
USA	$16.95

Printed in Canada